Table of Contents

Foreword from the First Edition

I wish I'd had a book like this one available to me when I started teaching 25 years ago!

While most books on Aikido are focused on a particular point of view and fairly narrow in scope, this book is quite open in its approach to the teaching of Aikido exercises, the operation of a school and myriad details that many forget.

Drawing on experience in the Virginia Ki Society and past martial art studies, as well as international associations created through the Internet and the Aikido-L ListServ, the author has woven a rich tapestry of Aikido and related topics which is easy to read and surprisingly easy to comprehend.

Sources for observations, suggested approaches, and additional resources are liberally quoted and referenced. While this work clearly reflects the impact of Master Koichi Tohei and Ki Society teachings it also includes information from physics and anatomy, from Judo and other Aikido systems (such as Aikikai and Yoshinkan) to help the reader to better understand the material.

The author has an easy writing style with a flair for detail which should satisfy even the most discriminating of readers. While the book was written primarily to help people who are new to Aikido, it will be a valuable resource for more senior students and teachers of the art.

A fitting adjunct to the author's first volume, *Ki in Aikido*.

—George Simcox, November 1999
Virginia Ki Society
Merrifield, Virginia

Preface

The first rule of writing is to "Know Your Audience" yet you will notice that this book switches relentlessly between "you the student" and "you the instructor."

This seems to me to be a fairly accurate analogy of any Aikido class.

Student is teacher.

Teacher is student.

What we know we can teach to another and we must never stop learning.

This book is not intended to teach Aikido. It is certainly not intended to teach the One True Right Way (of many right ways) of doing exercises or techniques. It does not represent official teachings or procedure of the Ki Society or any other style. It is not intended to teach throwing techniques beyond basics.

It is intended to provide exercises and insights into the processes and tools of training and learning, regardless of style. A ball is useful for demonstrating spherical movement whether you are coming from Karate, Judo, or Aikido.

And, while nothing replaces practice, *understanding* speeds the process by eliminating errors, misunderstandings, and other pointless blocks to progress. Oddly enough, many Aikido students and instructors ignore written reference materials. This approach is often defended on the grounds that martial arts skills are Traditional Arts and so should be taught in the traditional manner.

Consider that music, mathematics, and civil engineering are also Traditional Arts, yet few of us would consider taking on these complex disciplines without books and other reference materials, nor is there any need to do so in Aikido as excellent texts are available.

Keys in the following material refer to reference materials from Ki Society, Aikikai and Yoshinkan. *Aikido and the Dynamic Sphere* is the long-time standard Aikido textbook, composed prior to 1970 when Tohei (founder of the Ki Society) was Chief Instructor at the Aikikai Honbu dojo. Gozo Shioda's *Dynamic Aikido* and *Total Aikido* (Yoshinkan textbooks) are radically different in approach and appearance, but offer beautiful explanations of body mechanics which apply to *any* style.

As Casey Stengel *sensei* put it, "You don't have to belong to a ballteam to steal their signals."

If you are trying to discuss a technique in words (with names that vary between styles) over the Internet, it can be very useful to have these books on hand.

- **ADS**: *Aikido and the Dynamic Sphere* (Adell Westbrook & Oscar Ratti, 1970): This is the classic Aikido text, written when Koichi Tohei (founder of the Ki Society) was Chief Instructor at Aikikai headquarters. It is a standard found in most Aikido libraries.
- **BA**: *Best Aikido — The Fundamentals* (Kisshomaru Ueshiba and Moriteru Ueshiba 2002): From Aikikai headquarters, standing, rolling, and basic techniques presented by son and grandson of the Founder Morihei Ueshiba.
- **DA**: *Dynamic Aikido* (Gozo Shioda, 1977): A primer on basic Aikido skills. The large clear photos include reference grids to clarify body position and clearly illustrated lines of force. The physics and body mechanics behind joint locks and unbalancing (*kuzushi*) are the same regardless of style. In theory, replaced by *TOT*, but both are uniquely valuable.
- **KIA**: *Ki in Aikido* (C. M. Shifflett, 2009): *Ki* exercises for balance, coordination, and focus in step-by-step format including detailed directions for testing.
- **KDL**: *Ki in Daily Life* (Koichi Tohei, 1978): Basic exercises applied to Ki-Aikido and to daily living. The rationale behind the exercises is carefully presented. This is the source-book for Ki Aikido written by the founder of the Ki Society.
- **TOT**: *Total Aikido* (Gozo Shioda, 1996): Yoshinkan-style Aikido with illustrations and clear instructions. Information on "How Not To" is as carefully presented as "How To" with common mistakes.
- **ZC**: *Zen Combat* (Jay Gluck, 1997): The late Jay Gluck was the first American exchange student to post-WWII Japan. Stories and tales from the formative years of Aikido.

Also note the following abbreviations in the text:

LH = Left Hand, **RH** = Right Hand, **LF** = Left Foot, **RF** = Right Foot

Acknowledgements

Many thanks to the late George Simcox, former Chief Instructor of the Virginia Ki Society, and Father of Books.

Thanks also to Kjartan Clausen of Norway, maintainer of the Aikido FAQ and Jun Akiyama of Colorado, U. S. A., maintainer of the Aikido-List (begun by Gary Santaro) on the Internet. They are responsible for a world-wide web of Aikido friends and contributors who grumble about "trivia and lack of useful material on the List," while helping me to write this book a line and a thought and a nugget of information at a time.

Thanks to fellow travelers, helpers, and contributors including:

Philip Akin,

Jim Baker, Margo Ballou, Trudy Barnum, Mike ["Insert Quote Here"] Bartman, Kevin Beck, David Berger, Jan Beyen, Leonard Bohanan, Bruce Bookman, Peter Boylan" the Budo Bum," Chris Brogden, David C. Buchanan,

Ben Calvert, Gloria Campbell, Vicky Chiang,

Mark and Margie Dean, Kirk Demaree, Katherine Derbyshire, Serban Derlogea, Guy de Wolf, Emily Dolan, Jay Dunn,

Suzette Hayden Elgin, Matt Firor, Tony Fitts,

Robert E. Gardner, John Garner, Tarik J. Ghbeish, Stephen Gilligan, Tim Gion, Jay Gluck, Cady Goldfield, Chuck Gordon, Dale and Franklyn Gorell, Paul Gowder, Tim Griffiths, Wendy Gunther,

Judy Halloran, Daniel M. Henry, Julie Herbert, Dennis Hooker,

Patrick L. Jones, Carolyn Johnston,

Beate Kawelke, Ed Keith, Steve Kendall,

Neil McKellar, Wiley Nelson, Monica Norman,

John Oldenburg, Greg Olson,

Robert Pavese, Hilda Perkins, Minh Pham, Chris Pierce, John Pinkman, Will Reed, Janet Rosen,

Karl Schmidt, Yael Shahar, Dex Sinister, Michael Speece, Hal Singer, Stefan Stenudd, Chizuko Suzuki, Ben Swett,

Jim Templeman, William Thorndike, Jr., Joseph Toman, Lisa Tomoleoni,

Laura Walton, David Wang, John Wiley, Steve Wolf, Maxine Wright, and

Joel and Janice Zimba.

CHAPTER 1   *Introducing Aikido*

Aikido is a relatively new martial art dating from the 1920s when its founder, Morihei Ueshiba (*O-Sensei*[1]), began to develop what he eventually came to call *Aikido*[2], "the way to harmony with *ki*."

It is rooted in the Japanese *samurai* warrior tradition and incorporates concepts from swordsmanship. It is also based on Ueshiba's nearly 20-year study of *Daito-ryu jujutsu* which was gentled and transformed by his attachment to the Omoto religion and its celebration of life, creation, and loving protection of others.

Aikido replaced the maiming and destruction of the classical battlefield martial arts with control and compassion. Its goal is to subdue and control a situation, protecting both the attacker and the attacked. Aikido is, for example, the only martial art recommended to the parents of abusive children.

Ideally the Aikidoist does not punch or kick to injure or harm unnecessarily, does not block or resist attacks but blends with, redirects and transforms the attacker's energy, maintaining the flow. The result is devastating softness, invisible technique and an art that makes no sense to most observers accustomed to force against force.

There are surely more questions about the hows and whys of Aikido than for any other martial art. Some thoughts on these follow.

---

1. "Honored Teacher."
2. Aikido, Judo, Kendo, *Daito-ryu*, and Karate (Okinawan rather than Japanese) are all *gendai* ("modern") styles rooted in *koryu*, the traditional ("old flow") schools of classical *budo*. The division between traditional and modern is the end of the Shogunate and the Meiji restoration of 1868.

Some Common Questions and Observations

Q. Isn't he just falling down for her?

A. It depends.

An Aikido throw can look so improbably and impossibly smooth and effortless that it is easy to believe that it is faked.

It isn't. It's physics.

The laws of physics are just as strictly enforced at Aikido schools as they are on motorcycles or on ski slopes. If you have ever been a beginning skier, you know from painful experience just how devastating the forces of physics can be. Saying that the attacker fell down "for" the Aikidoist is like saying that the beginning skier fell down "for" the mountain. The advanced cyclist or skier has learned to use these forces; a small shift in weight or position is the difference between crashing into a tree or swooshing effortlessly through a turn and down the slope.

An accomplished skier flying across the snow is as wildly improbable to the frustrated beginner as an accomplished Aikidoist flying across the mat — but neither one is faking. Skiing is real and motorcycles are real.

As long as ski slopes are littered with the bodies of fallen and frustrated beginners, as long as motorcyclists drop their bikes[1] and as long as Aikidoists align with the law of physics and the universe, Aikido will be real.

Q. Does he *have to* fall down?

A. It depends.

Uke falls when balance and structure dictates that it is no longer possible to stand.
You can prove this with a simple experiment:

1. Stand in the middle of your dojo, on the mat.
2. Jump into the air.
3. Try not to fall back to earth.

If gravity dictates that you fall, you can't keep from returning to the ground.
It isn't a matter of speed or strength or submission to pain.
It is a matter of simple physics.
Apply this simple principle to all your Aikido techniques.

—Wiley Nelson

---

1. It is said that there are three groups of bikers: those who have dropped their bikes, those who haven't yet, and those who lie about it. Bikes fall on the street for exactly the same reasons that ukes fall on the mat. See "On Zen and The Art of Motorcycles" on page 82.

Q. What is Aikido?

A. It is . . .

Walking 10 steps down a flight of stairs when there are only 9.
Pushing a door just as someone opens it from the other side.
Reaching out to shake someone's hand just as they step back.

—David Buchanan, Ki Society

Did you ever . . .
Pull a chair out from under someone just as they were sitting down?
Try to kiss a girl on the lips just to have her turn her head at the last moment so the kiss landed on her cheek?
Hold something out to someone and snatch it away at the last moment?
Lead an animal around using bait?
Hold a child's hand to keep him from straying off?
It's not a touch you develop, it's a feeling you hone.

—Dennis Hooker, Aikido Schools of Ueshiba

Origami with people, instead of paper.

—Kjartan Clausen, Aikikai

The art of hitting people with planets.

—Anon.

Love at first flight.

—Randy

Combat yoga.

—Gregory Ford-Kohn, Ki Society

I've got you, I've got you, I've . . . oh Noooooooooooo!

—Many new students

Actually, I have had people look at me oddly when I say I study Aikido and ask "Isn't that one of those Japanese dogs?"
I have learned to reply with a straight face: "Yes. This is an art in which, when someone attacks, you pick up a dog and hurl it at them. Very effective."

—Janet Rosen, Aikikai

Aikido is a way of unifying the world.

—Morihei Ueshiba (*O-Sensei*)

Q. How is Aikido different from karate?

A. In the variety of responses and the end goal.

> In many martial arts there is really very little choice, since the techniques themselves and the methods by which they are employed . . . are intended to injure if not actually destroy an attacker . . . in Aikido the student is given the freedom and responsibility of choice.
>
> —A. Westbrook and O.Ratti, *Aikido and the Dynamic Sphere*

Because Aikido uses the energy and motion provided by the attacker, there must be a wide variety of possible responses to the wide variety of possible attacking energies and motions. Hal Singer gives this demonstration based on a single wrist grab.

Attack	Karate	Aikido
Pull wrist in, response is:	Punch/Kick	*enter (irimi)*
Push wrist in, response is:	Punch/Kick	*turn (tenkan)*
Turn wrist in, response is:	Punch/Kick	*shiho-nage*
Turn wrist out, response is:	Punch/Kick	*sankyo (wrist-lock)*

And so on . . . with a different response to every different attack.

In the end, because the Aikidoist is blending with the motions, they are easier to deflect, to redirect, to neutralize and control the attacker without the necessity of actual harm. And with far less input of energy and effort by the attacked.

Q. But what if he . . .

A. It depends.

Dennis: OK, but what if the other guy has a tank, and you're on foot and unarmed?

Wendy: Yeah, well what if my guy has a flame thrower, is mounted on a horse, and you are on the space station Mir?

Janet: It depends. What day of the week is it?

—Aikido-L

The possibilities of attack and defense are unlimited. Aikido 101 is like Math 101: we present a specific problem, and then stage a specific attack with specific energy to practice a specific response or its variations.

Calculus or *randori* free-style with infinite variables and possibilities comes later.

For now, give the appropriate energy, respond with the appropriate response. This is how we learn. It is never wrong to ask questions or experiment, but meanwhile, do, practice, test and learn what is presented. (See "Nage and Uke — Partners in the Dance" on page 177.)

Q. How can it possibly work? It's too much like dancing.

A. Dancing is controlled motion. So is Aikido.

> The genius of Aikido is to transform the most violent attack,
> by embracing it, into a dance.
>
> —George Leonard, Aikikai

> I think [Aikido] is the most difficult of all the martial arts to learn.
> Its demands for skill, grace, and timing rival those of classical ballet.
>
> —Jearle Walker, Physicist

Consider Fred Astaire and Ginger Rogers, the two moving in harmony, whirling around the floor in perfect control.

What would have happened to Ginger if Fred had let go at a critical moment?

She would have gone flying across the room and fallen.

What happens when the Aikidoist lets go of an attacker at a critical moment? The attacker goes flying across the room and falls.

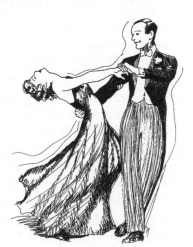

Yes, it is like dancing, but so is everything else.

Conversation is like dancing.

Teamwork is like dancing.

Any form of cooperation is like dancing. You can do it well or you can do it badly.

Yes, Aikido is like dancing[1].

Yes, it works.

---

1. See KIA pp. 233-245 for possible roots of Aikido in Argentine Tango, and the applications of *yin-yang* to Aikido in "The Solid-Empty Game."
   See also the original Japanese version of *Shall We Dance?*

Q. Why protect an attacker?

A. For his sake — *and* yours.

> Whoever fights monsters must beware that in the process he does not become a monster. For when you look long into the abyss, the abyss also looks into you.
>
> —Nietzsche

> The doors of heaven and hell are adjacent and identical.
>
> —Nikos Kazantzakis

It is often gratifying to think that an attacker deserves anything you can dish out. From both legal and practical standpoints this is untrue[1].

Legally you are limited to a type and degree of defense appropriate to the incoming attack, to do what is necessary to control the situation and keep yourself safe.

Practically, you are more likely to face assault from someone you care for, such as a drunken friend or relative, than from a malevolent stranger.

Aikido *skills* allow you to deal with either one but you must practice for both.

Aikido *attitudes* are practical self-defense against ending up in jail yourself for assault or murder. Regardless of who the attacker may be, do what is necessary to control the situation and protect all those concerned. No less, no more.

As Hollywood knows so very well, hatred, fear, vengeance and anger are exciting, exhilarating and energizing. Because they invoke mankind's favorite mind-altering drug of choice — adrenaline — these emotions are extremely seductive and they are the fast track to the Dark Side. Those who feed on the thrill of violence and assault are little different from those who relish and feed on the thrill of vengeance and hatred.

Destroying an attacker because "he attacked and therefore deserves whatever he gets" *is not* "self defense." What is? The late Bruce Tegner wrote an essay on this topic that is remarkable for its grace and good sense[2].

> One way of defining self-defense is to explain what it is not. Personal self-defense is not warfare; it is not vengeance; it is not an art; it is not a sporting event; it is not a movie or television fight scene.
>
> [It] is training to learn and use appropriate and effective physical actions if there is no practical available alternative. Many victims of assault are victims not because they lack the capacity to win fights but because they have been given absolutely no preparation to cope with this special kind of emergency.
>
> The old-fashioned view that self-defense instruction is training to reach a high level of fighting skill has the effect of eliminating those individuals who have the greatest need. It is precisely those people who are unable or unwilling to become fierce fighting machines who benefit from practical self-defense instruction to the greatest degree.
>
> Our capabilities ought to bear some relationship to real-life objectives. People learning to defend themselves against assault ought not to be trained as though they were preparing

---

1. See Sullivan, Edward F. (1993) for street realities.
2. From the introduction to *Self-Defense Nerve Centers and Pressure Points for Karate, Jujitsu and Atemi-waza*. Reproduced by kind permission of Thor Publishing Company, Ventura, California.

for warfare. The legal and moral definition of self-defense expressly limits the degree of force to the least which can be used to avert, stop, or escape from an intended assault. In old-style self-defense, every assault is viewed as a very vicious assault. Real life is different. There are degrees of danger. Assault intentions range from mildly threatening to the intent to do great bodily harm. More important, there are mildly threatening situations which, if handled properly with assertive self-control, can be prevented from escalating into physical violence.

There must be a full range of responses to correspond to the range of possible situations. Otherwise there is only the all-or-nothing response, which is not a choice — it is a dilemma. The person who cannot cope with a mildly threatening hostile act does nothing, or responds to the mild threat as if it were a vicious assault. If the intended victim is passive, it encourages the assailant and assaultive action is more likely to occur. Reacting to a mild threat as though it were a vicious assault is inappropriate. The objective of ethical self-defense instruction is to teach appropriate and effective responses.

—Bruce Tegner

Q. Isn't Aikido too passive? I may need killing blows.

A. Why? And what will they do to *you*?

Many that live deserve death.
And some that die deserve life. Can you give it to them?
Then do not be too eager to deal out death in judgment,
for even the wise cannot see all ends.
—Gandalf, *The Fellowship of the Ring* (J.R.R. Tolkien)

Whoever kills one innocent soul, it is as if he killed the entire humanity.
—*The Koran* (Chapter 5, Verse 32)

Protect an attacker for his sake — *and for yours*.

Contrary to popular fantasy, martial arts do not dwell in remote mountain temples of spiritual enlightenment. They do not float cloud-like high above the civil and criminal laws of State and country.

It isn't practical to spend several nights a week for 20 years studying deadly killing blows because someday you might be attacked On The Street while "just minding your own business." You're far more likely to trip over your feet while day-dreaming about such things and end up in the ER with a broken wrist or collarbone[1]. If you are actually attacked, you must still behave in a disappointingly rational manner.

Why? For effective *self defense*.

Real-Life laws on self-defense are thick with words such as "justifiable," "intent," and "reasonable." Self-justification of the worst possible intent is a common human talent, but if there is injury and especially if there is death, you will not be the one with the final say on whether your actions were reasonable and justifiable. You won't even be the one to decide whether they truly qualify as self-defense.

---

1. These two accidental injuries are the most common reasons for ER admissions aside from bad judgement with power tools.

If you behave badly, you may need to protect yourself from the perpetrator long after the fact. Professional criminals know more about the law than anyone else except the lawyers. It's their job. They know what their rights are and they know that if you took the opportunity of adding punishment to self-defense they can sue you for damages.

American courts consider self-defense to be a natural right of self-preservation. In general[1], a person is justified in using physical force upon another person in order to defend himself or another person from what he reasonably believes to be the use of unlawful physical force by that other person. Deadly force is for emergencies *only*. Under the law it is justified only if a person reasonably believes himself or another person to be in *imminent* danger of receiving serious physical injury, of being killed, kidnapped, or sexually assaulted.

So, yes, you can kill in reasonable self-defense. *However*, the emphasis is on *reasonable*. Deadly force is allowed only in situations where lesser force is not a reasonable option. That is, for a tiny 90-pound girl faced with a 250-pound body-builder attacker, whose only choices are to out-wrestle or shoot the attacker, shooting is considered reasonable self defense. However . . .

- You can't claim "self-defense" if you started the encounter as by taunting or provoking another person into stupid or violent behavior.
- You can't claim "self-defense" if you are assaulting someone and a third party comes to his/her aid. Assaulting this other person in turn is *assault*, not self-defense.
- You can't stage your very own "No Holds Barred" knife fight then claim "self-defense" when the guy you beat is badly injured or dead. The only exception to this is if the initial aggressor sees the error of his ways and makes it clear that he wants out of the situation, but the original victim continues to act in an aggressive manner.

Bottom line: You can claim "self-defense" only as long as it *is* self-defense and response matches the threat. Adding physical force to the point that the initial victim becomes the attacker and the former attacker becomes the new victim isn't self-defense either. When two combatants face off, there's nothing more common than for the loser to claim he was attacked and for the victor to claim self-defense. The police know this very well; no matter who ends up in the hospital they will be out looking for the other guy.

Feeling deadly? Make sure your reasons add up, because in the final analysis, what is *reasonable* will not decided by you. *Reasonable* will be decided by judge and jury.

The school or teacher or student who ignores this is in favor of martial arts fantasy and legal delusion is in for serious trouble.

As Bruce Tegner said, "There must be a full range of responses to correspond to the range of possible situations."

Aikido offers an unusually full range of responses for a wide range of situations to protect the attacker — *and to protect you.*

---

1. Most State statutes are available on the Internet. Many assume that Western laws are more "wild and woolly" than sissy Eastern ones, but there is little difference between Colorado and New York.

Q. Does Aikido work "On the Street"?

A. Why do you ask?

If you have a fantasy of becoming the invincible ultimate fighting warrior, learning a martial art won't help you achieve it. That's a fantasy, remember? To become "effective" first you have to drop the nonsense and meet Mr. Reality. He's the only one you have to defeat. Unfortunately, he always wins.

Aikido isn't a quick course in self defense. It takes a while before you could use the techniques.In Brooklyn, we'd answer this question with, "Look, you live in New York City. Sometime in the next five years you'll probably be mugged. They'll take your money, and maybe they'll hurt you.

Or you can study Aikido. Here we will take your money every month, and guarantee to hurt you every time you come!"

— Jim Baker, Aikikai

Q. How come it didn't work? (1)

A. Did your technique not work? Define "Working" or "Not Working."

Aikido works. Your Aikido doesn't. Don't confuse the two.

—Hiroshi Ikeda, Aikikai

It is useful to define what you mean by "it worked" or "it didn't work."

If someone grabs you and you prefer that he not do that, you have many options. Some techniques (especially those known as *kokyu-nage*) depend on the attacker holding on to the defender; the attacker is in danger of being thrown only so long as he holds on. If he lets go, you have no throw. But, if your purpose was to persuade the attacker to let go and he did, then the technique "worked." You do not have to put him on the ground to achieve that purpose.

When the purpose is to learn a technique, you are not there to fight, you are there to learn. The technique may proceed too slowly to "work" as a *throw*; it "works" as patterning and as part of the learning process, just as you would learn a new dance step.

Unfortunately, new students commonly see throwing as "winning" and falling as "losing." The attacker (*uke*) may counter every move that the thrower (*nage*) makes, or let go as soon as they feel themselves in danger of falling. They then confuse the cessation or change of their own attack with failure of the technique — and of Aikido.

In Aikido, falling is not "losing." It is *uke*'s time to practice *ukemi*. *Uke* is not loser but teacher[1]. The ability to fall safely is a valuable self-defense technique and a valuable tool for helping your partner to learn. We learn to give the appropriate attack and we learn to fall so that we can help others to learn. You "win" by being a good teacher.

Winning means winning over the discord in yourself. Those who have a warped mind, a mind of discord, have been defeated from the beginning

—Morihei Ueshiba

---

1. See "Nage and Uke — Partners in the Dance" on page 177.

Q. How come it didn't work? (2)
A. Aikido is defensive. Were you defending or attacking?

Aikido is primarily a defensive technique. It counters, neutralizes, and redirects attacks; it rarely offers them. Because the defender uses the attacker's strength and inertia, rather than his own, a smaller defender has a tremendous advantage — so long as he avoids a weight and strength contest.

When someone at home or office asks what Aikido is about, new students usually invite the questioner to "grab my wrist." They "do" something, the "attacker" counters, and it often ends up as wrestling match, not Aikido. Why?

- The attacker is feeling apprehensive and isn't really attacking so there is limited energy to work with.
- The student is trying to "do" a technique from a limited repertoire, rather than what might be most appropriate for the energy given.
- When the attacker blocks the technique, the student tries to force it, and the attacker forces back — a weight and strength contest, not Aikido.

"Real Aikido techniques" require and deal with real attacks. But on the street or on the mat, there should only be *one* attacker.

Q. Is Aikido really practical for self-defense?
A. Yes.

What we are all striving for is complete control over an attacker, a perfect combination of timing and sensitivity and power that allows us to go untouched as we "move" our attacker wherever we want. This may be onto his head or this may be simply to the other side of the room where he is, temporarily, no longer a threat — your choice. But at that level of control, you have that choice. Aikido suggests what you do with that control.

—David Berger, Aikikai

Practical is exactly the right word.

We go to see wildly impractical fantasy adventure slice & dice movies with Bad Guys and crazed psychotics, where the only hope of survival is superior firepower, and where the monster never dies.

In most Real Lives, an attacker is much more likely to be someone you know and care about, where firepower and death-dealing blows are not desirable or sensible options. While most martial arts are designed to kill or maim, Aikido offers the choice of control and a range of options regardless of the attacker.

The word "attacker" usually conjures up the movie version of the crazed stranger. Far more likely in Real Life are:

Drunken Buddies. A *Tae Kwon Do* blackbelt came to us because of drunken fraternity brothers who came home throwing punches and kicks so he would "show them his moves." Because "his moves" were designed to smash and kill, they were not an option. Meanwhile, his unwillingness to harm people he cared about was getting him beaten up. We showed him *tenkan*. He stayed.

Abusive Children. When my 12-year-old stepson came to live with us, he hit, slapped, or kicked me at every opportunity. When I spoke to him, he "wasn't doing anything" or he was "just playing." Not surprising. He loves his Mom and loves his Dad and although they had already been divorced for over seven years when I first met his father, it is obvious to a child that if only this strange other person would *just go away,* then Mom and Dad could get back together again.

Very wrong, but very understandable. Problem was, the "kid" was as big as I was, weighed more, and was being abusive. What was I to do?

- Yell "Just wait 'til your father gets home!" at every incident? — an abdication of authority and responsibility.
- Pull out my handy sidearm and blow him away?

Obviously neither of these were options. Aikido was.

The next punch got him flipped onto the couch. The next grab got him rolled across the rug and the next slap got him a firm *ikkyo* plant with pin. Any combination of these got him out of breath (as he was also fighting gravity) but he was allowed to live and I was not arrested for child abuse or murder. When he began purposely doing these things for the *fun* of getting rolled across the rug or flipped onto the sofa, we enrolled him in Aikido class.

Think of a favorite uncle who's had a bit too much to drink at the party, the wedding, the divorce, the layoff. This is your child, your brother, your friend. This may also be your attacker. Are you going to:

- Smash and destroy a person you care for?
- Be rendered completely helpless by unwillingness to harm? (While your attacker takes full advantage of your kindness).
- Be effective — and very glad that effectiveness and control come with the option *not* to smash and destroy?

How you *train* is how you will *do* Aikido. Choose a *range* of appropriate tools. And train for that.

. . . . Thus the attacked is saved from harm, and the attacker is saved from sin.
—Morihei Ueshiba

Q. Can a woman ever beat a man?

A. Yes.

Most of my Aikido heroes were under 5'4" and 130 pounds, and over 65 years old. Our friend Vicky is about 4'9" and threw a beefy prison guard so far that he asked if it qualified him for frequent flyer mileage.

—Jim Baker, Aikikai

I've often heard men gravely discuss some encounter with a hostile fellow "who must have been heavier by 20 pounds and at least 2 inches taller" while his listener nodded seriously in sympathy. It's strange to hear big strong fellows worry about a few inches and a few pounds when women, who have been assaulted by men a couple inches to a couple feet taller and heavier by several pounds to several hundred pounds, are often dismissed with the suspicion that they didn't "Just Say No" firmly enough.

In Aikido the tables are turned. Aikido uses the attacker's own weight, inertia, strength, and energy in such a way that smaller persons actually have an advantage. It may seem impossible but it is very real. [1]

Vicky is Chinese Cuban, has a *sandan*, rows like *O-Sensei*, does bookkeeping, teaches *reiki*, weighs 80 pounds, measures 4' 9", and in my presence beat up a Rikers Island prison cop who benches 300+ who had decided to learn Aikido. There was nothing he could do about it, either. And she giggled off and on as she did it.

He came over to me after about the fifth fall.

"Did you see that?"

"Yes, Mike, I saw it."

"I was flyin'!"

"Yes, Mike, you were."

He went back, and she beat him up again.

Sometimes the terrifying downswing on her muscleless *irimi-nage* reminds me of a story Hal once told me about falling so far, for so long, from one of Sugano *Sensei's* throws that he had time to actually begin to worry that there was no ground, that he was on the descent into hell and was going to go on downward forever; and when he did hit the mat, he almost kissed it, he was so grateful it was there.

—Wendy Gunther, Aikikai

---

1. See "A Brief Ki Class" on page 55 for the physics of Aikido and the power of small or large bodies.

Q. But doesn't size matter?

A. No.

You humans! When you gonna learn that size doesn't matter?
—Frank the Dog in *Men in Black*

I spent ten years getting my ass kicked by Japanese people who weighed one-third of what I did. There's not one person I fear more than anybody else. Size or sex have nothing to do with it.
—Terry Dobson, *It's a Lot Like Dancing*

One day I received a shipment of fan-foot geckos, small lizards about six inches long. Suddenly, while I was digging around in the box, one of the lizards ran up my arm and clamped itself onto the skin right over my carotid artery. Startled, I clamped my hand over the lizard, and sat up suddenly.
But the back of the chair that I was sitting in was broken. I fell backwards out of the chair, in the process, kicking the box, sending a couple dozen lizards airborne in a diffuse pattern that covered most of the room. I ended up on the floor, clutching my throat, in a futile attempt to defend myself from this one-ounce lizard who had quite cleanly thrown and pinned me and who even liberated his comrades in the process.
—Wiley Nelson

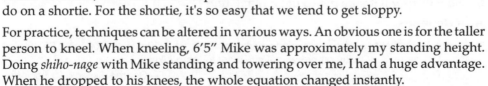

In Aikido size usually does *not* matter (except that shorter folk usually have usually have the greater advantage). Some techniques are awkward for partners of radically different sizes. Height differences cause problems due to different perceptions of "up" and "down." A very tall person may think he is dropping down but his "down" may still be "up" to a shorter person while the shorter person's "up" is still "down" to him[1].

For example, *shiho-nage* involves ducking under *uke*'s arm, difficult for a tall person to do on a shortie. For the shortie, it's so easy that we tend to get sloppy.

For practice, techniques can be altered in various ways. An obvious one is for the taller person to kneel. When kneeling, 6'5" Mike was approximately my standing height. Doing *shiho-nage* with Mike standing and towering over me, I had a huge advantage. When he dropped to his knees, the whole equation changed instantly.

Sometimes techniques must be subtly altered. Rather than trying to control the head, a shorter person may concentrate on control of wrist and fingers that control the arm, then torso, then head. Working with these differences is one of the many advantages of having practice partners of various shapes and sizes.

---

1. See comments on Kokyu-Nage Basic on page 214 for problems of insufficient up and down.

Q. What about physical disabilities?

A. They can be adapted.

Almost everyone has some sort of disability. In the end, it isn't the particular condition that matters as much as determination and persistence.

A young woman apparently doomed to life in a wheelchair was somehow dragged into Aikido. She went on to become a *nidan* with her own *dojo*. (See

One of our students, Jim Templeman, has no arms and he has taught us so much. No one has a more compelling *tenkan* than Jim! He isn't distracted by trying to muscle *uke* to the mat with his arms like the rest of us.

> Jim started out taking classes in Ki Development and Mind and Body Coordination. One evening at the beginning of the second hour I started to teach *ryokata-tori* techniques — both of *uke*'s hands holding onto *nage*'s *gi*. I got a *gi* top from our closet and invited Jim to participate in the first three techniques since they don't use arms. The rest is history.
>
> We don't change the class much to accommodate Jim but I usually work with him and his partner after the general instruction and figure out how to use the principles being taught with the "technique of the hour" into something Jim can do. He now has his 5th Kyu and is working toward 4th Kyu. Last month he was a member of a demonstration group for a local middle school and wowed the kids with his skill. Jim has taught us much about our art and ourselves. Blessings come in many shapes and guises. Jim is one of ours.
>
> —George Simcox, Ki Society

> My (now former) mother-in-law, over 50, portly, with persistent myalgia, asked me to teach her some Aikido. I was touched and honored. We went to the pool, and worked on *tenkan* from same side grab, spinning each other in the warm water. We also did some gentle releases and wrist locks. She cannot sit *seiza* on land, her knees aren't strong enough. But she can do it on the steps in the pool. I taught her how to rise properly so she can practice it with the water's support. "Pool-kido" for those with physical obstacles has potential to bring principles of efficient movement to those not able to withstand the rigors of "normal" Aikido training. It's also a lot of fun!
>
> —Emily D. Gordon, Kokoro Ryu Jujutsu

Q. How long will it take me to get a black belt?

A. It depends.

> There's a martial arts store nearby and you can pick one up in 10 minutes for about $6.00. On the other hand, if you want to learn Aikido . . . .
>
> —George Simcox, Ki Society

> How long is a piece of string?
>
> —Emily Dolan, Seidokan

> How long does it take to catch a fish?
>
> —Michael Bartman, Ki Society

Q. I've heard it takes 3-4 years to be proficient . . .

A. . . . Which is typical of real stuff that real humans do.

Think about it. Does a person with a two-year junior college degree know as much as one with a four-year degree? What does the job market say to that?

If you want to learn cooking, how good are you in six months? Decent, but nobody's going to hire you into the kitchen of a four-star restaurant, are they? With just six months of experience, nobody's going to hire you to run the microwave at the local diner because in just six months you are not yet good enough to go pro. Whether you want to learn how to restore old cars, shoot skeet, or run a business, how good are you in just six months?

Most real things take people about four years to get moderately competent at, and several years later they get some degree of mastery. (Aikido, being more complex, kind of up there with ballet or pro basketball, takes a few years longer.) But we all have this fantasy that somehow self defense is going to come faster than other human endeavors. Why? Because we might need it sooner? Hey, I can hear Mr. Reality laughing at us!

What would you think if you heard I was going around to medical schools, saying, "You tell me I can get an MD in four years, but MediQuick U. has offered me one in three. Can you promise to give me one in two and a half?" Then when your HMO assigns me to you against your will as your personal doctor how happy are you going to be if you find out I did just two and a half years of MD training, and went straight from that into practice?

Why should a black belt be any different from that? In *any* art?

It takes several years to get good at Aikido, just as it takes several years to get good at basketball, skiing, piloting a plane, or learning a language.

That's because Aikido is *real*.

—Dr. Wendy Gunther, Aikikai

Q. What if I need a self-defense class now?

A. Take a self-defense class now.

Martial arts are a long-term investment in time, money, and effort. Aikido does not provide instant self-defense. Neither does any other martial art. Neither does signing up for Drawing 101 or Basic Auto Repair make you an artist or a mechanic.

An excellent short-term self-defense series is the renowned Model Mugging (now called IMPACT Self Defense) which features full-impact training and skills in attitude, response, and technique[1].

Meanwhile, be aware of your own strengths and weaknesses. If you were a mugger, who would you pick and why? Professional muggers have repeatedly stated that their choice of target is heavily dependent on walk and carriage.

Women wobbling along in tight skirts and high heels[2] (the Western version of Chinese bound feet) are natural targets, as are men who walk in a vague, foot-flopping sort of

---

1. Classes emphasize women's stronger hips and legs while training the types of attacks which women are more likely to face. Classes are also available for children and men and all feature full contact with a fully padded attacker.

2. Silly shoes can invite a mugging. They can also kill more directly. "On 9/11, women were almost twice as likely to get injured while evacuating . . . a question of strength? Confidence? Fear? 'No,' says lead investigator Robyn Gershon. 'It was the shoes.' Many women took off their heels halfway through the evacuation and had to walk home barefoot. Survivors reported tripping over piles of high-heeled shoes in the staircases." Ripley, Amanda (2008).

way, or persons inattentive to surroundings and those with a poor sense of personal space. If in doubt, attackers will actually "interview" potential targets to confirm their potential as low-risk victims but the initial selection takes about seven seconds.

In a classic study[1] prisoners convicted of street assault were shown videos of people walking down the street and asked to rate their vulnerability. Those rated as highly vulnerable shared the following basic characteristics.

- Abnormally long or short strides.
- Placing the whole foot on the ground rather than using normal heel-to-toe motion.
- Moving same-side leg and arm at same time, rather than opposite arm and leg. While this appears to describe the "samurai walk" (page 44) it also describes the walk of severely overweight persons whose legs must roll around one another rather than directly past.
- Moving upper body independent of lower body, random arm and leg movements; not moving from Center.

Your best short and long-term self-defense?

Awareness, mind-body coordination, and confidence.

What we learn in Aikido.

Q. If you aren't here for self-defense on the street, why are you here?
A. Because there's more.

When I was in my third year of theatre school we got a new voice teacher. He had individual sessions with each student to evaluate their voice work. I went in and did my best big, deep, full theatre-resonant type voice. Beautifully supported and all.
He looked at me and said, "Well that's very nice, Philip. What else can you do?"
I have kind of adopted that as one of my mottoes.

—Philip Akin, Aikido Yoshinkai Canada

There's more to Aikido than self defense. People who have studied for more than a year or so seem rarely to be still in it only for application "On The Street." That was on the list initially, but not at the top. It is now pretty much at the bottom, and may be dropped entirely. So why study? A lot of reasons.
It's different from everything else I do, and I often need to be boosted out of my rut. There are aspects of it that I can't explain, and I love puzzles. I find the basic principles satisfying. They fit well with my outlook on things, and I love the way they are simple yet subtly complex. I can use any exercise, but I hate gerbil-like activities like stationary bikes and treadmills.
I've found things I learn at the dojo useful in all areas of life, including working with my boss, undergoing surgery, opening heavy doors, not falling on ice, and falling down a flight of stairs without getting hurt in the least (not even a bruise!) Being around the sort of folks who show up at the *dojo* is pleasant and relaxing. They are friendly, cheerful, helpful, kind, and interested in at least one of the things I'm interested in: Aikido!

—Michael Bartman, Ki Society

---

1. Grayson and Morris (1981). See "The Interview Language of Physical Attack" on page 247.

Q. Is Aikido the Ultimate Martial Art?

A. No.

Thermonuclear warfare is the Ultimate Martial Art, followed by long range artillery, armor, guns, knives, and large guys named Bubba. If you want to defend yourself in the street, buy a tank. Aikido isn't about that, neither is real *Budo*.

—— Jim Baker, Aikikai

Q. What if this were a *real* attack?

A. Make it a real attack now.

Although what happens on the mat is staged practice, the attacks should be quite real in terms of an attack having a particular direction, force, or momentum. Hence "real" is probably best interpreted as: "What happens in an attack or counter with a different direction, or force?"

Good question. Try it and see. Practicing different possibilities and options will raise your techniques from the level of staged Aikido to Real Aikido.

Not all attacks to the hand are the same and the different techniques are designed for different types of energy. You can practice all the *katate-tori* techniques to develop a repertoire of techniques for apparently similar attacks.

One technique designed for a wrist grab may deal with pulling forward, another with pulling back. Practice the alternatives. Every Aikido technique can be countered. In fact, the advanced Aikidoist will often set up a situation that invites a counter. These are known as "conversions" and are part of the fun of advanced Aikido.

Q. But instead I could . . .

A. Yes, but please don't.

We start by practicing basic attacks, basic skills and basic solutions to basic problems. Practice what you are practicing.

New students sometimes want to spend time debating intricate nuances of this or that, theoretical or *movie-do* comparisons with other styles, or pronouncements on why the basic technique they've been assigned to practice couldn't possibly work in the Real World. Better to get up and practice. There are things about driving a car with a manual transmission which simply cannot be explained in words to someone who has never driven anything but an automatic — or who has never driven at all.

Please practice what your teacher is teaching. Mat time is short and precious.

I think training hard, often and diligently is the only philosophy. After 23 some-odd years (some of them very odd), I find that the more I talk about philosophy, the more it eludes me. As long as I train, all that takes care of itself. Ki, harmony, love, whatever. All the same. All useless without good training to take you there. Without a solid foundation in the basics, nothing else is really pertinent anyway.

Talk about it and it slips away. Ignore it and it comes to you. Kind of like a cat.

—Chuck Gordon, Kokoro Ryu Aiki Budo

Q. But it's all staged. It isn't real!

A. Neither is Terminator, Freddy, Rambo, or James Bond.

> The trick, Fletcher, is that we are trying to overcome our limitations in order, patiently. We don't tackle flying through rock until a little later in the program.
>
> —Richard Bach, *Jonathan Livingston Seagull*

New students can't help but compare their first beginning steps with what they have seen in carefully choreographed movies. They aren't the same. Movies have the advantage of rehearsals, a set script, multiple shots, deceptive camera angles, stunt men, safety equipment, skillful editing, and few surprises. Learning Aikido is like learning other skills, from piano to basketball. Here's how it works in Real Life.

Level 1: Beginning Practice

> In school, it's learning to print big block letters and do basic arithmetic. In motorcycle class, it's the "duck walk," learning balance and how to shift gears. In skiing it's the bunny slope and "snowplow," proper foot position, weighting and posture.

In beginning Aikido, attacks are staged and static; techniques are done slowly and haltingly with emphasis on following the lines of force and leading energy. The purpose is not to smash *uke* to the ground, but to progress through the technique to its conclusion at which point *uke* is given the opportunity to practice *ukemi*. It is not the time to carp about how the situation would be handled in other martial arts or to list the reasons why this or that would or would not work "On the Street." In truth the technique may not yet "work" as a technique, because there is little movement, little reason for *uke* to be off-balance[1]. The task at hand is not so much to make *uke* fall down as it is to learn the letters and the alphabet of Aikido that will later be formed into words, and still later into entire sentences and stories.

> The alphabet of fencing . . . is as fixed and immutable as any other alphabet. Its characters are ascertained and definite motions, which are combined in accordance with the structure and balance of our organism, the natural action of the muscles and the flexibility possible to the limbs and body.
>
> —Baron César de Bazancourt, *Secrets of the Sword*

> Practice is like honing a knife. You start with a ragged piece of steel. You put it on the grinder, but two or three passes won't do the job. It has to be honed and honed and honed. Even then you aren't done, because with use, you still have to hone and sharpen. It is a never-ending process.
>
> —William Thorndike, Jr.

> The more I train, the more I realize that there are no "advanced techniques," just basics applied well.
>
> —Peter W. Boylan

---

1. See the physics of traffic on page 76. Consider walking through that curve or racing through the curve at full speed — in a fully loaded dump truck. The forces will be very different.

Level 2: Intermediate Practice

Printing becomes more fluid as the student is thinking and writing in words rather than individual letters. This child can also walk and run, but is amazed by older children on bicycles and skates. In motorcycling it is developing balance and the ability to lean into a curve and apply brakes without falling over. In skiing it is learning to carve (rather than force) turns but no idea how to handle moguls.

In the intermediate levels of Aikido, the student begins to grasp *processes* and *sequences* rather than one-step operations. This level emphasizes moving and leading *uke*'s center and balance. The "real" effects of flow and centrifugal forces begin to appear. Many throws still do not work in the sense of unbalancing. Many throws do.

Level 3: Advanced Practice

Calligraphy and calculus. Knowing the forms and building blocks, challenging them, enjoying them, playing among them. In motorcycling it's motocross. In skiing it's flying through the mogul fields that are so terrifying to beginning skiers — and loving it.

Advanced Aikido combines leading and moving in response to dynamic, forceful attacks. Minute adjustments in position and direction lead and move *uke* into positions that align with powerful forces of the Universe, of gravity, centrifugal force, inertia, and balance or loss of balance.

Q. But "On The Street . . ."

A. . . . Is mostly Hollywood and is mostly bunk.

Bad things happen and yes, some of them happen On the Street. However, most of them happen in Hollywood.

- *Do not* base training on a theatrical scenario designed to sell adrenaline and tickets.
- *Do not* use these scenarios to excuse or cultivate a mindset of justified vengeance and murder or to shortcut or alter techniques on the mat.
- *Do* consider a little statistical reality. Contrary to the popular media, most deadly injuries are not due to muggers with handguns. They are due to motor vehicle accidents and they are due to falls, usually at home or close to it.

What's really On The Street is cars. You may be in a hurry, lost, angry or frightened — and so may the other person. Therefore practice *ma-ai,* patience, awareness, flowing and blending. Practice good etiquette, good manners, good sense, kindness and consideration. Observe the laws of physics to keep yourself and others safe.

What's really on the street is concrete. You may trip on the curb, slip on the ice, miss a step, break a wrist, an arm, a leg, a head. Therefore practice your rolls and *ukemi*; it can save your life as it once saved mine.

The leading cause of death in America? It isn't psychopathic killers, gangs, or drugs, although you'd never know it from the movies. It is automobile accidents[1], barbecue

---

1. Amazingly, this is true even for policemen.

and "biscuit poisoning." That is, too much speed, too little awareness, too much fat, too much sugar, too little exercise, too much alcohol, too many power tools, and too little good sense. It is sticking your head in an alligator's mouth and yelling: "Bite me and you've had it!" when caution would have been the far better part of valor.

In Real Life, almost one-third of all accidental deaths including homicides, suicides, fire, and traffic deaths, are tragically visited (apparently as a random violent act of the Universe) upon persons who just happen to be legally drunk at the time.

Similarly, an amazing number of men are injured while trying to kiss rattlesnakes.

During Hurricane Floyd in 1999, a medical worker in Gainesville, Florida, reported that trauma cases fell into three distinct groups.

1. Three-car pileups suffered by people racing to get out before Floyd hit.
2. Chainsaw accidents from people who weren't familiar with chainsaws and who decided to go out and chainsaw down trees leaning against their homes, sometimes after several beers.
3. Later, as the storm was passing, elderly ladies with broken hips who had decided to go out into 40 m.p.h. winds on slick, rain-covered surfaces, in bathrobes and bedroom slippers, to get the newspaper down by the mailbox.

The real causes of death in the U.S. in order are:

1) Heart disease, 2) cancer, 3) stroke, 4) chronic lower respiratory diseases, 5) accidents especially *falls* (page 127) , 6) Alzheimer's disease, 7) diabetes, 8) influenza and pneumonia, 9) kidney disease, 10) blood poisoning, 11) intentional self-harm, 12) chronic liver disease and cirrhosis, 13) hypertension and hypertensive renal disease, 14) Parkinson's disease, 15) assault (homicide).

Behind this list you will see the results of bad diet, smoking and alcohol, and death by over-the-counter and prescription drugs. Notice also that you are more likely to kill yourself than to be killed by someone else.

Effective self-defense is not merely an issue of showing up at the dojo; it isn't an issue of how many bricks you can break or how many belts you've earned. It's a matter of surviving daily life using *all* your tools.

It is careful driving, seat belts, and using your body as it was designed to be used.

It is soap and water, good food, good rest, and recreation.

It is doing your homework, paying bills on time, dealing honorably with others.

It is batteries in the fire alarm, knowing how to swim, balancing your check book, and avoiding assault by banks, credit cards, payday loan sharks, and many other smiling attackers who can be far worse than the growling ones.

It's all the bits and pieces that make up daily life. *Real* life.

Aikido is just one more way of being responsible for yourself.

Practice Aikido on the mat, on the street, and at home.

Practice good sense and sensible living.

Q. Isn't Aikikai too hard? Ki Society too soft? Yoshinkan too stiff?

A. It depends.

> With softness and relaxation come responsiveness.
> —Bruce Bookman, Seattle Aikikai

Technique largely depends on the *practitioner* . In working with advanced students who presumably represent their respective styles, the most softly effective technique I ever felt came from Aikikai, the hardest and stiffest from Ki Society, one of the most graceful and flowing from Yoshinkan.

Yoshinkan is usually considered to preserve Aikido as it was up to WWII, Aikikai as it was up to *O-Sensei's* death. Ki Society split from Aikikai in part to include a new teaching tool (Ki Development Exercises) based on yoga.

These different styles offer different emphases, different approaches to teaching and learning. Yoshinkan and Ki Society, for example, are more *methods of teaching* than *styles* of Aikido technique. As a Ki Society practitioner, the most remarkable technical difference I have seen between the three styles is that Ki Society tends to emphasize rolls over breakfalls, and Yoshinkan techniques always move forward, never backward. Other differences are seen between individual instructors.

Few of us embody the pure philosophy of our particular style or made our original choice of style strictly on that basis. Choice of *dojo* is usually based more on rush-hour traffic patterns and rapport with other students than on philosophy.

But how different are the various styles of Aikido really? In 1998, members of the international Internet Aikido-L mailing list cyberdojo resolved to meet, to compare differences and perhaps to showcase the superiority of their particular styles — only to discover that while they were all different, they were all practicing Aikido. Another happy result of this gathering is a tremendous increase in visits and exchanges between dojos and seminars.

Before, "Not my style."

Now, *Aikido Friends*.

Q. Won't seminars be too confusing?

A. Seminars are valuable sources of supplemental information.

Shady martial arts schools are notorious for forbidding students to attend seminars or study Aikido magazines or books on the grounds that it will "confuse them." In reality, such persons are often less concerned about confusion than fearful that they will be revealed as frauds when their students realize that what they are doing bears no resemblance to real Aikido.

This is quite different from legitimate instructors feeling a tad annoyed with those who return from seminars having Seen The Light and announcing that "so-and-so does it this way and *your* way is wrong." Very often what they have seen are stylistic differences which can be greater between instructor and instructor than between named styles.[1] Being aware of variations can actually help to reinforce understanding of the underlying fundamentals. On the other hand, one's understanding of the basics themselves may undergo an epiphany.

Years ago I fell in love with the Paraguayan harp. In the course of attempting to teach myself to play, I learned that it was a true folk instrument with little or nothing written down. The traditional course of study (as in many martial arts) was to visit the instructor daily and memorize the lessons without written text or materials.

By wonderful coincidence, I met a Paraguayan harpist in town for the summer without her harp, willing to trade lessons for practice time. On learning that she couldn't read music, I offered to teach her. She adamantly refused for fear it would "stifle her creativity" (a common concern of play-by-ear musicians). She had another odd concern: the colors of the strings and their sequence. Fortunately, mine were the "proper" configuration and so we began with the traditional beginner's piece, *La Llegada*.

"Be patient!" she urged. "Don't give up! It took me six months to learn this but stick with it and practice, practice, practice! Eventually you will get it."

And so I did. While she played the music through, I transcribed it to staff paper. Within 10 minutes I had a fairly presentable rendition of what she had needed six months to learn. It needed work, of course, but notes and timing were correct because I had the advantage of reading them off the page rather than having to memorize everything at once by rote. She was stunned and I think a bit distressed. And so was I when I realized her problem with colors of strings.

People are surprised to see that harp strings are colored. "Is that a *beginner* harp?" they ask. Colored strings on harps are not like training wheels on bicycles. Just as the 88 notes on the piano are separated into black and white keys, harp strings are colored to help locate a single note among so many possibilities.

The colored strings mark the Tonic (I), Fourth (IV), and Fifth (V) (the most important notes on the scale) or a variation on those intervals. The Paraguayan harp is tuned to F so colored strings usually indicate F (I), B-flat (IV), and C (V).

She had been taught a finger position that was *off by one string*, hence moving the Tonic (I) from F down to E. Attempting to play in the key of E on a harp tuned to F means an extraneous B-flat and several missing sharps. It would sound terrible and require a massive retuning (no trivial undertaking on a harp). A comparison of good written texts (had there been any) or a few minutes with a more experienced teacher would have eliminated years of the error and confusion now being passed on to others.

Often seminars are not a matter of new information at all, but merely the opportunity to see or hear the same old things in a slightly new or different way. Sometimes slightly different words, sung to a slightly different tune can make all the difference. This is your wonderful opportunity at summer camps and seminars.

Learn! Enjoy!

---

1. Will Reed comments on the supposed differences in techniques between Aikikai and Ki Society which split off via Koichi Tohei. "What differences? I was at *Honbu* before the split. How you did a technique depended on who happened to be teaching class that afternoon."

Q. Is it always so bloody frustrating?

A. Yes.

Came back from class today having gotten something right maybe three attempts in two hours. I think not only have I not learned anything so far, I've actually unlearned things I may have already known (like how to do a *nikyo*, which I did successfully in the long ago *jujutsu* days, but cannot manage now). Is everybody this screwed up when they begin, or can some people just not learn it?

—Paul Gowder, Ki Society

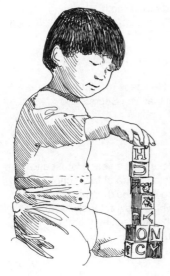

Great! You're right on track!

And the advanced students say the same thing.

Can some people just not learn it? Only the ones who give up. Sometimes they're the natural athletes accustomed to being good at every sport they try. They just can't believe Aikido can be so alien, which may be why we tend to retain more turtles than gazelles. Former turtles are now beautiful Aikidoists because they stayed when other more athletic and coordinated types fled in frustration.

The grace and beauty and rhythm and flow that you see in the senior students come from years of playing and dancing on the mat — from coming back when the others did not.

In essence, you have signed up for courses in classical ballet with a physics minor. Do not be shocked if you aren't ready to dance at Carnegie Hall after a few short months of study. Remember the old joke per the lost tourist who asks the old man on the street how to get to Carnegie Hall: "Practice! Practice! Practice!"

A poster that hung on our *dojo* wall for many years showed a little child carefully piling a tower of his first building blocks. The caption read: "The expert in anything was once a beginner."

Many times students would step off the mat, go to that picture, look long and hard, take a deep breath, turn around and go back to practice. I know because I was one.

Just keep doing and you will learn.

Meanwhile, I guarantee that you have learned more than you know and right now you can help new baffled persons coming in the door.

They will have questions you can answer.

Q. If it's so simple, how come it's so hard?

A. It's very simple, but the simplicity of it may not be easy.

They're all very simple concepts. We render them complex because we're unwilling to believe that it is really so much easier than we believe.

One of my first teachers told our beginning class that on the last day of class he would reveal The Secret of Aikido. When that day arrived, he revealed to the few of us that remained that The Secret of Aikido was . . . showing up and practicing.[1]

—Tarik J. Ghbeish, Aikikai

I've heard Saotome Sensei refer to the "Secrets of Aikido." He keeps meeting people who want to know these secrets, and he keeps telling them that The Secrets are . . . everything you learned in the first week of your training.

—Jun Akiyama, Aikikai

[Dad] is in his early 50s and has been in Tae Kwon Do for less than a year. He used to come home from practice and tell me that he had trouble doing some of the techniques, so he told his instructor he couldn't do it because he was too old! And then he wondered why his instructor yelled at him. I was flabbergasted. The whole reason I took Aikido classes was to learn Aikido. If I already knew how to do it, I'd be teaching them! I suppose some people think that if you aren't a "natural" you can't do it, which is [nonsense] that needs to be weeded out of the collective psyche.

—K. A. D.

Q. How often should I come to class?

A. It depends.

For beginners, we recommend three days a week. Twice a week is too long between classes for beginners, but may be adequate for experienced students. At one day a week, you will barely remember a thing from one class to another. Beginners who plan to come *every* day tend to burn out.

Three days of class throughout the week gives you training, repetition, reinforcement, and a rest in between.

Homework is another matter. You should spend at least 15 minutes to half an hour *daily* on basic exercises, even if it is only turning *tenkan* in the kitchen or while waiting for the elevator. Off-mat practice makes on-mat training time more efficient and rewarding. (See exercises starting on page 235 as possibilities for individual practice).

My Aikido sucks, but every day I try to suck at a higher level.

—Janet Rosen, Aikikai

---

1. "90 percent of life is just showing up," says Garrison Keillor. He attributes his success in radio to having an alarm clock to awaken him for the early morning show that no one else wanted.

Q. How is Aikido "non-violent"? Isn't throwing attackers around a bit violent?

A. It depends — on the appropriate tool.

"Do you think," said Candide, "that mankind always massacred one another as they do now? Were they always guilty of lies, fraud, treachery, ingratitude, inconstancy, envy, ambition, and cruelty? Were they always thieves, fools, cowards, gluttons, drunkards, misers, calumniators, debauchees, fanatics, and hypocrites?"

"Do you believe," said Martin, "that hawks have always been accustomed to eat pigeons when they came in their way?"

"Doubtless," said Candide.

"Well then," replied Martin, "if hawks have always had the same nature, why should you pretend that mankind change theirs?"

"Oh," said Candide, "there is a great deal of difference; for free will . . ." and reasoning thus they arrived at Bordeaux.

—Voltaire, *Candide* (1759)

Much of the problem of "violence versus pacifism" is in the definition of what is, in the end, merely a *tool*.

Pacifism is not the same as *passivism* and it is not the opposite of *violence*.

Pacifism is the opposite of *belligerence*.

As *tools*, violence, pacifism, and passivism can all be *appropriate* or *inappropriate*. A peaceable man may use violence where it is appropriate, just as he would use any other tool. The belligerent man is the one who uses or prefers to use violence[1] when it is appropriate — and when it is *not*. There may also be misunderstandings of life realities, available options, morality, and focus.

Life Realities. There are bad people in the world. Ignoring that fact does not change the reality although some try. For example, a religious university proposed a conference for members who had served in some of the grimmer areas of the world and those less traveled to discuss issues of violence and self-defense. It was the untraveled ones who were certain that gentle non-resistance was the answer to everything, that murderers faced with Christ-like patience[2] would be shamed and inspired into piety and good manners. They extended this delusion to the point of insisting that their brothers who had direct experience of a very different reality be forbidden to speak.

Available Options. A common perception is that there are only two:

- Kill, murder, destroy.
- Lie down and play doormat.

---

1. The most belligerent, vicious behavior may be disguised in verbal, rather than physical, violence. See the soft-spoken Kai Winn of *Star Trek DS9*. There are many Real Life earthlings like her.
2. The image of "Gentle Jesus, meek and mild" may be theologically traditional but historically shaky. Someone who tells the religious and governmental authorities of his day that they are clueless fools, assaults the clerks and officers of the First National Bank with a whip, and arms his followers with swords when necessary to ensure that only He is taken away, fits no standard definition of "meek and mild." It is a holdover from centuries of Christianity as State Religion when a meek and mild populace was much encouraged by those who would rule it.

There are other options and Aikido offers many.

One of the Hard Sayings of the New Testament is "Resist not Evil."[1] This is often taken to mean that Evil should be allowed free-rein, that we are to drop our defenses against it, embrace it, or harmonize with it. More likely it was first, an injunction against being an automatic stimulus-response machine, and second, an issue of *focus*.

For example, I have heard Model Mugging/IMPACT Self Defense courses dismissed by some Aikidoists as "too violent" (by people who went on to recommend a solution based on firearms). IMPACT is strongly karate-oriented because that is where it came from. I saw several situations that could be handled far more easily and efficiently with Aikido or Judo techniques. But students are trained to go for an effective knock-out and to get away; they are not trained to rip out lungs or eyeballs, maim or kill.

Dismissing it as "too violent" dismisses useful skills while focusing a lop-sided protectiveness on the perpetrator. It ignores behavior that made defensive skills necessary in the first place. It ignores the victim. Look at the victim.

Focus. A renowned example of focus is that of the pacifist French Huguenot village of Le Chambon. During World War II it threw itself into the work of rescuing fugitive Jews from the Nazis. Le Chambon is often cited as a triumph of pacifism over violence, but that is incorrect. Nothing done there helped to end the war. But rather than following the Resistance focus on the aggressor (with assassination and terrorism), Le Chambon focused on the equally hard and dangerous work of rescuing the persecuted. Nor did they work alone. Unknown to Le Chambon, the little town had its own "Schindler" in the person of German Major Julius Schmahling, who worked to keep Le Chambon safe to do its work. Had Le Chambonoise resorted to violence and destruction, he would not and could not have continued. But what mattered to Le Chambon and to Schmahling was not "death to the enemy." What mattered was *life*.

Morality. It is always important to investigate nonviolent solutions to problems. But confusing *pacifism* with *passivism* in the "I -will-do-nothing-because-it-is-more-saintly-of-me" sense is not necessarily the moral high-road, is usually unhealthy in practice and is often an evolutionary dead-end. The career criminal or predator does not rob, rape, and kill out of desperation, but as convenience, or simply because he enjoys it[2]. Consider the concept of passive non-resistance from the attacker's point of view: *convenient* and *contemptible*.

The sacrifice of self or others to such a perversion of right and reason *is not a moral act*.

---

1. "A *very* Hard Saying for me," says an old soldier, "for I have seen what Evil can do."
   Much psychopathic behavior can be traced back to brain injury with loss of inhibition circuits for impulsive behavior or acting out of early abuse. *Guilty by Reason of Insanity* (Lewis, 1998) exposed the past child abuse and brain injury found in all death row inmates that they interviewed but also clarifies the need to halt the cycle, not by passive resistance but by compassionate action.
2. See *Inside the Criminal Mind* (Samenow, S. E., 1984), for a chilling but practical dose of reality.

Ray Bradbury's classic *Fahrenheit 451*[1] is the tale of a totalitarian regime where books are systematically burned and the job of "fireman" has a whole different meaning. Former fireman Guy Montag joins a band of outlaw scholars whose strategy for protecting their books is to *memorize* the book, keeping the precious ideas and memories safely hidden away in mind and body until the day when they can once again be safely written down.

Essentially the person *became* the book.

"I am," says Montag, "*Ecclesiastes.*"

Who are you?

You are everything you've thought and done, places you've been, people you have known, skills and talents and loves and joys, creativity and points of view, tales and songs and stories, and all the things that will be lost without you.

You are an absolutely unique creation of yourself and others.

You are many books. Treasure them and protect them — and others.

> Is it worthwhile to be the owner of so many talents, youth and strength, a cultured mind, a healthy body, and yet not even to know how to defend your life? . . . I am reminded of the story told of a certain General. One of his officers, who disagreed with him on . . . some strategic movement, had said:
>
> "Well, General, when the time comes I will show you that I know how to die."
>
> "Don't be a fool, Sir," replied the General. "Your duty is not to see that you get killed, but to take care that you don't."
>
> —Baron César de Bazancourt, *Secrets of the Sword*

---

1. The title refers to the ignition point of paper. The book was published in 1953 at the height of the McCarthy hearings.

Q. Is Aikido a religion?

A. Not unless you make it one.

Founder Morihei Ueshiba was adamant that his Aikido was not a religion[1]. Should his students become Shinto or Omote because he was Shinto or Omote?

Absolutely not! He felt that Aikido should not make them anything except *better* Christians, Buddhists, Muslims, Jews — whatever they were already.

Unfortunately, too many people flock to worship Power or The Unknown. Too many others are willing to worship or be worshipped on that basis alone.

"See my great *nikyo*? I shall, therefore, be your spiritual Master. Sign here."

"Oh yes Master!"

This is as foolish and perhaps even less sensible than Goat Worship[2] which I suspect was developed by dwellers of arid areas on observing some interesting powers of goats and desperately desiring those powers for themselves. It is little different from persons desperately concerned with self-defense or the prestige of being a "master of mystic oriental secrets," desiring those powers for themselves and indulging in all sorts of worshipful nonsense to get them, from the simple mindlessness of herd behavior to the very worst kind of cultism.

Aikido is not a religion, however, Aikido and *ki* exercises can be used to demonstrate what all the great religions have preached. In so many ways Aikido forces us to confront secret desires of the heart, fears and hatreds, and to be aware of the physical effects of internal attitude and orientation.

Hopefully one day, students realize that it isn't about having power over others, or about allowing others to have power over us.

It isn't even about being really good at hitting people with planets.

There is a Bigger Picture.

Miss that picture and one day you may discover that all along you have actually been worshipping a goat.

Worship a worthy God.

Then practice Aikido for the fun and the joy of it.

---

1. For what Ueshiba was trying to accomplish see Ellis Amdur's beautiful essay: "Aikido is Three Peaches" at: www.aikidojournal.com/?id=744.
2. Horns radiate heat, regulating body temperature and when water is scarce, goats (like their camel relatives) can store water for days. To a human who lay dying of thirst beside a dry water hole, the sight of goats frolicking merrily on the rocks must have seemed nothing short of supernatural.

Getting Started

Customs differ from one dojo to another, but here are some general guidelines of interest to beginners, from clothing and equipment to etiquette and basic skills.

Clothing and Equipment

Few Aikido schools require you to have a uniform for your first class or classes. You are usually welcome to wear any comfortable sportswear. However, snug jeans restrict movement, you will be in positions where big balloony shorts were never intended to be viewed, and fashionable aerobics-class gear is just inappropriate.

Sweatpants provide freedom of motion and protect the knees from abrasion on a canvas mat or from sticking on a vinyl one. A long-sleeved T-shirt will protect your elbows and forearms. For attacks and grabs, however, shirts that are too stretchy or flimsy will be a problem to you and to your partner. Whatever your choice,

- **Wear clean, untattered, appropriate clothing**. Sweats and T-shirts are fine for those trying out a class, but no leotards or extra-stretchy tanks or Tees please.
- **Keep nails trimmed**. Toenails and fingernails can slice and cut.
- **Tie up long hair**. Long, loose, flowing hair in this manual appears under special artistic license to indicate flow and motion. In real life, long loose hair can get tangled in the course of a throw, stepped on during *ukemi* or caught under your partner's knee in a pin. In a high speed spin it can catch a bystander in the eye. Tie it up for the safety of all.
- **Avoid heavy make-up and heavy scents**.
- **Remove jewelry**. It can cut or injure you or someone else. Dangling wire-pierced earrings are particularly dangerous for the wearer. No watches, barrettes, rings. Rings with cut stones, prongs or fancy settings can slice a partner but even the plainest of rings can be a danger to the wearer. Swelling of a finger injured by jamming or a weapon strike may make it impossible to remove a tight band just when it is most critical to do so[1].

Dogi

The standard Aikido uniform is the white cotton *keikogi* ("practice clothing"). Two types are used but the choice between the two is usually personal[2].

- **The heavy-weight Judo style**. Helps to cushion falls and rolls. Those who sweat heavily tend to favor the thicker jacket because it absorbs more moisture.
- **The light-weight karate style**.[3] No appreciable padding, but cooler in summer, easily supplemented in winter, and easily packed for travel.

---

1. Pliers may work in an emergency, but petroleum jelly and a small flat file with a toothed edge will do the least damage to ring or wearer. Both are valuable additions to the *dojo* first-aid kit.
2. The heavy Judo jacket is often favored by men, especially in cold weather, because the Western men's knit undershirt is considered inappropriate (not a traditional Japanese garment). They absorb more sweat but, being heavier and thicker, may also make you sweat *more*. Feeling clumsy and uncoordinated? The heavier *gi* may actually help you learn via increased sensory feedback.
3. The light kimono top is used for Karate; punching under the weight of the heavy reinforced Judo jacket is exhausting.

Always buy cotton for comfort and buy large, as cotton tends to shrink. Unbleached "natural" garments will shrink more than the white ones that have already been subjected to the bleaching process.

1. Pull on the jacket, left arm first[1].
2. Remove street pants and step into *gi* pants (with loops in front), left leg first.
3. Snug the drawstrings through the loops and tie.

To put on a Judo jacket

1. Wrap right side over body.
2. Wrap left side over right side.
3. Secure with belt (page 31).

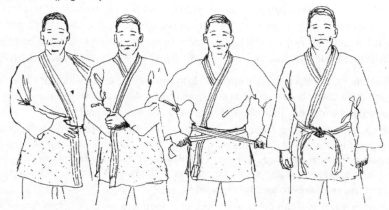

To put on the karate jacket

1. Wrap right side across body.
2. Tie right front outside tie to left inside tie.
3. Wrap left side over the right.
4. Tie left front tie to right side tie.

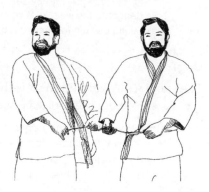

Jackets will gap. Ladies will need a camisole or some sort of fastener. A safety pin can snap open with painful consequences during hard practice but a small tie or strip of Velcro sewn down the inside surfaces is simple, safe, and secure.

The jacket closes like a man's shirt (left over right) so you can slip your right hand into the opening, a handy place for a small cloth.[2]

---

1. In the East, "left side first" is the traditional starting point for nearly all actions, so even the act of dressing mindfully is good practice for what will happen later on the mat. In *taigi* competition, points are lost for stepping on the mat with anything but the left foot. This is opposite to Western tradition. To the ancient Romans, especially, "starting off on the *right* foot" meant exactly that.

2. At a time when "to be civilized" meant "to be like the Chinese," Japanese clothing styles followed Chinese clothing styles. When the Japanese court moved to Nara in 1710, it adopted dress rules based on the Tang clothing code which specifically mandated that all robes cross left side over right side. The Chinese (and hence the Japanese) considered right-over-left to be the sure sign of a barbarian (Dalby, 1993) — or a dead person (see page 57).

Belt

Unlike beginning Karate students who must earn the right to wear any belt at all, beginning Aikido students wear a belt from the very beginning.

The belt is wrapped around the body from front to back and front and again and tied with a square knot.

1. Put center of belt at front of your waist. Wrap ends around your body bringing them back to the front crossing right over left.

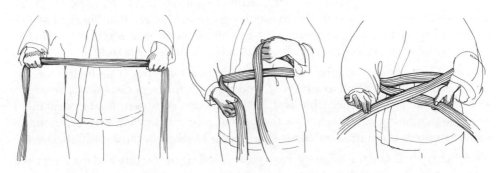

2. Pass the top (right) end around the entire belt and out again.

   The tie that was on the right is now on the left. Pass this left-hand tie over the right to form a square knot. The "arrow" of the knot should point to the left.

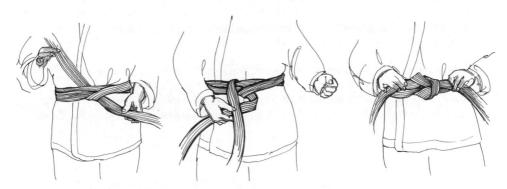

3. Align the folds of the belt to conform to the knot.

   The knot that is "folded" rather than forced will last longer and the weight of ends hanging down helps somewhat to keep it in place. During hard practice it will invariably work loose and need to be tightened.

   If knot comes loose, proper etiquette is to turn to the wall and make adjustments as discreetly as possible.

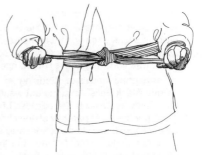

Hakama

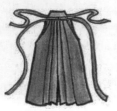

The *hakama* is a traditional lower garment worn by the Japanese *samurai* and others. The *andon hakama* (used in archery and religious ceremonies) is a skirt. The version used in Aikido is the *umanori hakama* (horse-back riding style) is actually voluminous pleated pants.

A common modern belief is that it hid feet so that opponents could not use foot position to anticipate movements. This is as likely as playing soccer in a full-length evening gown to hide ball handling skills from the opposing team. In fact, in action or bad weather, the *hakama* was hiked up to the belt so as not to encumber feet, catch on obstacles, or drag in the mud.

Because a long sweeping *hakama* can indeed conceal footwork from instructors, in class it is usually restricted to advanced students. In some schools, *hakama* are worn only upon reaching black belt (first *dan*). In others, women are permitted to wear them from the beginning supposedly for the sake of modesty[1] and the tradition that a woman in pants is not dressed. Some styles permit *hakama* at third (or higher) *kyu*.

Wearers may find that the *hakama* gives a greater feeling of stability and may improve awareness of One-Point. It certainly offers the advantage of keeping the belt firmly in place no matter how wild your practice may be. It is good etiquette to offer to fold the instructor's *hakama* after class — and good practice for learning to fold one's own when the day comes.

If you are in a dojo where *hakama* are worn by beginners, make sure that a first-time wearer knows how to wear the garment[2]. Aikidoist Philip Akin who played in the *Highlander* TV series tells of an incident (in "Eye for an Eye") in which fellow actor Stan Kirsch ("Ritchie Ryan") was hobbled and thrown by his *hakama*.

> "I was showing him how to wear one while putting mine on at the same time. I only noticed that he had it wrong after we had nearly finished the shooting. Those *kendo* shots to the head (which were not pulled, by the way) were all done with him in one leg.
> —Philip Akin, Aikido Yoshinkai Canada

---

1. Americans may recall that in the U. S. through the 1940s and 1950s, women in pants were considered improper or downright immoral. In some areas this is still true. However, to many Aikidoists the "women's *hakama* for modesty" rule seems a tad odd when ladies sit cross-legged (inappropriate to older, traditional Japanese) or change after class into shorts and tank tops.

2. A correspondent tells of attending an "Aikido Demonstration" at a local Martial Arts Academy. The "Aikido Black Belts" all came out wearing *hakama* backwards, *koshiita* in front. When he asked as innocently as possible the purpose of the hard thing in front he was seriously told that it was "to block punches." Apparently all they knew of Japanese arts was from watching Bruce Lee's *Chinese Connection;* the wicked Japanese all wear their *hakama* backwards (and their evil master is made up to resemble Toshiro Mifune). For the record, the *back*board goes in *back* and like any other pair of pleated pants, pleats go in front.

Miscellaneous Equipment

In Aikido most of what you bring is yourself. We don't use extensive equipment other than uniform and wooden sticks. You may, however, want to add pads and some basic supplies to your Aikido bag.

- **Toiletries**. Nail clippers and talcum powder can save injury and discomfort.

- **Eyewear**. There seems to be a large population of students with poor eyesight in Aikido. Many consider poor eyesight to be an advantage. Someone who cannot see well enough to focus on the hand or on details must take in the opponent as a whole and focus on his motion and direction as a whole in a way that sharper-eyed students may not. Many of course, successfully wear contacts. Sport goggles are always safe and secure. Many wear their regular street glasses if made of shatterproof safety glass and flexible frames.

- **Pads**. Volleyball or skating pads help knee exercises. Wear under your *gi* pants.

  Pads are also great for rolling practice. Female students in particular often begin forward rolls by falling down onto the shoulder (see why on page 138). I've never known anyone to suggest shoulder pads to help beginners through this awkward stage. Give it a try. Dense foam (from fabric or sports stores) can be inserted into the *gi*; even socks or a washcloth can be taped to the shoulders. You might even consider learning to roll in a motorcycle jacket or protective gear for skating. (See page 82). Pads are sold separately from the jackets and are specifically designed to protect the wearer from impact.

- **Washcloth**. A washcloth, bandana, or other small cloth is extremely useful during hot sweaty summer months and can be slipped into the fold of the *gi* top. It also has many uses as a training tool. (See page 234).

- **Weapons**. Most established schools will have a supply of wooden practice weapons, but you will soon want your own. They are stocked by martial arts supply houses and available mail-order.

  Note that these are *wooden* practice weapons. Don't even think of showing up at class with "Genuine Special Collector's Limited Edition 420 Stainless Steel" movie or series reproductions! Despite high prices and glittering advertisements they are usually of dangerously shoddy construction (for example, no *tang*—meaning that the blade can fly off the hilt and go flying across the room). Even if "real," a three-foot razor blade does not belong in the hands of beginners or in the vicinity of other beginners.

  - *Jo (wooden staff)*. It need not be an expensive weapon handcrafted from rare tropical woods. Most students start with a broomstick or a dowel from the hardware store, but these may be weak and splintery softwood. Instead, consider a replacement handle for a hoe or other tool, of strong and splinter-free hickory. Cut to chest (nipple or armpit) height. Check for straightness and for any rough, uneven, or weak spots where the *jo* might shatter if struck.

  - *Bokken (wooden sword)*. Best bought in person to check weight and balance.

  - *A note on travel:* At the airport, never ever refer to these items as "weapons." Call them "sticks" or you may miss your plane. For carry-on, try packing them in a length of PVC pipe with a cover and drawstring.

Dojo Etiquette

From ancient times one dictum of budo has been: "Begin with etiquette, conclude with etiquette." The etiquette taught in aikido [is] mutual respect, consideration for others, cleanliness . . . Etiquette is an important aspect of practice for all aikido students.

—Kisshomaru Ueshiba, *The Spirit of Aikido*

Budo without courtesy is just a lame excuse for mutual abuse.

—Stefan Stenudd

Upon entering the *dojo*, bow to the *shomen*[1] at the front of the room. Shoes usually go on a shelf near the door, and are never worn inside or on the mat. Sandals (*zori*) may be worn inside but left at the edge of the mat (toes facing outward).

Bowing is the traditional Japanese expression of respect, courtesy, and thanks. The standing bow (*ritsu-rei*) inclines the upper body to about 45 degrees. (The kneeling bow is described on page 42). Bowing is polite but also practical; it helps to stretch and limber muscles which may have tightened in the course of practice.

- Bow (standing) when you enter and leave the dojo.
- Bow to the *shomen* before getting on or off the mat.
- Bow to partners and teachers.
- When in doubt, bow.

To get on the mat,

1. Remove shoes.
2. Bow to *shomen* before stepping onto the mat. Be seated quietly. You may wish to do some warm-up, limbering or stretching exercises before class begins. Or sit quietly in meditation. Class is about to start when the instructor steps onto the mat.

To begin class,

1. The instructor (*Sensei*) and students sit in *seiza*, the formal Japanese kneeling posture (see page 41) facing the *kamiza* at the front of the *dojo*. During this period sit in silence.[2]
2. *Sensei* and the class bow to the *kamiza* in unison. *Sensei* then turns to face the students.
3. The class bows to *Sensei* who returns the bow.

   You may hear the phrase o-*nagai-shi-mas* (usually interpreted as "please teach me"). Class now begins, usually with warming or stretching exercises.

To get on the mat if you are late and class is in progress,

1. Sit in *seiza* at the edge of the mat.
2. Wait for a bow from the instructor.
3. Return the bow and step onto the mat.

---

1. The focal point of the room, perhaps with a photograph of The Founder, calligraphy, flowers. For the "religious significance" — or not — of bowing see page 42.
2. Different schools have differing seating protocols. Some line up strictly by rank, others do not. Some clap before or after bowing to the *shomen*, others do not.

To work with weapons,

1. Keep the weapon to your left when sitting.
2. Keep swords (*bokken*) or knives (*tanto*) with blade out.
3. Replace weapons in the rack with blade up.

   Blades out while sitting and blades up in weapons rack are appropriate for the martial intent of a *dojo*. In a home or in company, or in a less martial *dojo*, weapons are placed blade-side in (or down). Placing weapons blade out (or up) in inappropriate environments is considered extremely rude and threatening.

To observe a technique,

1. When *Sensei* halts practice (usually with two claps) to explain a technique, stop what you are doing at once.
2. Be seated (to allow everyone a clear view) in *seiza*.

   By extension, *do not clap in the dojo during class!* Confusion will result.

To take a test when *sensei* goes around the room testing,

1. Take your test.
2. Sit down and wait for the others to finish and class to resume.

To help demonstrate a technique,

1. *Sensei* may ask you — with a bow and *dozo* ("please") — to serve as *uke* to demonstrate.
2. Return the bow, then rise and come forward.

If Sensei stops the demo to lecture,

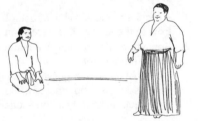

1. Be seated in *seiza*, facing the instructor and side wall. Your part of the demonstration is over when *Sensei* dismisses you with a bow.
2. Return the bow and return to your place.

To ask a question or work with another student,

1. Indicate your request by bowing.
2. Your partner will accept by returning the bow.
3. Take turns serving as *nage* (the one doing the throw) and *uke* (the attacker). Switch partners with each technique.

   Usually, techniques are practiced 2-4 times (on right and left) by one partner, then 2-4 times by the other partner and so on. Repeat the cycle as often as possible in time allotted matching your practice to the time available.

To practice a technique,

1. Do only the technique demonstrated.
2. Be as gentle and cooperative as possible or as necessary — you're next!

To indicate discomfort or pain,

1. *Uke* should slap the mat or body. If no free arm, slap or kick with a leg.
2. On hearing the slap[1], *nage* should release the pressure immediately.

---

1. In a crowded class or a seminar, a slap may be hard to hear. Add the visual channel by slapping in *nage*'s sight. If he still doesn't notice, slap *nage*'s arm, leg, or body.

Aikido techniques are designed to control while avoiding damage to the opponent, hence injuries are rare compared to many other martial arts. Nevertheless they do occur. In the general population the most common injuries are broken wrists and collarbones. In the dojo where we practice the arts of war, the most common are stubbed toes (often from catching toes in the seams between mats).

To deal with injuries,

1. Tape any stubbed fingers or toes or tie a red cloth or bandanna[1] around an injured arm or part to signal partners to take special care.
2. Report injuries to *Sensei*. If you have any bleeding injury, get off the mat to bandage it. Do not bleed on the mat. To tape a toe,

   - Rip 3-4 inches of athletic tape in half lengthwise.
   - Use one strip to bind adjacent toes together. Add the remaining strip for padding. Wrap snugly enough to move with you but not tightly enough to cut off circulation. End the wrap *between* the toes. If it ends on bottom or top of foot, it will pull loose.
   - Ice and elevate any swelling.
   - Optional: Wear a sock, tabi[2], or soft shoe that won't harm the mat). This keeps the toe safe and reminds others to watch out for it.

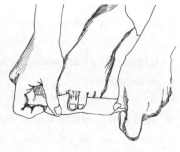
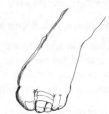

To stop or rest,

1. If required, check with instructor before leaving the mat. Bow to the *kamiza* before leaving.
2. Bow yourself back onto the mat (or await permission) when ready to return.
3. Do not stand idle or gossiping on the mat. Practice time is limited; make the most of it. How often can you do a technique accurately in the allotted time?

To end class,

1. *Sensei* and the class will again face the *kamiza* in *seiza*.
2. All bow in unison.
3. *Sensei* will turn and bow to the students who bow to him; but this time you will hear "*Thank you, Sensei!*"
4. *Sensei* may respond with "Please thank each other!"
5. Turn and bow to everyone with whom you have practiced.

To leave the mat and the dojo,

1. Bow again towards the *shomen* before stepping off the mat.
2. Assist with any mat cleaning or equipment storage following class.
3. Bow again before leaving the dojo.

---

1. Often it's better to flag the *opposite* side. Many people are subconsciously attracted to it (the "target fixation") rather than noticing that they should stay away.
2. The Japanese split-toe sock is worn indoors even when shoes come off. You will see many old pictures of martial artists practicing in *tabi*.

Some Basic Skills

Words and Phrases

"The question is," said Alice, "whether you can make words mean different things."
"The question is," said Humpty Dumpty, "which is to be master, that is all."
—Lewis Carroll, *Alice in Wonderland*

On entering the dojo you may be overwhelmed by new concepts and ideas, a new vocabulary and new words. Most traditional schools use Japanese words and phrases in their classes. While this may seem intimidating at first, they are quickly learned. They also offer the opportunity to increase cultural awareness and understanding.[1] One example is the word for *Aikido* itself.

Ai means "to fit, to be in harmony or agreement with." The lower strokes form a square which represents a mouth or opening such as that of a teapot. The upper three strokes originally formed a lid or stopper. The combination suggests two things that harmonize or fit together, such as the lid on a teapot, the cork in a bottle, the round peg in the round hole.

Ki comes from the ancient Chinese character for *Qì*, steam, composed of elements representing sun and fire, the sources of steam. In this symbol the horizontal stroke with the curved vertical line represents a boiling pot of rice with a lid and a handle. The uppermost strokes represent the rising clouds of steam. The cross in the pot represents a stalk of rice with four individual grains, the food that gives life and energy to humans.[2] Together these elements compose a symbol which came to indicate vapor, spirit, breath, or "breath power."

Dô shows a human figure walking along a road or path. *Dô* (*tao* in Chinese) now means a road or path in the literal sense; by extension it can mean a course of study. There is a difference between a *jutsu* which implies a collection of "techniques," versus the *do* which implies a way of life.

---

1. See Glossary (page 265) for literal meanings and examples.
2. I once saw two elderly Korean hairdressers faced with the daunting task of hoisting a hefty customer into the chair. They succeeded. "Rice power!" they cried, exulting.

Some words which you will hear from the very beginning are:

- **Sensei**. Instructor, teacher, from *sen*, before, and *sei*, living or born. Literally it is "one who was born before you."
- **Nage**. The one who "throws" or responds to an attack. In Judo and Tomiki style lineages (and more widely used in Aikikai) this may be *tori*. In others such as Yoshinkan, it is known as *sh'te*, pronounced "shtey," literally the principal actor in a *Kabuki* play).
- **Uke**. The attacking partner who is thrown. This partner, in turn, performs *ukemi*, the ability to receive an attack and protect oneself while being thrown.

Techniques in this Japanese art are usually identified by Japanese names. Formal names for techniques are usually provided by the organization headquarters and so may differ from style to style.

A string of unfamiliar sounds can be intimidating, but the advantage of the Japanese names is that once the concepts are mastered the words come apart. Most technique names describe exactly what you are going to see and do. In the Ki Society, names break down into three parts: the type of attack, the technique you will use, and directions on how to move yourself into position. For example, consider *katate-kosa-tori kokyu-nage irimi tobikomi*. Its English nickname is *"Kokyu-Nage* Basic" but the Japanese name provides the following detailed instructions.

- **Attack**: *Katate* is "single-hand," *kosa* means "cross," and *tori* is an "attack." Hence this technique deals with an attack to the opposite wrist (his right hand to your right hand).
- **Technique**: You will deal with this attack using a *kokyu-nage*. *Kokyu* means "breath" (but may be interpreted as "timing"); *nage* means "throw" thus *Kokyu-nage* is a family of "breath-throws," techniques which depend on timing and balance rather than a joint lock.
- **Approach**: How will you move to begin the technique? *Irimi* is an "entering" motion and *tobikomi* means "jumping in." In this technique, you will move into the attacker's space (rather than around him).

Hence, loosely translated, *katate-kosa-tori kokyu-nage irimi tobikomi* means:

"An attack to the opposite wrist dealt with by entering the attacker's space, leaping into position, and performing a throw based on timing and sensitivity to the attacker's movement and position."

The same attack handled in almost the same way but with an added wristlock known as *kote-gaeshi* is called *katate-kosa-tori kote-gaeshi irimi tobikomi, hence:*

"An attack to the opposite wrist dealt with by entering the attacker's space, leaping into position, and performing a throw by unbalancing *uke* with a wrist-twist."

Guy de Wolf puts this all together.

Essay: Teaching by the Numbers

One of the biggest problems facing new Aikido students is learning the Japanese terminology. Those of us who have been around longer forget how many Japanese words we know and how baffling the exotic terms we use so casually among ourselves can be to novices. Back when I first started studying Aikido, our group met in a building with a parking problem. People were constantly coming in from outside and asking us to move our cars so they could get out.

"Please move the Honda."

"Somebody move the Mustang."

"We need somebody to move the white van!"

One evening when requests for vehicles to be moved had been particularly frequent, my *Sensei* said to me, "Get into your *hanmi*."

"Oh no, Sensei," I said. "I drive the Thunderbird."

Now that I am an instructor, I want to spare my students similar embarrassing moments. When new students come into the *dojo*, I like to expose them to some of the terminology of Aikido and at the same time give them an overview of the structure of our art. I choose one of the regular students to act as my *uke* and do a brief presentation that I call . . .

The 9 Basic Attacks, 9 Basic Throws, and 2 Basic Movements of Aikido

Before I begin, I reassure the new students that I don't expect them to memorize the terms as I go. The idea is not to make them feel pressured to learn everything immediately, but to expose students to the terminology of Aikido in the beginning to make it more familiar when they hear it again later.

9 Attacks

I categorize the nine attacks into 6 grabs:

1. *Katate-tori* ("wrist-attack"),
2. *Katate-kosa tori* ("cross-wrist attack"),
3. *Katate-tori ryote-mochi* ("wrist-attack with both hands on *one* of *nage*'s wrists"),
4. *Katate- tori ryote-tori* ("wrist-attack with both hands grabbing *both* of *nage*'s wrists"),
5. *Kata-tori* ("lapel attack"),
6. *Ushiro tekubi-tori* ("attack to *nage*'s wrists from behind") and . . .

3 Strikes

1. *Shomen-uchi* ("front-head strike"),
2. *Yokomen-uchi* ("side-head strike"), and
3. *Mune-tsuki* ("mid-level-punch").

I give the English translation for each of these terms, explaining that *kata-te* means "wrist," *tori* means "attack" and so on.

The 9 Basic Techniques

I do the same thing with the 9 basic techniques. I demonstrate:

1. *Ikkyo,*
2. *Nikyo,*
3. *Sankyo*, and

4. *Yonkyo,*

   . . . explaining that these exotic terms simply mean the "first-," "second-," "third-," and "fourth-technique." Then I move on to . . .

5. *Kokyu-nage* ("breath-throw"),
6. *Shiho-nage* ("four-direction throw"),
7. *Ude-oroshi* ("arm-drop"),
8. *Kote-gaeshi* ("wrist-bend"), and
9. *Zempo-nage* ("forward-direction throw")

   . . . explaining that each technique can be performed in response to a variety of attacks and that these combinations of attack and response make up the body of Aikido.

Two Basic Movements

My journey through the basics of Aikido is completed by demonstrating the "Two Basic Movements" of:

1. *Tenkan* ("turning") and
2. *Irimi* ("entering").

I show students pairs of techniques that differ only in these two basic movements.

For example,

- Shomen-uchi IRIMI versus
- Shomen-uchi TENKAN

presented in pairs makes Aikido terminology meaningful in the students' minds.

Finally, I explain how techniques are called out, as a combination of:

1. Attack,
2. Response, and
3. Technique.

I demonstrate some of the techniques whose names follow the rule but also point out names that *don't* follow this rule. The term *kokyu-nage*, in particular, requires additional explanation. I tell students that, unless some other throw is also given as a part of the technique name, it will be a *kokyu-nage*, a "breath" or "timing throw."

Presenting attacks and techniques in terms of families and explaining the rationale behind the technique names gives students a structure or mental framework where they can hang their new knowledge as they acquire it. Educational theorists refer to these mental frameworks as *schema* and many believe that *schema*, either constructed by students themselves or supplied to them by their teachers, are vitally important in learning.

Ultimately, Aikido students must construct their knowledge of the art for themselves as they progress, but we instructors can give them a head start. When I spend part of an evening categorizing techniques and then teaching by the numbers, I'm giving my students not only a lesson in Japanese terms but also the beginning of a personal understanding of the art that we all study together.

— Guy DeWolf , Ki Society

Sitting and Standing

Seiza ("correct-sitting") is the formal Japanese sitting or kneeling posture. To kneel and to rise, remember "left down, right up."

To go from standing to *seiza*,

1. Drop left knee to mat (right knee is up).
2. Drop right knee to mat and sit back on lower legs.
3. To sit resting, rest hands lightly on thighs, and cross right big toe over left big toe. To sit in *seiza* but prepared for movement and action, stay up on toes ("live toes").

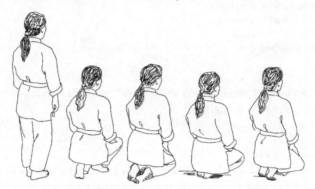

- Forehead and weight of head are over your center[1] rather than over feet.
- Lower back curves gently in.
- Knees are approximately two fists apart.
- Posture is softly erect.

When pressure is applied to the chest, *seiza* position allows you to transfer the force to the tailbone which, being pushed into the mat, just makes you more stable.

It is common to lean too far forward or too far back. A partner usually provides a test for proper position, but you can easily test yourself. Proper position of torso is the point at which you can stand up without first shifting your weight forward.

You may have problems with *seiza* if your quadriceps (thigh) or other leg muscles are too tight and pull painfully on the knee. Beginners find it impossible to believe that they will ever sit comfortably in this position. You will, but meanwhile, pay attention to leg stretching exercises, especially for front thighs. Transition can also be eased by using a pillow under the hips or a *seiza* stool.

When you reach your limit of sitting *seiza* in class, bow to the *shomen*, then relax into cross-legged sitting (*anza*). Shoulders are relaxed, weight slightly forward and hands rest on knees slightly forward of ankles. Weight is properly distributed relative to Center when a partner has difficulty lifting your knee[2].

Return to *seiza* if class is called to attention or when you need to bow.

---

1. In Ki Society this is referred to as One-Point. For discussion, see page 64.
2. See BA, pp. 24-25; KDL pp. 40-41; KIA, pp. 23-25. For knee pain see page 114 of this manual.

To rise from *seiza*,

1. Bring right knee up, while bringing left toes up and forward.
2. Push off with legs (no hands!) and the *toes of the back foot*.
3. Left leg down while rising keeps leg safe while drawing a sword.
4. Adjust stance as necessary.

    Why left knee down? The sword is on left, drawn across leg and body with right hand. Drawing a sword across a raised left knee could have horrible consequences.

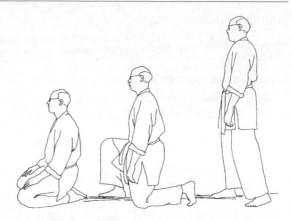

Variation

- In rising from *seiza*, compare doing so with "live" toes vs. extended toes.
- Compare the strain on your knees.

Bowing

Sometimes there is great anxiety over the "religious significance" of Eastern bowing.

We rarely think of the "religious significance" of Western bowing because we've mostly forgotten it. In the U.S., bowing still survives in the Catholic church[1], on stage, and in Southern beauty pageants and "court" festivals[2]. All around the Western world the bow or curtsy (the female bow) was a standard greeting until World War II.

The Eastern bow is equivalent to the Western handshake or tipping of the hat with variations overlaid with social information on status and intent. It is *not* worship.

Nevertheless, a student who truly believes that it would be a sin to bow should not bow. And leaving rather than discussing your concerns with the teacher in the belief that they would not be understood is a tad presumptuous. I've never heard of a school that refused a student for refusing to bow. Such concerns are not rare and certainly

---

1. *Curtsy* comes directly from "courtesy." To *genuflect* is literally "to bend the knee" from L. *genu*, knee + *flectere*, to bend. With the continuing loss of etiquette and tradition in the U.S., you will often see people flip-flopping into church in Bermuda shorts and sandals — but they still genuflect.

    Non-Japanese Aikido students are often heard debating the "one proper way" to bow. Actually there are many versions, depending (as always in Japan) on rank, sex, intent, and the message to be conveyed. Kurosawa's *samurai* adventure movie *Sanjuro* is wonderful fun on its own. But watch it again just to count and observe the many different versions of bows.

    For a review of Western bowing, see *The Student Prince in Old Heidelberg*. This gem of a film was set in 1902, but made by a German director on a U.S. movie lot in 1926 when the bow and curtsy were still very much a part of the etiquette of daily life. Observe the constant bows, curtsies, and tipping of hats, with a gentle spoof of a fellow who doesn't know the rules for when to stop. See also the superb modern BBC productions of *Pride & Prejudice* or *Sense & Sensibility* filmed with British actors who, if presented at court today, would still bow or curtsy to the Queen.

2. The "Texas Bow" or "Full Court Bow" involves a full kneeling bow, actually touching the forehead to the floor. It certainly isn't a part of daily American life, but pageant hopefuls study bowing for months in the homes of sponsors in what can only be described as *uchi-deshi* training.

aren't limited to one particular religion. We have had Muslim and Orthodox Jewish members in our club who, strictly speaking, are forbidden to bow; we have also had fundamentalist Christians who chose not to. They sat quietly during the bow then went on with the rest of the class in learning this wonderful Japanese art with its other cultural trappings.

Unlike the traditional Karate bow (eyes warily fixed on the opponent lest he make a sudden move), in Aikido, the kneeling bow (*zarei*) is done by lowering head and eyes to the mat, a formal gesture of courtesy, honor, and trust.

From *seiza*,

1. Bow forward from One-Point by sliding both hands simultaneously from thighs to mat.
   Hands form a triangle and should be closed, no space showing between the fingers.
   Head is not held stiffly at top of spine, but rolls forward, like a ball rolling off a table.
   Forehead is held a few inches above the hands, parallel to the floor.
   Eyes follow direction of head.
2. Hold this position for three seconds, then rise.

Variation

Uke may test stability by:

- Pushing *nage* from side during the bowing down and the coming up.
- Standing behind, holding *nage*'s shoulders to prevent bow.

Back is rounded so that back, neck and head form a continuous curve[1]. If you try this version of the bow with a straight flat back, you will topple forward. Instead, bow into a curve, bending and relaxing (a nice stretch for back muscles) from One-Point.

The bow can also be a throw.

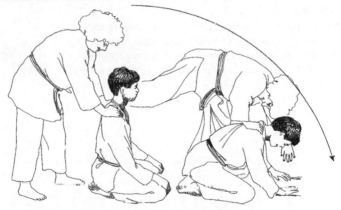

---

1. This bow is used in Ki Society, the tea ceremony, and Zen Buddhism. See BA, p. 24.

Standing, Stepping and Stance

Kamae means "posture." Linguistically it conveys no particular stance. It's also used in the phrase *kokoro no kamae* which means "(the) heart's posture." I think that the latter of the two is perhaps as important if not more important than the physical *kamae*, because if you don't have the proper "heart posture," your physical posture will betray that fact.

—Michael Hacker

The width of your feet limits you. It makes you strong in this forward dimension. But it makes you tremendously unstable to the side. Next time you're brushing your teeth, reading in the bookstore, look down and notice how your feet are. That's normal, natural stance, the natural way that you've evolved. That's the best thing for you. That's what we want to get to in Aikido. Then you'll be asked to bend your knees and make different kinds of adjustments from it. But the starting and returning points are always your normal natural stance.

—*Terry Dobson*

So now you're standing on the mat. You may notice that some students are standing rather differently, at an odd angle. What is this and what exactly are they doing?

Hanmi (meaning "half-body") comes from Japanese sword tradition.

In most styles, the distance between front and back foot is quite small. Stability comes from Center, not just the geometry of foot position.

Traditionally the "*samurai* walk" was a moving version of *hanmi*, an erect version of knee-walking (*shikkyo*)[1]. Although it looks and feels awkward at first, it isn't quite as alien as may first appear.

- It is how children make a Teddy Bear, doll, or other toy walk, pivoting from side to side.
- In the Western world, this is the "Glamour Girl" walk, leading with a hip, a side, presenting at most a three-quarter view. The martial arts and women's fashion are two very different forms of traditional warfare, but the purpose is the same — to expose the least amount of body bulk to view while sending a distinct message to the viewer.

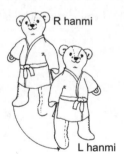

R hanmi

L hanmi

---

1. The foot moving in alignment with the arm also provides more stability under load than normal walking. In *Samurai Trilogy II*, there is a scene of farmers dancing to celebrate the arrest of the brigands. Notice the striking *hanmi* stances, the "*samurai* walk" performed by farmers who may themselves have originated it for its value in surviving hard labor. Rotating the pelvis under heavy load strains the quadratus lumborum muscle, one of the most common causes of chronic lower back pain (see page 120). Some say that *Daito-Ryu jujutsu* (from which Aikido was derived) used this method of walking and that the success of its techniques depend on this stance.

Left hanmi means standing with *left* side of the body and *left* foot forward.

Right hanmi means standing with *right* side of the body and *right* foot forward.

Different styles of Aikido use different foot positions, but in general the forward foot is pointed directly forward or slightly out; the back foot is at an angle up to 90-degrees to the line of the front foot.

Hanmi looks nonthreatening but offers ease of motion and dynamic stability.

The classic Karate stances provide a solid platform for outgoing punches and kicks, and a brace against incoming force but they are unstable against lateral forces. The Aikidoist simply moves easily out of the way.

To rise into *hanmi* from *seiza*:

1. Push off with legs only, left knee still on mat, right knee up and foot forward (page 42).
2. Rise up on toes.
3. Lower heels to floor without shifting weight backwards.
4. Stand comfortably, with attention at Center/One-Point.

To return to *seiza* from *hanmi*, reverse the process above putting:

1. Left leg down, then
2. Right leg down.

The following stances are used in all Aikido styles although names may vary. Note that Yoshinkan uses what appears to be a very pronounced forward stance which may *appear* to be off-balance. The practitioner is very balanced, with most weight on the forward leg and less weight on the back leg which serves as a sort of outrigger and lever arm for powerful turns which come directly from the hip.[1]

- **Shizentai.** Sometimes referred to as "natural stance." Feet are aligned shoulder width apart, knees and ankles relaxed and slightly bent.

- **Ai-Hanmi ("Harmonious" or Mutual Stance).** The partners' legs "fit" together. That is, both *nage* and *uke* have L feet or R feet forward. Seen in *katate-kosa-tori* ("cross-hand grab") techniques, page 213.

R hanmi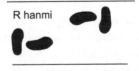

- **Gyaku-Hanmi (Reverse Stance).** Partners' feet are in opposition: *uke* has RF forward, and *nage* has LF forward. Seen in *katate-tori* or "same-side grab" techniques (see page 221).

L hanmi   R hanmi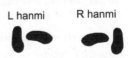

---

1. See TOT for illustration and detailed explanation.

Practicing smooth, balanced transitions between sitting, bowing, and standing has as many lessons to teach as do other Aikido techniques. Observe what happens if you attempt to stand with Center too far forward or too far back.

To practice stance and standing,

1. Practice all stances with a partner calling out their names.
2. From *seiza*, practice standing up and sitting down repeatedly.
3. From cross-legged sitting, shift to *seiza,* bow, then rise.

You can also combine the exercises above with weapons.

With *bokken in obi*, combine sword practice with:

1. Standing up and sitting down,
2. Drawing sword, striking, replacing the sword in your *obi*,
3. Sitting down again.
4. Stand and sit repeatedly. Strive for balance and smoothness of motion.

Combine with *kata* (forms), with *bokken* sheathed in your *obi*,

1. From *seiza*, rise into *hanmi* while drawing sword,
2. Assume ready position with sword and go through *kata*.
3. Resheath sword in belt.
4. Return to *seiza*.

With sword or *jo* at left side placed parallel to the body,

1. Grasp weapon in center at balance point.
2. Rise into *hanmi* drawing sword or extending *jo* to ready position.
3. Return weapon to L hand, again grasping weapon in center.
4. Return to *seiza* and return weapon to its position on the mat.

Internal Stance

What we call "attitude" can be thought of as internal stance and what we do on the mat can be considered internally as well.

Is your internal stance rigid? Unyielding? Too far forward? Too far back? Can you evaluate which stance of so many options is the appropriate one?

An interesting features of the science-fictional *Highlander* TV series was the repeated demonstration of effective internal stance and the ability (and process) of evaluating the situation.

We are inspired by our animal brains and tribal roots to be suspicious and assume the worst —Bad Until Proven Good.

We are exhorted by our political system and our current perception of good to always assume the best — Innocent and Good Until Proven Guilty.

The correct stance for a warrior or any other form of survivor is neutral.

The 400-year-old Duncan McLeod demonstrates this stance again and again. He refuses to trust or assume good of someone or something until trustworthiness or good has been clearly demonstrated and validated[1]. He does not condemn for trivial reasons, he does not trust for trivial reasons.

It is an interesting contrast between the notion of "niceness"[2] which requires that the practitioner automatically assume that "everyone is just as nice as they can be and really means well" versus the notion that "everyone is malicious and dangerous and intends harm."

In dangerous situations, a person subscribing to the first behavior will not survive.

For the second, life would hardly be worth living.

> The warrior's internal stance is neutral in the sense of no prejudgment without evidence. The key is readiness to see either black or white and act on it instantly.
> Philosophical gray (New *Maya*, "the delusion of relativism") is neutral in the sense of not believing there is any black or white, and/or believing that it is wrong or futile to judge anyone or anything.
> Those who subscribe to this doctrine are never ready.
>
> —Col. Ben H. Swett

---

1. In contrast to our Guilty/Not Guilty, the Scottish legal system allows three possible verdicts: "Guilty," "Not Guilty" and "Not Proven."
2. "Nice" is a social strategy, a tool, and possibly a weapon. See "Charm and Niceness" on page 247.

On Learning

Here are some suggestions that many find useful in the journey.

- Enter the work with humility and an open mind.
- Keep a journal for your class notes, observations, memories.
- Practice with senior students, *with emphasis on your ukemi* (following and rolling).
- Work with many different skill levels and sizes of partners.
- Practice with eyes closed to pattern movements via other sensory pathways; use images, feelings and sensations, sound or stories to shape concepts.
- Practice at home, off the mat.
- Watch for circles and patterns, angles, triangles, lines of force.
- Break down longer techniques into smaller parts.
- See how softly and smoothly you can do techniques and rolls.
- Apply class concepts and principles to daily life.
- Breathe!

Aikido is a complex discipline. It is never so uncomplicated as simply punching an opponent. In any given Aikido technique, there are at least three different things going on. And that's just at the beginning levels.

Yet many new students assume that they should be able to stroll onto the mat and perform a throw perfectly the first or second time they try it. If unable to do so, the problem is that Aikido is "too difficult."

Actually, the problem is the underlying assumption. The beginning math student does not start with calculus. The beginning skier does not start on the black slopes. The beginning music student quickly learns that the best way to learn music is not to struggle and crash through the entire piece.

Although any student will want to see and hear the entire form to understand just where it is going and how it should be approached, not even the most superlative musician will tackle a complex work in its entirety.

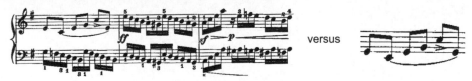

Instead it is broken down into workable segments. A few notes, a single phrase, then a single measure. Then a new phrase and when this is correct, adding it onto the first and continuing only when these — and all their parts — are correct.

When the individual modules have been mastered they are combined and practiced. Then another measure is added, then another and another . . . .

When I began piano lessons at the age of seven, standard equipment on the piano was the music, the metronome, and five pennies.

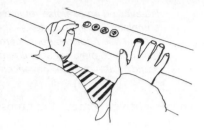

Each practice segment had to be done correctly five times.

On playing one measure correctly, one penny moved to the other side of the piano.

On playing it correctly a second time, the second penny moved to the left and so on through five correct renditions. If I stumbled or made an error, all the pennies went back to the right and the process began all over again.

In Aikido, it is tempting to practice by zooming through an entire technique before the individual components are mastered or even understood. Continuing through to the throw is as satisfying as whipping through the written music to a crash-bang finale but the end result is years of poor technique and poor performance. On a very practical note, this approach decreases your practice time by unnecessarily tiring even the most helpful of partners.

> *Quality* of training is important, not just quantity. There is value to pushing through the exhaustion, the pain. But also important is truly focused intense training. And this type of training comes in many flavors — "hard fast through the mat," "slow and conscious," "smooth and connected," "big movement," "small movement," and many many more.
> I can train for an hour very slowly and focus on one or two points only, and be just as tired, if not more so, than throwing through the mat for an hour.
> —Lisa Tomoleoni, Shindo Dojo, Tokyo

When learning new skills,

- **Know your goal**. See the entire form. This includes the test list, the syllabus. Writers are advised to start with the back cover copy, never with Chapter 1.
- **Break techniques into smaller component parts**. This approach has the added benefit of allowing work with injured partners who cannot take falls but can "dance" the individual sections. With multi-step skills, such as *taigi*, start at the *end*, work *forward*.
- **Practice!** Not 3 or 4 attempts followed by chit-chat, but *real practice*. Having trouble with the "Standard Response"? *Tenkan*? Rolls? Don't just *try it* 4 or 5 times, *do it* 40 or 50, or 400 or 500 times. Was it perfect? Were you able to handle variations in direction and speed and flow? If not, do it again.

  Some new students (especially those who never studied music!) try techniques a few times and when all does not work perfectly, conclude that it's "too hard." Traditionally the beginning *jujutsu* student was assigned one thousand rolls. After one thousand rolls you will know how to roll. And you will no longer be a beginner.
- **Create skills with exercises**. They build new brain connections, allow you to integrate movements, to take them out of conscious control to the realm of unconscious automatic skill. Instructors of musical background often mention the endless scales and arpeggios practiced by musicians. Boring, perhaps. But these skills are the building blocks used to create the breathtaking music of Beethoven and Mozart.
- **Maintain skills with exercises**. The late guitar master Frederick Noad told of "a very famous concert guitarist" conscripted into the army and afraid of losing his technique.

He evolved an exercise routine covering the main aspects of playing, which could be completed in forty minutes — the maximum time he felt sure of being able to secure daily without fail. After two years of military service he found that he had not only maintained his ability to play, but actually improved it. As he said afterwards, technique seldom stands still — it either advances or retreats.

The repetitive themes of composer Antonio Vivaldi often sound remarkably like drills and exercises for music students. And this is precisely what they were. For most of his musical career, Vivaldi was employed by the *Ospedale della Pietà,* an "orphanage" for the unackowledged but well-funded daughters of philandering noblemen. The home was known for its superb musical training and many gifted graduates. Listening to a Vivaldi concerto it is easy to imagine the violin master urging his students through drill after drill after drill.

"But Master," they might have asked, "What do we *do* with this?" I imagine he might have twinkled as he told them "You take the individual parts and you put them all together of course! — and then you have *The Four Seasons.*"

As a beginner you will suffer a constant barrage of humbling experiences. You will feel like two left feet and the fifth wheel on a horse. You will feel like the world's greatest bumbler. We all do. Aikido is difficult if only because you are relearning how to sit, how to stand, how to walk, and even how to breathe. A big order. And that's before you even get to the throws. If you feel foolish, don't worry. We all do and you won't progress if you're more worried about dignity than about learning.

Natural and Unnatural

Until I became a parent, I thought children just naturally knew how to catch a ball, that catching was an instinctive biological reflex that all children are born with.

But it turns out that if you toss a ball to a child, the ball will just bonk off the child's body and fall to the ground. So you have to coach the child. . .Thanks to this coaching effort, my son has advanced his game to the point where, just before the ball bonks off his body, he winces.

—Dave Barry

Although we talk about the "naturalness" of the moves, the motions and emotions which accompany them are not at all natural. That is, if someone threatens to smash you over the head with a stick, it is not natural to step into it and be delighted with the amount of force and commitment. The point is to practice until it *becomes* natural, to remove the need for conscious thinking.

This can be accomplished only through endless repetition and an attitude change that makes them natural.

Catching a ball is not natural either, but it can become very natural indeed.

On Teaching

Nothing is so hard for those who abound in riches
as to conceive how others can be in want.

—Jonathan Swift

Keep in view from the very first the importance of inspiring confidence in the unpracticed fencer for confidence alone implies some sort of self-possession and reacts immediately on nerve and muscle. He soon begins to feel somewhat more at ease. Some slight modifications are all that is required to correct the glaring faults that are most obviously dangerous.

—Baron César de Bazancourt, *Secrets of the Sword*

Teaching ability is not a function or reward of rank, experience, or mat time. The minute that you know one small thing you can pass it on to another. Good teaching, however, is a learned skill like any other.

- **Remember what it felt like to be a beginner**. Almost the starting point. If you can remember the confusion and bafflement, the clumsiness, the feelings of stupidity and incompetence, structure your classes and your teaching materials accordingly.

  If you can't do this, consider signing up for a class of overwhelming complexity in which you have no experience, say, organic chemistry. Review and re-experience the feelings of total incomprehension. Worst case, you may end with a new skill.

- **Study "How to Teach."** Observe an experienced teacher whose classes and teaching techniques you enjoy and admire. What exactly is this person doing and how?

  What exercises were taught, demonstrations given? How were these tied to techniques? What were the time frames involved, the pacing, the timing, the proportion of lecture to exercise? How were errors corrected? What kind of feedback given or received? There is a great deal of material available on teaching techniques and styles applicable to any coursework.[1] Aikido does not exist in a vacuum.

- **Relate to the Known, then build on that foundation**. When a student learns something, no matter how simple, you can build on it. This may simply mean stepping through the first few steps of an exercise. When that is done, then add a few more. Only then add hands or other details. This is how innumerable other skills are taught.

- **Correct in the positive, avoid the negative**. Our subconscious minds do not recognize the verbal negative. What the mind actually hears in "Do NOT do X" is "DO X." Even worse things happen with repeated negative encounters. Psychologist John Gottman found that just 15 minutes of verbal interaction allowed 90 percent accuracy in predicting whether the relationship would endure. One marker: the ratio of positive to negative must be at least 5:1. (See "Life Etiquette" on page 249).

- **Be aware of the learning process**. Learning involves several distinct steps.

  - *Experiential learning / Recognition*. This is a step-by-step process in which the student must concentrate on every movement, every position. Actual learning ("saving to file") takes place when the student can say "Oh that's how you do it!" This initial stage must be reinforced by repetition.

---

1. For a great start on positive versus negative reinforcement, see *Don't Shoot the Dog* (Pryor, 1999). Also highly recommended, *Secrets of the Sword*, by Baron César de Bazancourt, an 1862 sword manual where you will find the same teaching dilemmas as today. See also KDL, pp. 120-127.

- *Repetition*. The new skill or movement must be practiced until it becomes automatic, routine, reflexive. This concept was beautifully illustrated in the *Karate Kid*. Mr. Miyagi promises Daniel emergency training for an upcoming tournament. Daniel shows up expecting to start Karate. Instead, Miyagi puts him to work polishing cars and painting miles of fence with careful instructions on the exact movements to be employed. Daniel is furious and resentful then stunned to realize that these simple movements are actually blocks[1] now made automatic through repetition.

- **Emphasize basics and drills over flourishes and frills**. Drills and repetition in Aikido are the scales and exercises of music. It's more fun to jam with the jazz band than to practice the timing, touch, rhythm and flow of scales and finger-strengthening exercises — but the basics are what make up the most advanced techniques. The notion that they are somehow separate (like *hitori-waza* from throwing techniques) is nonsense but common nonsense. In works by Bach, Beethoven, Mozart (and everyone else) you will find pages of scales and arpeggios. Building blocks are important to even the most advanced students and so is playtime.

- **Tie the basics and drills to the actual technique**. Basics are important, but always be ready to answer the unspoken (or spoken) question: "Why do I care?"

  It is always useful to show the music student that the passage that he wants to play in a beautiful sonata is actually the E-flat scale that he thinks he doesn't. It is always useful to show the Aikido student that the magical throw he is yearning to do is merely the arm-dropping and spinning exercises that he thinks is merely warm-up or a waste of mat time.

- **Observe and employ the range of sensory modes**. Visual imagery is highly regarded in our culture and common in Aikido. Unfortunately, for many students, the standard instruction to "see a glowing white light at your center" is a non-starter. Why?

  Incoming information must be processed via the sensory systems (sight, hearing, touch[2], taste, and smell). Most people have a preferred sensory system. [3]

  - Visuals use Sight. ("I see what you mean). On the mat, "watch for circles!"

  - Auditories use Hearing, ("I'm just not hearing this" or "Sounds good!") Does a technique go *zip-zip*? does it go *whoosh*? Or make Donald Duck noises?

  - Kinesthetics use Touch ("I don't get it" or "That feels right to me!"). They do better if encouraged to close their eyes and just *feel* the technique.

  Useful information or just trivia? It turns out to be extremely important. Normally we can shift from mode to mode, but when uncomfortable or stressed we tend to lock into one preferred mode. Not only do we have difficulty *expressing* ourselves in another sensory mode, we also have difficulty *understanding*.

  To decrease emphasis on the visual, simply turning out the lights and practicing in the dark can change everything. Classes held during power failures have been some of our most memorable experiences. Awareness of surroundings actually improves when students must rely on alternate senses[4].

---

1. This 1984 movie is the origin of the now famous phrase "wax on, wax off."
2. Information processing styles (sensory modes) are also referred to as "Visual," "Auditory," and "Tactile-Kinesthetic." Oddly enough, closing eyes can help even Visual people to "see."
3. Think of the little Arkadian Prince driving his humanoid transport vehicle in the movie *Men in Black*. For more on sensory modes in teaching and communications, see page 243.
4. At a seminar by Nadeau *Sensei*, my *Sensei* asked him what he thought was the biggest problem with Aikido students. Nadeau *Sensei* said: "They're blind, they're deaf, and they practice what they did yesterday." Next class, *Sensei* was pulling up people to do techniques, then asking: "What did you see? What did you hear? What did you smell, or feel?" — Tim Griffiths

- **Make images, feelings, and examples Real.** Is *shikko* like connecting ankles with a bungee cord? Provide a bungee cord and try it. Is rolling like curving over a big beach ball? Provide a ball.[1] Is *funekogi-undo* like pushing a lawn mower? Go mow the grass.

  There is a common notion that adults are familiar with all these concepts simply by virtue of being adults. Not only is that untrue, but providing physical examples and hands-on demos allows students to process information in ways that may have been missed before. Terry Dobson was notorious for using tools and toys in classes, one of the reasons his classes were so memorable. These reinforce the physical concepts.

The *dojo* "too traditional" to consider these approaches should note that the very old styles did not "teach" as we understand it. Students were expected to watch and observe and "steal" the technique from their teachers. *Teaching* in the Western sense (via exercises, drills, and even explanation) is a very recent development.

In Japanese martial arts it began in the late 1800s with educator, reformer, and Judo founder Jigoro Kano who introduced Western styles of teaching to Japan via Judo; it continued with Ki Society founder Koichi Tohei who, startled by the questions of American students in Hawaii, introduced Western teaching styles into Japanese Aikido. A student of *koryu* comments:

> Classical Japanese *budo* masters are not remembered for their great teaching skills. They would demonstrate techniques, but most often they would not show you how they were doing it. Students were expected to "steal" the technique from the teacher themselves. In the classical *jujutsu* dojo, there really was no instruction, silent or otherwise. Kano Jigoro Shihan was the first person to actually teach techniques. He did this by mixing Western learning theory into the *budo* pot. One reason Judo spread throughout Japan so quickly was that students could learn the techniques so quickly.
>
> In *koryu* schools today, I find the teaching atmosphere better than in most *gendai* schools. There is more camaraderie, and everyone is more relaxed. The teachers are generally excited to have *any* students. (When I left, Kiyama Sensei was so disappointed to be losing a student that he actually said something about it. This is almost unheard of in Japanese males of his generation!)
>
> My teachers talk, but not much. The emphasis is on learning to see what you are being shown. Matsuda Sensei always looks disappointed when he shows something several times and the student (me) still has no idea what he was looking for. Then he will say a few words to help me figure out what to look at, and show me again. Koryu *budo*, just like everything else in the world, changes over time. A teacher who tried to teach in the old style would have no students. What I find amusing is how many of the *gendai* schools insist on trying to prove they are traditional by using the brutal old-style methods.
>
> —Peter W. Boylan

---

1. See "Weapons, Tools, and Toys" on page 227.

The Dark Side of the Course

> Men you meet in the fencing room do not as a rule come there to sit at the feet of the professor, and imbibe the mystic lore of scientific theory which he expounds, but rather to be drilled and disciplined in the practical use of the sword which he holds in his hand.
>
> —Baron César de Bazancourt, *Secrets of the Sword*

Poor instructors (especially with New Black Belt syndrome) can dwindle a thriving class down to nothing in a heartbeat. Some confuse mat time with stage time to show off flying kicks or drone on about Being at One with the Universe while oblivious to Being at One with the direction and needs of the people sitting right in front of them.

It is useful to observe and analyze these classes as well. What's wrong here? Why? And how can it be done differently? For starters, the position of Instructor must never be confused (by instructor or by students) with the right to replay old internal "parent tapes," pass an abusive personal history by inflicting it on others, or use a captive audience to feed hunger for attention, adulation or prestige.

The first two behaviors appear in teaching styles heavily based on "No, no! *Don't* do that, *don't* do this, you're doing this *wrong* and that *wrong* and . . ." The punchline is often a gracious and beaming "There now, that's *much* better!" — but it's often really congratulations from the instructor to the instructor for such a fine job of instructing.

The last behavior is common in newbie instructors disoriented by what they see as graduation from student to instructor. They often talk too much, practice too little. Sometimes they need to be patiently waited out. Sometimes they need to be dealt with more directly. Those who do not recover sometimes give rise to what is known as the "Spontaneous Shihan." Those who lie about their credentials and abilities are lying to their students and are doing what they are doing for their own benefit. The student is there only for food or income[1].

Good teaching is not "Get." Neither is it purely "Give."

Ideally it is a two-way flow: Student is teacher. Teacher is student.

> It is one of the most beautiful compensations of this life that no man can sincerely try to help another without helping himself.
>
> —Ralph Waldo Emerson

---

1. Some hilarious examples of trolling for students or even *uchi-deshi* can be found on the Internet (and in real life). Don't rely on expansive claims, certificates, photographs, or belt-buckle size. Check with the headquarters organizations and Aikido groups such as Aikiweb.com.

   Many independent schools are absolutely legitimate. Others are "independent" because they know nothing about Aikido (consider the "Aikido Blackbelts" on page 32) but set up shop anyway because they are intrigued by its current popularity and potential income. Basically, one cannot claim to be a high ranking Yoshinkan, Aikikai, Ki Society, or Tomiki instructor if one does not belong and has never belonged to that organization or has only studied gymnastics, Karate, Judo, dance, or videotapes. All of these are valuable endeavors, but they are not Aikido. Be especially wary of those claiming to have "taught the SEALS," police, or Special Forces. They may be very real, but check them out. The real thing will have no objection to your doing so.

CHAPTER 2

A Brief Ki Class

Ki was, for example, the essential principle of harmony . . . the source of creativity expressed in the form of yin and yang (Lao-tzu) the vital fullness of life (Huainan-tzu), the courage arising from moral rectitude (Mencius), the divine force that penetrates all things (Kuan-tzu).
—Kisshomaru Ueshiba, *The Spirit of Aikido*

The hand is the cutting edge of the Mind.
—Jacob Bronowski, *The Ascent of Man*

For many Aikidoists, *ki* is a sticking point.

Some ignore the laws of the physical world and hasten to attribute everything to *ki* or spiritual power.

Others dismiss the power of mind, explain everything as pure physics, feeling that *ki* defines some sort of "magic" and, since they do not believe in magic, *ergo* they can not believe in *ki*.

Likely the truth is somewhere in the middle — part mind, part body.

Ki can be defined as "attention" or "mind" or "intent." Yet many who emphasize *ki* training insist that *ki* is not magic at all, that it is a culmination and a continuum of:

• **Mind** (Awareness, focus, and goal, attitude, neurology and psychology and
• **Body** (Good physics and good body mechanics).

In 1919, Tempu Nakamura, who had studied in Nepal, introduced yoga[1] to Japan as *Shin-Shin Toitsu-Do*, The Way of Mind-Body Unification.

In 1974 Koichi Tohei, an Aikido student of Morihei Ueshiba and yoga student of Tempu Nakamura, founded what we know in English as the Ki Society, in Japanese, *Shin-Shin Toitsu Aiki-Do*, "Aikido with Mind-Body Unification."

---

1. See this history in Chapter 1 of KIA. From the Sanskrit root, *yeug-, yoga* is a system of exercises designed to promote mind-body union. Related words in English (*yoke, jugular, junta, conjugate*) all reflect this concept of "joining," "unification," or becoming as "one."

Mind

> In my humble opinion, "intent" would be the very best way of looking at *ki*, at least for starting to grasp it: *the dimension and dynamics of intentions.*
>
> —Stefan Stenudd, Aikikai

In Aikido, just as in gymnastics, dance, golf, or baseball, the image is integral to the technique. The human brain differentiates very poorly between fantasy and reality; imaging helps or allows the body to respond in ways that are quite impossible when working from the intellectual mind. Learn the feeling that the images invoke — then reproduce that feeling.

In the real world, mind-body coordination presents itself in many ways, from stage-fright and blushing to sleep and nutrition. For example:

- **The classic experiment by Russian physiologist Pavlov.** In collecting saliva from dogs for research, he knew that dogs would salivate when offered food. He soon learned that if he rang a bell *before* offering the food, the dogs would salivate in *anticipation*.

- **Visualization.** At nearly every "human potential" seminar, the speaker invites you to imagine taking a fresh, juicy lemon from the refrigerator and holding it for a moment cool against your cheek. Feel its smoothness and texture. Now imagine taking a sharp knife, placing that lemon on a thick wooden cutting board, slicing into the smooth yellow skin. Smell the clean, fresh scent, see the spurt of juice as it is cut. Pick up half of that lemon, heavy with juice, in your hand, and raise it to your nose. Inhale the sharp lemon smell. Put it to your mouth, sink your teeth in and take a big cold bite of that juicy lemon . . . as mouths pucker throughout the room. (And did you notice any reaction just now?)[1]

- **Ability to awaken at a specific time without an alarm clock.**[2] Sleep is regulated by hormonal cycles; researchers measured hormones in sleeping volunteers who had been told they would be awakened at a specific time. About one hour before subjects were due to be awakened, adrenocorticotropin surged indicating that anticipation, long considered unique to *conscious* action, pervades *sleep* and the *unconscious* as well.

- **Food absorption.** Greater when meals are pleasurable and attractive than if the same fare is presented in an unattractive manner, say, run through a blender to make mush.

- **Pain perception.** Researchers have identified a powerful new approach to pain control: looking at a painful limb through the wrong end of binoculars. The smaller the apparent size of the involved limb, the less the apparent pain. Even the *measurable* swelling decreased. (Conversely, the larger the image, the greater the reported pain). Why this works is unknown, but may relate to how the brain perceives danger[3].

- **Somatopsychic responses.** Under hypnosis, subjects can develop "burns" (red and blistered skin) when told that they have been touched with a burning cigarette (but in fact touched only with a finger or an ice-cube).

    A related phenomenon is fire-walking, the failure to develop burns despite strolling across hot coals. Skeptics insist that the coals can't really be all *that* hot, or surmise that walkers must be protected from 3,000-degree coals by insulating ash or perspiration (which

---

1. In a similar exercise, a speaker facing an audience of fellow psychiatrists, who were skeptical and hostile towards the then-revolutionary concept of mind-body interaction, proceeded to read a selection from *Lady Chatterley's Lover* — to the growing distress of his listeners.
2. Jan Born *et al.*, *Nature*, January 7, 1999.
3. *Moseley, G. L. and others (2008).*

would form steam!). Unfortunately this will never be properly tested until a matching group of skeptics with no preparation but skepticism agrees to walk across the same hot bed of coals as a control group. Strangely, this does not seem to have happened.

Physics aside, what may be most remarkable is the *willingness* to stroll barefoot through a barbecue-pit by subjects who might have been halted in their tracks by a piece of paper or a T-shirt on the mat (see "Mind-Body Coordination" on page 79 and "Obstacle Course" on page 152).

- **Death and survival rates**. "Psychosomatic illness" is a familiar concept but there is also "psychosomatic health" and "psychosomatic death." The well-known placebo effect and "expectation" are behind many remarkable recoveries and/or drops in death rate before birthdays or special holidays. The reverse is true in situations that do not fit a purely physical model. Cancer patients have developed and "melted" tumors based on their beliefs, hopes, and fears[1]. If, as some claim, all of these cases can be explained away as misdiagnoses, our medical system is truly in deep trouble!

Cultural Clues. In Japanese clothing, the one exception to closing a garment left side over right side is for the dead. Health-care workers in areas with high populations of elderly Japanese are carefully trained in this tradition because of the problem of patients of good prognosis dying apparently from reading too much significance into the way that a Western nurse happened to close their garment. (See footnote on page 30.)

How Long Can You Tread Water? During World War II, when German submarines were torpedoing British shipping with devastating efficiency, two basic groups of sailors went into the water:

- Grizzled old salts with years of smoking, drinking, and bad food, and
- Strapping young men in their prime of life and peak physical condition.

One group lived, one group died at rates entirely beyond expectations[2]

Apparently the young men hit the water thinking: "*Oh no! This is the most terrible thing that has happened in my entire life!*" They were right, and they died of shock and terror. Apparently the older men hit the water thinking: "*Oh no! Not again!*" and knowing they had survived before, they survived once again.

A military historian comments:

> This pattern is not fantasy or wishful thinking. It is part of the official record of every war. It has been observed repeatedly that persons with the tools and resources of experience (a power of mind), who have persons and places they love and care about have higher survival rates than those who do not, even when compared to persons younger and physically healthier.
> —Frank R. Shirer, Historian, U.S. Army Center of Military History

---

1. See Becker, R. O. (1985). See Siegal, Bernie S. (1990).
2. This sometimes backfires. Older people who have lived through previous floods and hurricanes often refuse to evacuate on the assumption that because they survived before, they'll survive again. They are often wrong (Ripley, 2008). Regardless of mindset and the most positive thinking, we are still subject to the laws of physics and biology.

Ki Testing and Exercises

Note that *nage* is the partner to be tested; *uke* gives the test[1].

1. *Uke* stands or sits perpendicular to *nage*.
2. With the palm or fingers of the hand nearest *nage*'s body, *uke* applies pressure *perpendicular* to *nage*'s chest, fingers parallel to the floor. Gradually increasing pressure is applied until *nage* *begins* to lose stability.
3. *Uke* observes degree of effort required to disrupt stability.

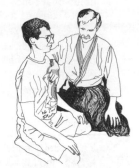

This configuration greatly reduces mechanical advantage so that the inexperienced *uke* can't knock *nage* over as easily simply through arm strength with body weight behind it. Fingers are parallel to the mat because hand tends to follow fingers. A test done with fingers directed upwards tends to go in that direction — a very difficult test.

Tests 1 and 2.

Standard testing is divided into three levels.

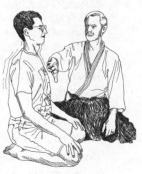

1. Test One: gentle or gradually increasing pressure.
   This is the basic test for beginners.
2. Test Two: applied with hesitation.
   In *nage's* sight, *uke* may bring a hand in rapidly as if to strike, stop, then proceed with the test. Or, *uke* may place a hand a few inches away from *nage*'s body and wait to see if *nage* withdraws or moves toward the hand in anticipation. This is the notorious "Magnetic Hand" — *uke* holds it out; *nage* is attracted to it like magic. The cure is for *uke* to immediately test from the back.
3. Test Three: testing with *ki*.
   Nage must extend out so that *uke*'s *ki* never even enters *nage*'s body. Or mind.

Variations

Possibilities are endless, but the following basics test for focus, relaxation, balance and body mechanics and can be applied at any time during exercise or technique.

With *nage* in *seiza*:

- Pressing from chest and back.
- Pressing shoulder from the side.
- Lifting knee.
- Lifting hand (not up from knee, but towards shoulder).

With *nage* standing,

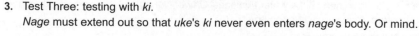

- Pressing from front (chest), back, and small of back.
- Pressing shoulder from the side.
- Lifting leg up from the ankle.

---

1. See KIA for details on testing and extensive exercises and demonstrations.

Testing the Tester[1]

In some schools there is a tendency for *nage* to pretend to break the laws of physics and for *uke* to pretend that *nage* has successfully done so. The best thing for this is unbiased test.

1. Test several times to experiment with technique, feeling, and results.
2. Repeat the tests with *nage* choosing the conditions — but without telling *uke*.
3. Verify results of *nage*'s internal choices with *uke*'s external observations.

For example, try telling a lie.

- My name is [*right name*].
- My name is [*false name*].

From the results, *uke* tries to guess which of the two *nage* was thinking.[2] *Nage* then confirms or corrects *uke*'s conclusion. This approach removes temptation for *uke* to load or skew the test in any way. It also provides essential reality testing for *nage*.

Ki testing is a team sport but it is not a win/lose sport. Many who try *ki* tests "fail" because *uke* saw himself as opponent and attacker, rather than as a teammate serving as a useful biofeedback device. The point is to test, observe, and evaluate. It is not to overwhelm, smash, or "win" by attacking. It is a *cooperative* effort in feeling and sensing that partners can use to help each other improve. It is like testing new ice for strength before putting your full weight down on it.

Ki exercises offer up-close Real-Time proof that setting goals matters, what we focus on matters, what we think about matters, and even good posture matters — more than most of us will ever know. The classic *ki* exercise is Unbendable Arm[3]. *Uke* tries to bend *nage*'s extended arm at the elbow while *nage* keeps the arm strong but relaxed. The secret is largely an issue of which muscles you use and which muscles you relax. Biceps bends (flexes) the elbow while triceps extends it. Tensing biceps and triceps at the same time isn't strong, it's *weak* for the simple reason that *you are fighting yourself.*

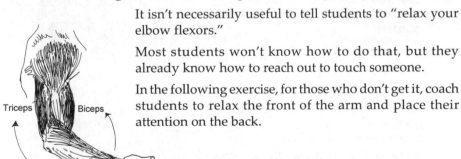

It isn't necessarily useful to tell students to "relax your elbow flexors."

Most students won't know how to do that, but they already know how to reach out to touch someone.

In the following exercise, for those who don't get it, coach students to relax the front of the arm and place their attention on the back.

Triceps   Biceps

---

1. See KIA p. 16 and Jan Bergen's essay on discovering the point of testing, KIA pp. 18-19.
2. In the movie *House of Games* a professional con-man refers to them as "tells" and explains their usefulness and applications as tools of the trade.
3. For history and observations, see ZC, pp. 212-214; KDL, pp. 31-32; KIA, pp. 18, 100.

Unbendable Arm

This exercise shows the power of a goal (beyond the immediate battlefield of the elbow), and the weakness of tension and fixation.

1. With one hand on *nage*'s bicep and other on *nage*'s wrist, *uke* attempts to bend *nage*'s arm. Test gently at first with steadily increasing challenge as *nage* learns the feel.

2. Quantify strength and duration by counting elapsed seconds ("one-thousand-one, one-thousand-two, one-thousand-three," etc.).

   Once learned, *nage* will be able to maintain Unbendable Arm, exhibiting a strength beyond all apparent physical capacity.

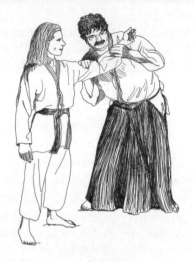

To help the feeling, *nage* may:

- Imagine a water pump at Center that pumps water up through the torso, through the arm and out the fingers.
- Imagine touching the opposite wall or the hand of a distant third person.

A smaller or weaker *uke* can,

1. Place *nage*'s hand on her shoulder.
2. Place her own hands on *nage*'s elbow joint.
3. Drop weight underside.
   The taller partner may kneel or sit.

Variations

- Note difference between "extending," and "stop *uke* from bending arm."
- How much effort is required to maintain "unbendable-ness"? Count seconds to compare.

Turning from One-Point

Another example of not-stopping mind, of extension and goal setting.

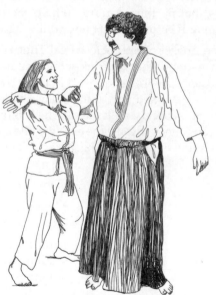

1. *Uke* places hands firmly on both sides of *nage*'s hips.
2. *Nage* attempts to turn hips while:
   - Concentrating on *uke*'s hands.
   - Concentrating on turning around a very small point at Center/One-Point.
   - Thinking of moving one of *uke*'s hands forward and around in a circle.

On Truth Testing

The problem with citing examples of mysterious deaths, remarkable recoveries, or fire-walking is that although they are very real, few of us know of them from direct experience. To most Americans, a topic far more near, dear and familiar than psychic or psychological research is sports wins and rankings.

"Thanks to Ki Development Exercises I feel so much more At One with the Universe"

or even

"My techniques feel stronger"

are both a tad vague. In contrast, baskets, goals, pitching and hitting are eminently quantifiable. Either you are pitching a no-hitter, batting 0.300, winning the playoffs — or you definitely, certainly, verifiably are not.

Basketball coach Phil Jackson[1] uses yoga, meditation, and visualization exercises in working with players, the very thing that tends to be dismissed as delusional or "fruity" in Aikido. His regular season winning percentages have set decidedly non-fruity NBA records, and his .730 playoff winning percentage (111-41) is the Number 2 all-time record. Koichi Tohei used *ki* exercises to train baseball star Oh Sadaharu and Hawaiian *sumo* champion Takamiyama.

Closer to home, professional baseball instructor John Pinkman uses *ki* training to develop pitching and hitting skills. Pinkman is confident that this approach creates better balance and better players, but for true effectiveness, the lines between imagination, wishful thinking, and hard reality must be clearly drawn, demonstrated, and evaluated. Does it work or doesn't it?

The only way to know is to actually quantify (measure) the results. Pinkman does exactly that.

Essay: Aiki-Pitching

To start, a radar gun tracks a series of 50 pitches. The results (balls, strikes, and scatter pattern) are charted on an X/Y axis under three different circumstances:

- **Under pressure**. Initially, speed and delivery for new students are erratic. When the pitcher calms, strike percentage rises.
- **Under controlled circumstances**. With calmness and mental control, pitching improves.
- **In a state prepared for success**. The student is relaxed, pitching one pitch at a time, understanding that every pitch is a whole new game. Balls are delivered at consistent speed from the same place. Balls go down, strikes go up.

For skill to *remain* requires cognitive awareness of body control, cause and effect. To alter body mechanics or muscle memory you must *know*, you can't just *do*. Body can only do what

---

1. See Alexander, R. (1999), "Jackson — Zen and Now" for yet another practitioner in the growing field of sports psychology and applied *ki* development.

mind already knows. On the other hand, for efficient motion you can't take time to think, you must flow. How to coordinate mind and body?

Enter the Tao of baseball, the Zen of pitching, and *ki* in its purest day-to-day form. Pinkman's pitching training begins with *ki* exercises.

1. **Downward *ki* flow**. We train *ki* flow "down into the ground" and ask parents to try to lift their child. After just 5 minutes of training these children are amazingly successful. Equally amazing are the expressions of Mom and Dad at their inability to lift a child who inexplicably seems to have just doubled in weight[1].
2. **Upward *ki* flow**. We train to reverse the *ki*, pulling energy from the ground up into the ball. Energy starts from the ball of the foot and flows into the ball. *Ki* begins in the foot when it comes in contact with the rubber and flows through the body and out of the hand and into the ball. At this point we teach . . .
3. **Biomechanics**. Understanding of the musculature and physics of throwing. Then . . .
4. **Passive Imagery**. Passive, non-movement visualization, moving to . . .
5. **Active Imagery**. Throwing with eyes closed on flat ground and then on balance beams, bringing the pitcher into a state of heightened sensory awareness.[2]

Understanding energy flow becomes much more real and easy to grasp once the student makes the sensory connection with the new experience of listening to their breathing, feeling the flowing arm motion and the path of the ball exiting their hand at a specific point in space.

In pitching, finding the release point is a critical skill. It takes players who are excellent players to the level of elite players. Shoulders are rotating at 2,800 degrees per second and the difference between high pitch and low pitch is only a few degrees. Finding that point involves feeling and sensitivity yet maximum energy. These repeated exercises give the pitcher the opportunity to relax, to practice and program the idea that "I want to release the ball *here*." But for a pitcher on the plate, doing these exercises *physically* would be considered a balk. So how to make a more relaxed, calm, and consistent pitcher in a "safe" manner? With breathing and visualization.

1. **Breathe**. Oxygen dilutes adrenaline and delivers energy to the entire system. Next,
2. **Visualize source**. Visualize where the pitch is *coming from*, starting from the foot, up through calf, hamstrings, shoulder, triceps. Another deep breath and . . .
3. **Visualize target**. Visualize where the pitch is *going to go*.
   Most people think that a ball is thrown with the hand and the eyes follow. We train pitchers to close their eyes and throw using the flow of their energy in their body to the target. There's nothing more thrilling than throwing strikes[3] with your eyes closed.

Pitching is physically and mentally demanding. In a typical outing a pitcher will throw 189 pitches (100 during the game, 40 in pre-game warm-up, and 49 (7 at a time) prior to each inning in a 7 inning game). During a game, exhaustion, drama and emotion interfere with *ki* flow and pitching. We drill body mechanics, but we also drill to create emotional instability, anger, and frustration while having the pitcher throw at a very small target (for example, a softball on a batting tee). The process is this:

---

1. See KIA Chapter 4 and the "Unliftable Body" exercise on page 94.
2. See the railroad track *suburi* practice described on page 233.
3. See PinkmanBaseball.com. Yes, Pinkman had me do it and I pitched a strike even though I hadn't had a baseball in my hand since 1967. Also consider that there are thousands of blind bowlers in the U.S. who must do the same thing. See Gaines (1999).

1. **Record performance with anger and anxiety.** The ball's velocity and accuracy are always inconsistent. Contrary to what many would think, anger limits ball velocity and scatters the location pattern. The term "he's lost control" applies to more than the pitcher's inability to find the strike zone. Graph the data as a learning tool. Then . . .
2. **Calm**. Lead the player, through quiet verbal and non-verbal instruction, out of a hopeless, anxious state. We structure breathing, mental images, starting point of *ki*, and flow.
3. **Record performance**. Velocity, mental composure, and target location increase. Always.

We must measure and be held accountable for results. Specifically, do players improve in the game after we work with them? And does that improvement remain as consistent skill performance? It does.

Our results-oriented training has produced an extraordinary success rate in educating pitchers. But this teaching method is not for the unusual player. It is normal instruction for pitchers in our school. I have done these drills hundreds of times over the years, always with the same successful results.

Ki is normal. It is daily and it is ordinary.

Ki can be used without understanding or even using the word.

Ki is not the product. It's the process.

—John Pinkman

Pinkman, like many other sports trainers and *ki* practitioners, believes intensely in the value of *ki* exercises. But notice that he is not relying on mind alone.

A player has both mind and body.

And as long as that body is on this physical earth, it must obey the laws of physics.

Body

Is Aikido "mere physics?" Perhaps. But there is nothing "mere" about good physics. The study of physics is the power and magic of the physical world and the physical body made replicable. In many ways Aikido is Remedial Physics for City Kids.

I had a useful refresher course while drying out a wet basement. The project involved digging a ditch 10 feet long, 3 feet wide and 7- to 8-feet deep to drain and repair a cracked and leaking wall and install a sump pump. A backhoe would have been awkward and damaging. I dug it by hand and I did it alone. Dirt, cinder blocks, gravel, rebar, and shoring all had to come in and out of that hole as efficiently and as safely as possible. Good physics and good mechanics are survival tools.

When muscling 70-pound buckets of mud out of a deepening hole became impractical, up went a hoist with block and tackle. The easiest way to lift that weight? Lift feet, drop weight. Not projecting out, not pulling with arms, but just dropping down, as close to 90 degrees down as possible, "in harmony with the laws of the universe" such as gravity. No 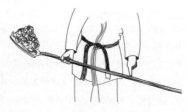 need to attack a gravel pile directly when a tweak of a blade at its base will fill it with stones sliding easily downslope under gravity. *Pulling* down requires strength and effort. *Dropping* down or *allowing* to drop down does not.

The physical building blocks of Aikido are the same tools of lever arms, rotation, and their vectors. Some basic physics concepts often presented in the specialized Aikido language are: One-Point, Weight Underside, and Relaxation.

One-Point

The story about the 255-pound instructor being thrown by the five-year old is about me, and took place at a Lee District kid's class. We were doing the katate-tori kokyu-nage in which nage stands beside *uke*, then takes a little back hop to do the throw. I was in the process of explaining the throw, when I said, "Now if Emily takes a big hop backwards right now . . ." and she did. It was like having a 30-pound bowling ball hanging off the end of my arm. I was looking in a different direction at that moment and the throw took me totally by surprise. It was one of those moments when the *ki* was just right.

—Kirk Demaree

Part of what Aikidoists call the Center, the One-Point or *hara*, physicists consider to be the center of mass of the body, the point where gravity acts on the body as a whole[1] hence "center of gravity." When standing upright in a normal posture, the center of mass is approximately between spine and navel at about the level of the hip joints. From the physical standpoint, One-Point is the body's center of gravity. The vertical location is commonly said to be about two inches below the navel (although this changes). It can also be the center point of rotation, the fulcrum of a lever.

---

1. In mechanics, the motion and behavior of this one point is considered to be characteristic of the entire object. But note that this Center Point of stability varies; see page 214.

In static conditions, that body is stable as long as the One-Point remains centered over its support — the feet. If center of mass moves beyond its support, the pull of gravity creates a torque that requires greater effort to control; failing that, a body may fall, regardless of size, weight, or muscle.

In Haiti, I watched a woman purchase a basket of goods so heavy that neither she nor the merchant who sold it to her could lift it alone. Only together were they were able to heave it atop her head; from there she strode away home. The following exercise illustrates the difference in effort between weight Over Center or weight Away From Center.

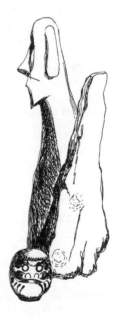

1. Hold a 10- or 20-pound weight at arm's length (past Center). Observe effort required to do so and how it feels while walking around.
2. Compare effort required to do the above with elbow bent. Observe the change in effort required if you shorten the lever arm by a few inches.
3. Put weight on your shoulder and then head. How heavy does it feel there?
4. What happens if you slump or bend over?

Exhortations by your instructor to bring *uke* in close, to drop everything to One-Point reflect this physical law: the closer you are to your Center, the longer your end of the lever, the more control and power you have, the less strain and struggle. You need not be constantly over Center to be balanced, but if off-Center you need support (even if it is motion or inertia) to maintain stability.

Weight Underside

Weight Underside is demonstrated in Japanese *daruma* dolls, Western punching clowns, Balancing Baby toys, and ancient engineering works from Celtic monoliths to the massive stone works of Peru. How was it possible to move the mammoth 50-ton statues of Easter Island from their quarry to the other end of the island, many miles away? Apparently they walked. Once levered to an upright position, the bottom-heavy figures could be rotated about their stable center just like the Teddy Bears or swordsmen on page 44.

In Aikido, Weight Underside is usually discussed in contrast to "weight upperside" which implies tension or placement of "mind" somewhere other than at One-Point in the abdomen[1]. Whether you are moving a 50-ton statue or a 150-pound *uke*, weight upperside or underside matters.

It matters because it changes the probability of you falling or *uke* falling because it changes the physical dynamics in strange and wonderful ways[2].

---

1. For relaxation vs. tension and the physical results, see KIA Chapter 3, and KDL p. 45.
2. For Weight Underside, see KIA Chapter 4.

Relaxation

A familiar line from various novels and murder mysteries is "the dead are heavier than the living." Actually, that would be the dead, the drunk or unconscious, and the unwilling two-year-old. Tension and relaxation are wild cards. Tension improves a lever arm, relaxation degrades it. The more tense and rigid, the easier *uke* is to throw, haul, carry. The more soft and relaxed, the more difficult and the more of an advantage you may have over a stiff, tense opponent. How is this possible?

When you are tense, you take up all the slack in your own body, giving *uke* a direct line to your center with lots of lever arms to unbalance you. You even get tired quicker. *Uke* is trying to lock you up and tire you out anyway. Tense up and you do it for him. If you prefer not to provide this service to your attacker, relax! You become invisible to *uke* (he can no longer feel exactly where you are), and harder to manipulate. Which is easier to lift and carry? A 50-pound rod or a 50-pound bag of rice?

This is the rationale behind the constant refrain: *"Don't be strong, be soft!"* but coming from Karate to Aikido I thought: "Har! Buncha wimps!" Very slowly I came to realize that the point of relaxed muscles is not to be weak and mushy, but to not waste energy or tighten lever arms which hand the advantage to the opponent[1]. I might have grasped the concept more quickly if rephrased as:

> "Tense" gives *uke* the gift of lever arms. "Relaxed" does not.

"Removing slack" also allows other forces to operate that cannot otherwise. You can see this in everyday examples such as rugs and towels. To shake a rug you can:

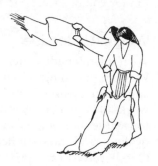

1. Hold it with hands together, the rug or towel hanging slack and limp. Shake it and you get no snap, only flop and flutter. For a small item, that may be enough. Or you can . . .
2. Hold snugly, hands pulling apart, slack out. Now you can snap that rug and send the dirt flying. The bigger and heavier the item, the more critical it is to take the slack out. Otherwise you have no control and won't get it moving at all.

Neither rugs nor towels (nor chains—see page 195) make good lever arms in their normal state, but with *slack out* they behave in completely different ways. So does *uke*[2]. Who would you rather have as *uke* for demo or test? The Tin Man or the Scarecrow? Tin Man would provide the easier leverage.

And it's all "just leverage" isn't it?

---

1. Stiffness isn't desirable in Karate either. You will never survive your black belt test if you don't learn to relax, if you don't learn the difference between appropriate tension and relaxation.
2. The locker-room rat-tail is a towel rolled and twisted to eliminate excess slack. This changes the normal physical properties of a towel; the whipping tail can actually split skin. Taking slack out of towel or rug is equivalent to taking slack out of a floppy flexible multi-jointed arm (even one of straw). It is the critical secret behind arm locks and how to *push* with a chain. See page 195.

Just Leverage

Give me a place to stand and a lever long enough and I will move the earth!

—Archimedes (287?-212 B.C.)

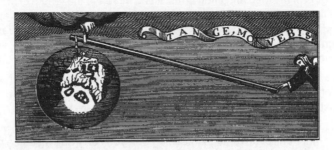

There is much popular nonsense over the pyramids of Egypt, too big, too heavy[1] to have been built by human hands. Yet those amazed that our ancestors could move blocks of such weight and size (with huge levers, massive work gangs and unlimited time and resources) are oddly calm at seeing a tiny woman single-handedly moving blocks of similar or greater weight and size — with the help of the small lever known as a "car jack."

A shovel is a lever. It is a waste of effort to lift a load with precious energy. It is so much easier to lever it up around the fulcrum of an arm that (as in *funekogi-undo*) need serve only as a connector. In Aikido, similar lever arrangements allow tiny bodies to throw large bodies across the room with great ease.

Essay: Levers and Leverage

There are three classes of levers, three different permutations of where you can place a weight, a fulcrum, and an opposing force on a lever.

1. First-class levers have the fulcrum between the weight and the force.

   In Aikido an example is old-style *sumi-otoshi*[2]. Your shoulder under *uke*'s elbow levers them up and over. *Koshi-nage* is the same action done with the hips.
2. Second-class levers have the weight between the force and the fulcrum. An example is a wheelbarrow, or the *ikkyo* or *nikyo* pin, where the shoulder joint acts as a fulcrum and the anterior shoulder muscles wrap up onto the arm to provide the "weight" when you stretch it.
3. Third-class levers have the force between the weight and the fulcrum, like the end of a *bokken* strike where the back hand acts as the fulcrum, the front hand is the force and the *bokken* is the weight (although not a point mass).

The difference between the three is like choosing a gear for driving.

---

1. The average-sized block in The Great Pyramid is about 1,200 pounds. Wow!
2. See Projection #10 ("Sumi Otoshi"), ADS p. 277-281.

First-class levers are low speed, high torque, if the effort arm (distance between force and fulcrum) is larger than the load arm (distance between weight and fulcrum).

Second- and third-class levers are really the same thing. Which one you have depends on the relative lengths of the load and effort arms. If you increase the length of the load arm from initially being shorter than the effort arm, you're trading how much force you apply for how quickly the load moves. With second class levers you must move through a larger angle to move the weight by the same amount but you need not apply as much force. With third-class levers you move a little to get a lot of movement, but you must exert a lot of force.

Once you have begun a technique, the reason you want to be close to your partner rather than at arm's length is efficient leverage. Standing far away puts you on the wrong end of the lever. Even "just leverage" works poorly (on your end) if you are holding *uke* at a distance.

If you're going to manhandle *uke* you want your effort arm to be longer than your load arm, so that you have a mechanical advantage, meaning that you can trade distance for force. You want to be up close so that *uke*'s arm, that beautiful lever, is under *your* control and not *uke*'s. So now you've made *uke*'s whole arm the effort arm instead of holding *uke* at a distance and making it the load arm. It's like very static *jo-nage*. You retain mechanical advantage by always controlling more than half of the stick.

Exhortations by your instructor to bring *uke* in close, to drop everything to One-Point reflect this physical law. The closer you are to your center, the longer your end of the lever, the more control and power you have, the less strain and struggle.

—Dr. Joseph Toman

Rotation and Its Center

In ancient *jujutsu* they taught that "when pushed, pull back; when pulled, push forward." In the spherical movements of aikido, this becomes: "When pushed, pivot and go around; when pulled, enter while circling." This means that one moves in circular motion in response to the opponent and while moving spherically, one maintains his center of gravity to create the stable axis of movement. And at the same time the opponent's center is disturbed, and when he loses his center, he also loses all power. Then he is subdued swiftly and decisively.

—Kisshomaru Ueshiba, *The Spirit of Aikido*

Rotation is "just leverage" in a circle. Observe the leverage in the following exercise. The lever is the side of the block, the back of the chair.

Cinder Blocks and Chairs

Cinder blocks are heavy to lift, easy to rotate. If you don't have a pile of spare cinder blocks in your dojo, use a chair or even a firmly packed gym bag. In real life these items become lumber, oxygen cylinders, file cabinets, or other items. Compare the effort required:

1. *To rotate* the item as opposed to that required . . .
2. *To lift* the item (especially at arm's length).

Variation

- "Walk" the chair across the room by rotating it around its two front legs, alternating from one front leg to another. This is the same motion behind *shikkyo* (see page 103).
- Sitting in a simple, light-weight, 4-legged chair, observe the effort required to lift yourself out of the chair compared to that required to tilt back or forward.

Laundry-Bag Tenkan

For details, see *tenkan* exercises beginning on page 147 of KIA.

1. Fill a bag with clothes or towels. Heave the bag as far as possible with one arm. Use linear energy and muscle power, no wind-up, no swing. Note where bag falls.
2. Keeping arms at sides (to limit size of circle), turn a partial *tenkan*, releasing bag to fly across the mat. Note new point where the bag falls.
3. Compare distances achieved via a partial turn, a full turn, two full turns. Compare also the effort required to move the bag, and the power generated in the course of doing so.

Joseph Toman continues:

Actually, this exercise does not describe the Aikido technique. You're not really tossing *uke* like a sack of potatoes off a wall, you're guiding him around the outside of a circle in order to have more time and distance. Why? Because the perimeter of a circle is 2 times the radius of the circle times *pi* or:

$$P = 2\pi r \tag{EQ 1}$$

In two-dimensional space, turning *tenkan* dissipates the initial attack over time and distance. It also encourages the attacker to over-commit to the attack by letting him think he is just about to get his balance back.

In three-dimensional space, you're also guiding him down and out beyond his One-Point ("tripping"[1]) and then back up and over ("clotheslining") once you've compromised his hip stability. You can add a little energy in *tenkan*, but not a lot because then *uke* gets wise to what you're doing and counters by pulling back or changing the attack altogether.

So, if *uke* is 3 feet away, and wants to grab you, in the linear world, the distance from *uke* to you is the radius *r* or 3 feet.

If however, you step off-line and lead him around in a circle, the distance he must travel around the perimeter (P) of that circle is not 3 feet but 2 x 3.14 x 3 or *12.56 feet*—with a corresponding increase in time.

To do *tenkan* properly, you do not push or drag *uke* in a circle, you allow him to drive himself. The following exercise demonstrates the difference.

Rag Doll Tenkan

In *tenkan*, the competitive or contrary *uke* may pull back (rather than extending forward) while the inexperienced *nage* valiantly attempts to *drag* the unwilling *uke*

---

1. See "Clotheslining and Tripping" on page 193.

around in a circle. This exercise allows *uke* to practice extending forward while *nage* practices accepting and aligning with the energy. In pairs,

1. *Nage* extends a wrist and stands with One-Point and Unbendable Arm.
2. *Uke* grasps the wrist and *pushes nage* around in a circle.
   A strange feeling? This is how it should feel.

"But On The Street," protests many a new student, "you wouldn't do a *complete tenkan*." Why? Because the student doesn't yet understand the power of circles and opts out for what has worked before (or what he imagines might work, having seen it in the movies: muscle and linear energy). Unfortunately, there's always going to be someone or something bigger and stronger. Consider tons of stampeding cattle.

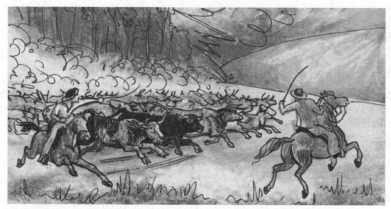

Few occupations are more cheerful, lively and pleasant than that of the cow-boy on a fine day or night; but when the storm comes, then is his manhood and often his skill and bravery put to test. When the night is inky dark and the lurid lightning flashes its zig-zag course athwart the heavens, and the coarse thunder jars the earth, the winds moan fresh and lively over the prairie, the electric balls dance from tip to tip of the cattle's horns, then the position of the cow-boy on duty is trying far more than romantic.

When the storm breaks over his head, the least occurrence unusual, such as the breaking of a dry weed or stick, or a sudden and near flash of lightning, will start the herd, as if by magic, all at an instant, upon a wild rush. And woe to the horse, or man, or camp that may be in their path. The only possible show for safety is to mount and ride with them until you can get outside the stampeding column. . . .

The moment the herd is off, the cow-boy turns his horse at full speed down the retreating column, and seeks to get up beside the leaders, which he does not attempt to stop suddenly, for such an effort would be futile, but turns them to the left or right hand, and gradually curves them into a circle, the circumference of which is narrowed down as fast as possible, until the whole herd is rushing wildly round and round on as small a piece of ground as possible for them to occupy.

—Joseph G. McCoy
Historic Sketches of the Cattle Trade of the West and Southwest (1874)

The process of running the cattle back into themselves to end the stampede was referred to as "milling" the herd. The root concept was rotation and redirection.

Vectors — Deflection and Redirection

On reading the paper ["Roundabout"] I was amazed to see
how long it took him to say, "Hey! It's all vectors!"

—Dr. Joseph Toman

Vectors describe and analyze forces. They are represented by arrows drawn to scale, plotted on graph paper, or by trigonometric calculations. The *length* of the arrow shows the *magnitude* of the force. The *direction* of the arrow represents the direction of the force. The end result of the combined forces is the *resultant*, the single vector which would have the same net effect as all the original vectors combined.

In a tale by 19th-century Russian fabulist I. A. Krilov, a swan, lobster, and a fish plan to haul a heavy cart by pulling from three different sides.

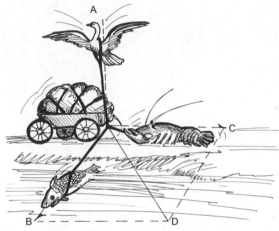

The swan flies straight up to the sky. The fish heads for deep water, and the lobster trudges ahead on land (although here he's moving backwards as lobsters often do.)

The traditional teaching point of the fable is that without cooperation, all their best efforts cancel each other out and the cart does not move. Vector analysis, however, suggests quite a different situation.

The swan, by rising up (A), reduces friction and stability of the load. Easier to move. Fish and lobster pull in directions B and C producing the resultant force (D). Hence the cart *will* move, although very inefficiently. It will end up in the river, not exactly where they really wanted it to go, but it will move.

Compare this image with *sankyo zempo-nage*.

1. The *sankyo* (*swankyo*?) locks *uke*'s arm so that you control his Center/One-Point and he is rising up, possibly teetering on tip-toe. Easier to move.
2. Forward motion is provided by shifting your Center, as you step forward. So far, so good. However, just as you prepare to lob *uke* across the mat . . .
3. Something fishy happens. Perhaps you pull *uke* in closer because you weren't close enough to start with. Perhaps you push *uke* slightly away because you're uncomfortable being so close to the attacker. Perhaps you tense up thinking "Uh-oh, how do I do this?"
    Uke will move, but not very efficiently, and not exactly where you really wanted him to go.

The concept of "blending" is the act of aligning with the force and direction that is offered. We talk about "using *uke*'s strength and power" but tend to be a bit vague about how exactly we do that.

In the example of the fish and the lobster, the most efficient way of moving a load is to provide pure forces in the desired direction. Fish and lobster will succeed in moving the cart, but not as efficiently as if they were directly aligned with each other, moving in the same direction. In the illustrations below, compare the degree of "harmony," "congruence," "blending," shared goals and direction between the two partners and their arms.

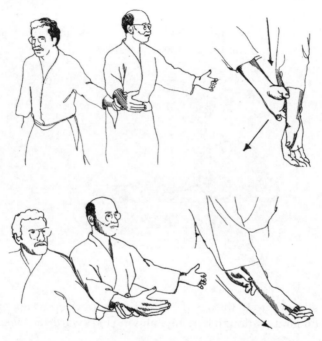

Try rolling up a car window with your arm aligned with the crank, or reaching over from the middle seat. What is the difference in efficiency and required effort?

Simply pulling in different directions distorts directions, but so does muscle tension which originates or transmits all sorts of spurious forces. Simply tightening fingers and clenching a fist and forearm almost certainly means that you are pulling back, no matter how slightly. There is a world of difference in feel and result in a *tenkan* where *nage* is leading forward, pulling back, pulling to the side, or any combination of these as opposed to a pure forward lead.

As aid to centering and direction (and also because of Aikido's sword tradition), Yoshinkan style Aikido uses a stance (*kamae*) in which hands constantly define the center line of the body and therefore direction of hips and of travel. Or, try pointing fingers into a V at waist and see how this changes your perception of position, and direction, and alignment of your own body and that of others.

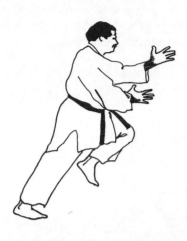

Much of the magic and flow of the adept Aikidoist is the ability to blend perfectly with the motion offered and with the desired goal.

In his classic paper "Roundabout," Jearle Walker comments on the hefty amount of force required to actually *stop* a punch compared to the mere fraction of effort required to *redirect* it. Applying a small force at right angles to the path of a punch applies a torque to the arm which deflects the punch.

The further away you are (*ma-ai*), and the more extended *uke* is, the longer his lever arm. This puts *uke* on the short end of the lever, you on the long end, and deflection or redirection of the fist at the end of that lever takes little effort.

A remarkable example is *shomen-uchi irimi* (page 172). *Uke* attacks with a powerful overhead strike. *Nage* appears to block *uke*, turning him completely around in *ikkyo*. The stronger the attack, the more forcefully *uke* is spun around. But despite appearances it isn't a ferocious block. It is simple redirection. Joseph Toman explains:

> Imagine a line connecting *uke* and *nage*. *Uke* delivers an overhead strike along that line. *Nage* moves laterally off the line omote[1] to *uke*, connecting with *uke*'s attacking arm. The lateral distance creates a moment arm.[2] When that is combined with the force of *uke*'s attack the result is that *uke* experiences *torque*[3] around *nage* and the pivot point where their arms meet. *Uke* is still going the same direction as he started out, but torque and anatomy combine to spin him around and make him travel backwards. It looks like a block because we assume that people travel in the direction they are facing, which isn't true in this case. The two variants on this throw are adding a step forward or a step back.
>
> - Stepping forward increases *uke*'s angular speed relative to *nage*, making the technique tighter and faster, but decreasing the energy *uke* can put into it.
> - Stepping back decreases *uke*'s angular speed[4] making it a slower technique, allowing *uke* time to put more energy into it.

The following exercises demonstrate a critical Aikido skill; the ability to align with, follow, and amplify the energy that *uke* provides, rather than exhausting one's own strength. You can think of Aikido as "arm" or "body" surfing. Just like the ocean surfer, you must align and flow. Going counter to that force is commonly known as a "wipe-out." Just as you can't steer a canoe effectively unless you are moving faster than the current, you can't move effectively through traffic unless you match its speed and direction, you can't lead *uke* unless you align and blend.

---

1. *Omote* or *irimi* mean "front, forward" or inside the line of attack.
2. From Latin *momentum*, from *movere*, to move.
3. *Torque*, from Latin *torquere*, to twist, is the tendency of a force to produce rotation around an axis, in this case, the tendency of *uke* to rotate around *nage*.
4. That is, "How big an angle will the *jo* move through in one second?" By analogy with baseball, stepping *in* requires *uke* to bunt; there is no time for a big swing of the bat and the result is a low-energy pop. Stepping *back* allows time for a full swing of the bat, perhaps a home run.

Aiki Arm Wrestling

"Aiki arm-wrestling" is a valuable exercise for illustrating just how Aikido works and how very different it is from preconceived concepts of strength and strategy.

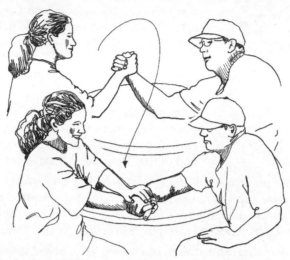

It is not collision, not resistance, not a weight and strength contest. It is aligning, accepting and following energy, until for *uke*, it's too late — and people have a very hard time comprehending this simple exercise. On table or lying on mat, partners assume the classic arm-wrestling position.

1. Start by pushing arms against each other, pushing/resisting as normal.
2. At some point *nage* ceases all resistance, allowing *uke*'s arm to crash to the mat. In normal arm-wrestling, this would be a "win" for *uke*. Here, *nage* uses the other hand to pins *uke*'s hand. By cooperating with *uke*'s strength and power, *uke* has now been "brought to the mat" and can't get up again.

The Bounce

If weighted down with a heavy backpack, groceries, or other load that makes lifting the weight straight up from a dead start difficult or impossible, try this exercise.

1. Raise up just a little bit, then drop right back *down*. Springy muscles and tendons in your knees will bounce.
2. Add enough muscle and effort to amplify the "bounce" and follow it *up*.

Parked on a slope? Rather than forcing the door uphill against gravity,

1. Push it a little ways, let it fall back down where it rebounds against the spring, and
2. Follow the rebound back up to close the door.

You will see these physical principles operating throughout Aikido and life. A good understanding of the fundamentals of physics gives you a big advantage in Aikido and everything else. And yet it is still difficult to believe that Aikido can do what it is said to do, as physicist Jearle Walker puts it, "make the strong equal to the weak."

Hence, Aikido is often of special interest to women who have been carefully trained to believe for years that they cannot possibly protect themselves, meaning (in part) that a Small Person cannot possibly deflect, redirect, or resist a Big Person.

A particularly absurd example of this notion appeared in the early 70s on a popular talk show addressing increasing assaults on women. Guests were a "Karate Expert" and an actor whose only apparent qualification for comment was a role in the TV show "Police Surgeon." Between them they solemnly agreed that since No Woman could ever resist Any Man, her best policy would always be "to submit." A common rationalization is that "fighting back is the worst thing you can do because it will just make him madder[1]." Situations differ, but contrary to popular fantasy and wishful thinking, police reports clearly indicate that women who fight, resist, and behave in the most unsubmissive and uncooperative manner possible are overwhelmingly likely to come out unharmed. It is the ones who are cooperative, passive, submissive, who fit an attacker's ideal fantasy victim, who allow themselves to be seen as a script, a cartoon, a fantasy scenario — something less than human — who are hurt, mutilated, murdered.

Bad Guys just love to hear this sort of advice offered; it does half their work for them. It is bad advice in daily life and it is great nonsense in Aikido where the stronger and more committed the attack the easier and more devastating the technique. In fact, the bigger the attacker the greater the advantage of the attacked.

Don't believe it? You see this daily, in highway traffic.

---

1. See page 61 for comments on what happens to ball pitchers who are angry and nervous.

Essay: Physics On and Off the Mat

A basic law of the universe with which we must harmonize is:

$$F = ma$$ **(EQ 2)**

In words this says:

Force = mass times acceleration.

As analogy to road traffic, consider:

- Small bodies/bicycles: 85 kg (~ 190 lbs)
- Medium bodies/ cars: 1400 kg (~ 3,100 lbs)
- Large bodies such as fully-loaded 18-wheelers[1]: 36,000 kg (~ 80,000 lbs)

First, linear situations. To simplify, we'll assume all of our examples are elastic collisions that will ignore friction. In these linear cases, *acceleration* (*a*) is the change in velocity divided by the *time* (*t*) of that change (the duration of the impact). Change is represented by the Greek symbol delta (Δ). So, if F = ma, then

$$F = (m\Delta_v)/(\Delta_t)$$ **(EQ 3)**

In words this is:

Force = mass times the change in velocity divided by the change in time.

If you are sitting still on your bike and are struck by an 18-wheeler going about 40 m.p.h. (18 meters per second), the truck will continue as if nothing happened but you will be hurled forward at 2 times the truck's velocity. Assuming the impact lasts about 1 millisecond, the force you would experience would be:

$$F = (85 \text{ kg}) (2^* 18 \text{ m/s}) / 0.001 \text{ second} = 3,060,000 \text{ N} = 688,500 \text{ lbs}$$ **(EQ 4)**

The truck, on the other hand, will feel almost nothing.

In some martial arts, attacks are dealt with by blocking or attacking with greater speed and force. Suppose you as small body attack the larger body linearly? if you ride your bike at 40 m.p.h. into the 18-wheeler while it is sitting still, the truck will essentially remain motionless and unmoved but you will bounce backwards at 40 m.p.h. Force on bike and rider would be:

$$F = (85 \text{ kg}) (18 \text{ m/s- (-18 m/s)0} / (0.001 \text{ s}) = 3,060,000 \text{ N} = 688,500 \text{ lbs}.$$ **(EQ 5)**

Again, the truck feels little or nothing.

What about an opponent of equal size? If you drive your car at 40 m.p.h. into a stopped car of equal size, you will come to a stop while the other car will be knocked away at 40 m.p.h. The force both cars experience will be:

---

1. An 18-wheeler flat-bed trailer may weigh 32,000 pounds fueled, unloaded. Its engine alone may weight 3,000 pounds.

$$F = (1400 \text{ kg}) (18 \text{m/s} - 0) / (0.001 \text{ sec.}) = 25,200,000 \text{ N} = 5,670,000 \text{ lbs} \quad \textbf{(EQ 6)}$$

which is even worse! Clearly, if you are smaller and dealing with oncoming linear energy, your best approach is to get off line and avoid these devastating forces entirely[1]. Otherwise, in none of these cases do you fare very well. But let's look at a circular approach. Imagine:

1. A tight circular curve on a freeway exit ramp.
2. The bicyclist zooming around the curve at 40 m.p.h. and the resulting forces.
3. The passenger car zooming around the curve at 40 m.p.h. and resulting forces.
4. The loaded 18-wheeler tractor trailer trying the same thing, and
5. *You* standing at the center of the circle turning around your center to watch these vehicles going by and the forces that operate on *your* action.

For a moving object to follow a circular path, it must exert a force towards the center of the circle (centripetal force), otherwise it will continue in a straight line and fly off that path, at a tangent to the circle. This centripetal force is defined as:

$$F = m\frac{v^2}{r} \qquad \textbf{(EQ 7)}$$

or in words,

Force = mass x velocity squared divided by the radius of the circle

Vehicles going around the curve of a tight exit ramp (with a radius of about 100 ft. or 30m) at 40 m.p.h. must exert an inward force through their wheels in order to maintain a curved path. For the small body (the bicycle) this force is:

$$F = (85 \text{ kg}) (18 \text{ m/sec}^2 / (30 \text{ m}) = 918 \text{ N} = 206 \text{ lbs} \qquad \textbf{(EQ 8)}$$

For the car:

$$F = (1,400 \text{ kg}) (18 \text{ m/sec.}^2 / (30 \text{ m}) = 15,120 \text{ N} = 3,402 \text{ lbs} \qquad \textbf{(EQ 9)}$$

For the 18-wheeler:

$$F = (36,000 \text{ kg}) (18 \text{ m/sec}^2 / (30 \text{ m}) = 388,800 \text{ N} = 87,480 \text{ lbs} \qquad \textbf{(EQ 10)}$$

The vehicle unable to exert the required force will go off the ramp[2].

Meanwhile, you stand at the center of the circular ramp, turning in order to watch the cars go around the ramp. Instead of your center of mass following a circular path as the vehicles above do, you are spinning about an axis which goes through your center of mass, so the

---

1. Similarly, if you are sitting in traffic and notice that a truck or car is coming too fast to stop in time, the best approach is *not* to slam your car into reverse, hoping to overcome its force with greater force. The best approach is to head for the shoulder, get off-line, don't be there, be safe, *ma-ai*.
2. . . . or suffer a blowout which may accomplish the same thing. Hence tough mylar racing tires on bikes and steel-belted tires on motor vehicles, designed to endure the enormous forces generated by speed and angular momentum. Another blowout known as a "herniated disk" may occur in circular throws such as Kokyu-Nage Basic if *uke* fails to step out of the throw. See page 213.

forces are computed differently. Assuming your body is roughly cylindrical, we can describe its motion with the following equation:

$$F = mr\,(\alpha/2)$$ (EQ 11)

In words, this says:

"Tangential Force = mass x radius of cylinder x angular acceleration divided by 2"

After exerting an initial force to start, you will spin at a constant rate and therefore having no change in speed, you have no angular acceleration ($\alpha=0$). Therefore you exert no force while spinning (except to overcome the friction between your feet and the ground). While the bike/car/truck must generate significant centripetal force to traverse the ramp, you only have to exert a minimal effort to spin and watch them go by.

Applying this to Aikido, *nage* stands at the center of a throw, maintaining One-Point and applying minimal forces. Meanwhile, *uke* is led into a circular path, in which significant energy must be expended to generate centripetal force to prevent flying off the road on a tangent.

—Karl Schmidt, Virginia Ki Society

And that is why a tiny 4'9" 80-pound woman can deflect, redirect, and throw a far larger, stronger partner, and how grown men were thrown by 5-year-olds and one-ounce lizards[1]. It's how a 76,000-pound 18-wheeler was thrown and pinned by a 4,000-pound Lincoln, equivalent to a 200-pound man being thrown by a puppy.

If lured into a weight and strength contest, the smaller body hasn't got a chance. (*Bambi Meets Godzilla* comes to mind[2]).

Staying offline, using the tools of leverage, rotation, and the power of the circle, the smaller body has the advantage.

That is the *physics* of Aikido.

But there is also Mind-Body Coordination.

---

1. See page 12 of this manual for 4'9" Vicky vs. the Riker's Island prison guard; see page 13 for the tale of the Aikidoist thrown and pinned by a one-ounce lizard; page 64 for the story of the 220-lb. Aikido instructor thrown by a 5-year-old girl. See page 178 of KIA for "The Trucker's Tale."
2. See Marv Newland's famous student film at www.YouTube.com/watch?v=tAVYYe87b9w.

Mind-Body Coordination

Koichi Tohei[1] offers the following four principles for mind-body coordination.

1. **Keep One Point.** A principle of mind and body that keeps a low center of physical and mental gravity and concentrates on Center and balance, rather than on muscular strength.
2. **Relax Completely.** A principle of mind, aware but calm, and a principle of body, relaxed but alert. It gives *uke* poor leverage while increasing sensitivity to his.
3. **Keep Weight Underside**. A principle of body that embraces both heaviness and floating, that is, movement from center and allowing physical bodies and actions to flow "in harmony with gravity" as a boat floats upon the water[2].
4. **Extend Ki.** A principle of the mind that extends attention, awareness, and focus, providing a goal, a purpose, a path to follow.

It is indeed possible to dissect out the individual elements but the whole point of Ki Development is "Mind-Body Coordination," or "Putting It All Together."

Like a sandwich.

Hey! you want mayo with that?

Maybe not. After all, mayonnaise is "only" eggs and oil and vinegar. But ladling raw egg and vinegar over a greased pig, a head of lettuce, and a tomato just isn't the same as the combination that make it all work together.

Visualization and other internal exercises for Mind-Body Coordination are practiced by all athletes — dancers, ball players, golfers, gymnasts, skaters — and studied intently in the new and growing discipline of Sports Psychology. Physicists who study Aikido affirm (with deep regret) that they cannot do Aikido simply by running the equations in their heads. And not even the most dedicated student of Ki Development can afford to ignore the physics. They work together.

In *Aikido for Life* Gaku Homma very reasonably "debunks" a number of physics tricks as "physics tricks," which is exactly what they are. However, later in the book Homma mentions having students roll over a piece of paper white on one side, red on the other. When the paper is laid on the mat . . .

- White side up, the students roll with no problem.
- Red side up — oops! Their minds are disturbed.

This is an excellent example of mind/body coordination (or loss of it), where visual input and mindset affect the physical outcomes, exactly the sort of thing that *ki* exercises are designed to observe and alter. If you have problems with the possibility that attention changes the equation, consider the flip side: *inattention*.

Studies by the U.S. Department of Transportation find that using cell phones in the car while driving impairs the driver to a degree equivalent to blood-alcohol levels of

---

1. Koichi Tohei was strongly influenced by his studies with Tempu Nakamura, a student of yoga. The Sanskrit *yoga* means "union," (related to the English *yoke*) and implies a union of mind and body, that of the physical and that of the spirit.
2. Compare to trying to *lift* that boat out of the water.

up to the legal limit and possibly beyond depending on the conversation. You can see a far safer demonstration of this effect, via a computer game such as *Tetris,* which like driving, requires recognition and manipulation of geometric shapes and spaces. To evaluate,

1. Play several games to establish a skill baseline.
2. Play several games while talking on the phone or to a partner.
   Do not discuss the game itself. Rather, emphasize personal matters or topics such as taxes or your favorite inflammatory political issue.
3. Observe what happens to your score; compare with baseline.

Attention and awareness translate into details and action in many ways. For example, millions of spaghetti cooks around the world believe that adding a few teaspoons of salt to a pot of water will raise the boiling temperature and cook the pasta faster or better. In fact, teaspoons or tablespoons of salt added to quarts or gallons of water *do* raise the boiling temperature but only by a few thousandths of a degree. There is no possible effect on cooking *time* unless you are measuring in microseconds. On the other hand, it may effect *taste* which is a great deal of what cooking is about.

The cook or Aikidoist who pays attention to details, who is aware of processes and who has a definite goal in mind will almost certainly turn out a better meal or a better technique than the one who merely threw it all together at random.

Goals matter, but they don't repeal physical law.

The Ki Door exercise combines *ki* with mechanics. If a door is not available, it can also be done with *uke* standing with an arm extended.

Ki Door

1. Try to push your way through a heavy door while placing your mind *behind* you.
2. Push through the door directing mind *forward*..
3. Repeat while extending, but try to push door from the *hinge* side.
4. Using the knife edge of your hand[1](not an open hand), inch back along the door towards the opening edge. Find the point where you begin to move the lever that is the door.

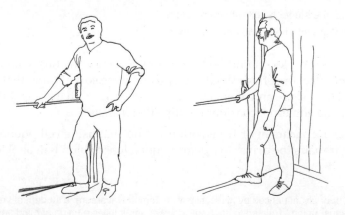

---

1. A thumb provides a point-source of force; a hand a spread of force and leverage.

Variation

The same principle of leverage above appears in *sankyo* and other wrist locks.

Grasping the knife-edge of *uke*'s hand,

1. *Nage* place thumb near ridge of left hand and turn hand.
2. Place thumb at middle of left hand and turn hand.
3. Place thumb in line with index finger of left hand.
   Which position gives most leverage?
   What happens if you think about how strong *uke* is and how impossible it will be to turn the hand?
   What happens if you rotate the hand in your mind — but with poor mechanical advantage?

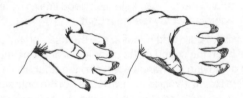

In general, we are controlled by two things: what we want and what we fear.

What is it that *uke* wants to do? Align with that. And consider what it is you fear (and why you are standing so far away).

Goals and intentions and the energy behind them are the vector quantities of spiritual orientation. And, as it is possible to align with physical energy, so it is also possible to align with the energy of life and human relationships.

Essay: On Aikido and Music

I sit before the looming black instrument struggling for composure. The notes on the page of music have turned to hieroglyphics and my fingers to stone. At the end of my performance the other piano students smile weakly and mumble false praise. My teacher tells me to work on rhythm and timing. I flee to the practice rooms, to a small cubicle with a battered old baby grand. Alone, I sit and play the music, this time flawlessly.

To succeed at making music at the piano requires the coordinated involvement of my whole being. Ears, eyes, fingers and feet (and every part they are attached to), heart, reason and soul. All the parts must work together in time, the present, past, and future seamlessly interwoven. How does one accomplish this? Without an audience the many parts of me come together and I succeed in making music. Under the pressure of judgement by my teacher and peers the parts scatter and the music fails.

A simple idea was introduced to me in college while I was struggling with performance anxiety at the piano. A friend described to me the process of "Keeping One-Point," something she had learned in Ki Aikido. She told me to put my mental attention at my physical center of balance in my lower abdomen. While I did this she pushed on me to test my balance. She could not budge me; I stood my ground against her force with no sense of physical effort.

Curiosity led me to try this mind/body exercise while playing the piano. To my amazement, I found that awareness of my One-Point helped me to not "fall apart" in front of an audience. The image of One-Point worked for me like a conductor coordinating the musicians in an orchestra; the many music-making parts of me came together to create music, overcoming the scattering effect of my anxiety.

The Musician's Mind/Body Coordination

One Point is one of the four basic principles in Ki Aikido for establishing mind/body coordination. Aikido, like music, is a series of events in time. Finding One-Point helps my timing, that is, the coordinated movement of all of the parts of my mind and body in a series of events in time, like playing Bach, hitting a golf ball, or doing an Aikido throw.

A symphony conductor leads the orchestra to play in time together by providing a beat that everyone follows. The relationship between a sense of timing, or feeling a beat, and mind/body coordination is circular. That is, I can establish good timing by finding my one point, and I can create mind/body coordination by feeling a beat.

A beat is a repeating cycle of build and release, like the rise and fall of a wave. When I clap my hands to express a beat, the sound of the clapping is only one moment in the life of the beat. The silent action of moving my hands apart and together again is as much the beat as the sound itself. Effective timing involves an awareness of the entire cycle, for the Aikidoist as well as the musician. The power of rhythm and timing in Aikido movement is in riding the wave of the beat as it builds and releases and builds and releases. See this demonstrated in the *ikkyo-undo* exercise (page 99).

And the Beat Goes On . . .

1. Mark a steady beat with your feet feeling the movement throughout your body.
2. Stop the *movement*, but continue the feeling of the beat. *Uke* test.
3. Stop the *feeling* of the beat. *Uke* test.

—Susan Chandler, Ki Society

On Zen and The Art of Motorcycles

Turn your head! Look into the turn before you turn!
No! No! Don't look down, look ahead! Mind and body follow eyes!
Look right, you'll go right. Look down, you're going down.
Relax the shoulders! Relax the arms! Breathe!
And while you're at it, smile! Have fun!

A "fruity" *ki-aikido* class?

No. A Motorcycle Safety Foundation class, where the skills, the physics, and even the instructions and imagery are uncannily similar to those heard in Aikido. Students often ignore solid physical principles because mat speeds at a beginning level cannot develop the forces that will later make the same techniques so devastating. High speed activities such as skiing, skating, or cycling make physical forces above and beyond muscular strength vividly real. You will learn to harmonize with the laws of the universe or you will face the swift and terrible retribution of the physics gods.

The Honda Goldwing is one of the largest motorcycles made. It weighs over 800 pounds empty, before fluids, rider, passenger and gear. Off its stand, it must be over its Center or supported by inertia at all times. The rider's physical strength doesn't matter. It is not possible to hold a half-ton of falling bike on one leg.

At low speeds you steer by turning handlebars in the direction you want to go. At high speeds, angular momentum of the wheel makes it difficult or nearly impossible to turn the handlebars. The bigger the bike, the more difficult this becomes and the more critical it is to use center, hips, balance, and weight shift.

For slow, tight turns, you lean only the motorcycle while keeping your own body straight and upright. For high speed turns, you lean with the motorcycle and "countersteer," pressing the wheel *right* in order to turn *left*. Countersteering makes no more sense to the beginning motorcyclist than does the idea that the most effective way to throw *uke* "down" is to first send him "up." But both are excellent physics.

Eye Direction

Eyes reveal conditions. They can also create conditions.

Most Westerners can't believe that eye direction (*me-tusuke*) could matter. Japanese consider it to be critical. To see the difference, experiment with eye direction on skates. If you try doing it wrong on a motorcycle under the watchful eye of an MSF instructor, you will hear about it. The standard instruction for turning on a motorcycle is:

Look right, go right. Mind and body follow eyes.

In MSF classes, points are deducted for not looking into the turn, or for looking down at a stop when eyes should be on the horizon, on the path of travel, on the goal. On rolling in class, focusing on the mat may take you directly into the mat. Instead try looking at your belt, your knee, your back leg, or where you want to go in these and other techniques. Running a slalom? Look at the goal, never at the cones.

- To do a U-turn in a MSF class, look at your own tail-light and turn. Similarly,
- To do a *tenkan*, look at *uke*'s tail light or look around your circle of travel and turn.
- Try doing the opposite and compare the results.

Falls

Motorcycling requires serious protection against falls. In Aikido, if you're having trouble learning to roll or are suffering from a bruised shoulder, try rolling in a motorcycle jacket. Shoulders, elbows, and back are protected with material that ranges from "padding" to outright "body armor." What keeps you safe on the highway will also keep you safe at mat speeds. You can feel the spots where you are not round enough, and will avoid bruises, bangs, headaches and separated shoulders. Padding can ease you into proper position and keep you safe until you are ready to roll unassisted.[1]

Off the mat and on the road, a standard recommendation for *ukemi* from a high speed motorcycle throw is essentially a breakfall —maximum surface area in contact with road surface, maximum braking due to friction, minimum amount of time spent travelling. In theory, you won't control a roll at 60 m.p.h. and the more time you spend rolling the more time you have to hit some other obstacle such as a tree, post or guardrail at high speed[2]. "In theory," says MSF Instructor John Garner, "but I disagree."

"Taking a breakfall at 60 m.p.h. with extended limbs (to maximize surface area) risks snagging said limbs on a pole or a tree; they may not continue on with the rest of you. I would roll. But, in fact, you should never be taking a fall that fast. If you're falling at 60 m.p.h. then you haven't already slowed and prepared, which means something has already gone terribly wrong. That something is usually *awareness*."

In *Aikido and the Dynamic Sphere*, the process of awareness applied to self defense is broken down into the following distinct steps:

Perception, Evaluation-Decision, and Reaction

MSF uses a similar approach:

Scan, Identify, Predict, Decide, Execute

Experienced Rider classes combine the steps to get:

Search, Predict, Act.

These are step-by-step strategies for awareness and action that can be used in Aikido techniques, whether you are on the mat or on the road.

---

1. No need to buy a motorcycle jacket just to practice Aikido; pads are sold separately. Pads are also available in skate supply stores. These can be secured to you or your uniform until you can fly and fall safely on your own.
2. Bicyclists can reach highway speeds, but do not dress to survive high-speed breakfalls. Racers are taught to "lay down" their bikes as soon as the fall starts and slide out of an accident rather than hurtling over the handlebars. The theory is that you lose some skin, but don't break anything.

ᴀikido Class

Aikido exercises are designed to enhance flexibility and coordination while patterning the basic motions of Aikido.

Warming and Limbering

A supple, flexible body is as much a part of self-confidence, safety, and self-defense as are throws. It is easier to throw (or to injure) a stiff body than a flexible one. A flexible body can move and adjust in ways that an attacker may not anticipate or control. It is the difference between trying to throw a rope and trying to throw a broomstick.

Drop the hand of a flexible partner to the mat and there may be little effect since that hand can go there very comfortably; another vector must be added in order to shift *uke*'s Center. Tight muscles present a very different situation. If *uke* cannot bend down, his own inflexibility forces his Center forward of his feet. *Uke* essentially throws himself[1] and might even tear something in the process. In daily life, inability to turn the head enough to check for oncoming traffic is a life-threatening situation.

Flexible muscles are also *stronger* than tight ones. Because muscle power is generated by contraction over the length of available contractible muscle, muscles are weak when they are already shortened due to lack of use, stress, or disease.

Shortened muscles can also be extremely painful, producing problems from knee pain and headaches to the tingling and weakness of nerve entrapment, including such symptoms as dizziness while rolling[2].

Stretch for flexibility, strength and good health but do it properly. Stretching is *not* a warm up. Stretching cold, stiff bodies (especially when combined with extreme bouncing and overstretching) strains muscles, ligaments, and tendons. The resulting "flexibility" is more accurately known as "joint instability." It sets the stage for chronic injury.

First activate and warm the muscles, *then* stretch.

---

1. For a demonstration, see "The Ma-ai of Balance and Flexibility" on page 189.
2. Sufferers, especially if over 21, are usually told they have "arthritis." In healthy individuals, true arthritis is far less common than commonly believed; tight muscles leading to pain and dysfunction are very common and largely avoidable. See www.round-earth.com/Myo-diagnoses.html

Large muscles of the legs are often the main target of stretching exercises but should always be worked and warmed *before stretching*. What happens if you try to stretch a frozen rubber band? Current research shows that for real gains in flexibility and injury reduction, serious stretching is best done *after* a workout.

The Three-Minute Ki Exercise for Health and the *hitori-waza / aiki-taiso* pattern Aikido skills and provide an excellent general warm-up[1] but there's more. They help rewire the brain's motor cortex by introducing new motor skills including the challenge of balance and controlled dizziness[2].

1. *Three-Minute Exercise for Health, page 87.*
2. *Tekubi-Kosa Undo* ("Wrist-Crossing Exercise") page 88.
3. *Funekogi-Undo* ("Boat-Rowing Exercise") page 90.
4. *Udemawashi-Undo* ("Arm-Dropping Exercise") page 91.
5. *Udefuri-Undo* ("Arm-Swinging Exercise") page 92 and
6. *Udefuri-Choyaku Undo* ("Arm-Swinging-Spinning Exercise") page 92.
7. *Sayu-Undo* ("Right-Left Exercise") page 94.
8. *Tenkan-Undo* ("Turning Exercise") page 95.
9. *Ushiro-Tori Undo* ("Rear-Attack Exercise") page 96.
10. *Ushiro Tekubi-Tori-Undo* ("Rear Wrist-Attack Exercise") page 97.
11. Ushiro Koshin-Zanshin ("Rear-Front-and-Back Exercise") page 98.
12. *Ikkyo-Undo* ("First Teaching Exercise") page 99; and Spinning Ikkyo-Undo, page 100.
13. *Zengo-Undo*, page 101 and *Happo-Undo ("Eight-Way Exercise") page 102.*
14. Wrist exercises, page 105.
15. Leg stretching exercises (beginning page 109) perhaps with supplemental stretches as desired, at end of this chapter.

---

1. Another excellent option is yoga's classic morning warmup, Salutation to the Sun.
2. They are remarkably similar to Cawthorne-Cooksey exercises, introduced in the 1940's for patients with vestibular problems, secondary to head injuries. The intent was to *provoke dizziness in a controlled manner*. The rationale was based on the observation that active patients recovered— rather than drifting into chronic invalidism (Herdman, S. J., 2000).

The Three-Minute Ki Exercise for Health

Ki Society classes often begin with this three-minute exercise of paired movements repeated four times. Emphasize gentle stretch rather than compression. For example, in tilting the head back, think of stretching the front of the neck rather than forcing the back of your head into your shoulders.

The exercise is counted in sets of 2 of 8 counts each.

The count comes before the motion.[1]

1. Lateral Arm Swinging (*udefuri-undo*)
2. Bending Side to Side
3. Bending Forward and Backward
4. Shoulder-Blade Exercise
5. Tilting Head From Side-to-Side
6. Tilting Head Front to Back
7. Looking From Side To Side
8. Knee Bends And Heel Raises
9. Knee/Hamstring Stretch
10. Arm-Dropping (*ude-mawashi undo*)
11. Dropping Both Arms
12. Dropping Both Arms While Dropping Center/One-Point.
13. Wrist-Shaking Exercise (*Tekubi-Shindo*)

Variations

- *Uke* test after doing the exercise once (for example, one arm swing rather than two). Repeat doing the exercise twice and compare stability.

  Baseball coach John Pinkman does the same, but why sets of two?

  For batting warmups, rather than mindless or random motions, Pinkman teaches players to clear the mind and focus on the ball through pre-programmed *ki* exercises.

  "We assume batting position, and visit this place twice to clue-in the body. Going there once is not enough for the body to understand what the mind wants the body to do. The mind does not already know. We have to send it a verification message. This is done by repeating the desired movement."

- Do the exercise while walking around the mat. If you do not return head (and eyes) to center you will become badly disoriented.

- Do the exercise in a motorcycle helmet. Does this change your posture and balance?

  Far-fetched? Consider traditional armor, helms, and other weighty military equipment. The heavier the load the more critical that it be supported by bones, not muscles, and the more important good posture becomes, as in the classically erect military bearing.

---

1. For Pinkman's use of *ki* development exercises in pitching and hitting, see page 61. For detailed instructions and count for the Three-Minute Ki Exercise, see KIA page 97. Instructions include a list of muscles involved in the individual movements.

Hitori Waza and Other Exercises

Hitori Waza is the term Koichi Tohei *Sensei* uses to encompass the body of exercises he teaches which are precursors to practicing technique. *Funekogi-Undo, Ikkyo-Undo,* and *Happo-Undo* are all classic exercises of Aikido, building blocks of good technique.

—George Simcox

The following exercises are known as *hitori-waza* in the Ki Society, *aiki-taiso* in other organizations. They are basic exercises of coordination, the fundamentals of Aikido.

Tekubi-Kosa Undo

ADS: Basic Exercise # 11, 12 ("Wrist-Crossing Exercise"), pp. 131-132; ZC p. 237.

Baffling and pointless to new eyes, *tekubi-kosa undo* is practice in relaxation while maintaining balance and proper alignment. It is also the precursor to many throws such as different versions of *kote-gaeshi*, wrist grabs and locks. Done from a rear grab it becomes *ushiro-tekubi-tori-undo* (page 97).

With feet shoulder-width apart and arms relaxed at sides,

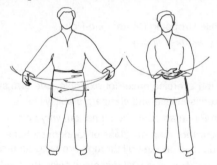

Mid-level (Joho)

1. Leading from fingertips, swing arms up to waist height, crossing wrists.
2. Drop arms to sides.
3. Repeat. Continue into . . .

Upper-Level (Koho)

The tendency is to tilt back from the waist as the arms swing up. Lead from fingertips, swing arms up to just below eye level and drop down as above. The challenge is to emphasize relaxation of the arms, a natural swing, and proper posture. To test this,

1. Instructor calls "Stop!" at some point and directs class to:
2. Raise the left foot (balancing on right).
3. Raise the right foot (balancing on left).
4. Observe any changes in your stability when you:

- Concentrate on your hands.
- Concentrate on your foot.
- Concentrate on Center/One-Point.
- Imagine holding onto a rope from the ceiling, a pole extending up through your body, or having your Center at mat level so just your eyes are above the mat.

Tekubi-kosa undo is actually the exercise or the motion which we are trying to recreate when we tell new students faced with a wrist grab, to "look at your fingernails," or "adjust your glasses," or "scratch your nose." These familiar activities reproduce the motion while eliminating the mindblock that it can't be done merely because there's an attacker holding the wrist. The following exercise is a spectacular demonstration of the motion and the mindset. In groups of four,

1. Two partners hold *nage's* wrists.
2. Third partner tosses a ball or bean bag to *nage*. Despite being held by the wrists, *nage will* catch it, not by struggling free of the restraining hands, but by focusing on catching the bean bag, an act even less self-conscious and more compelling than itches or glasses.

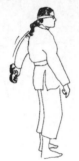
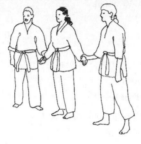

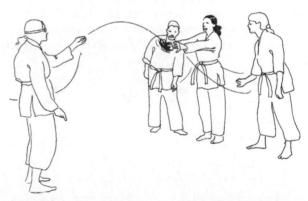

The classic martial arts exhortation, "Don't think, DO!" doesn't mean to be a mindless moron or a loose cannon. It means to catch the ball, rather than standing there thinking of all the reasons it can't be done. Turn off the analytical mind; let the automatic body skills take over. The first approach accomplishes great things. The second is like driving through life with your parking brake on. A fine example appears in the animated film *Kung-Fu Panda*. Panda Po desperately wants to study *kung-fu*, but appears hopelessly inept at learning the art. The situation changes radically when Po's attention is fixed on buns or cookies.

Funekogi-Undo

ADS: Basic Exercise #4 ("Boat-Rowing Exercise"), pp. 123-124; KDL pp. 56-57; ZC pp. 230-232.

Funekogi-undo is the workhorse of Aikido. A committed, energetic attack is a gift of motion and energy. The more aggressive the attacker, the less work for *nage* who need only transform and redirect. But how do you deal with the static attacker who offers no energy or motion to play with? *Funekogi* gets *uke* moving with the power of hips and legs; and, once started, almost any motion can be transformed. The pattern is:

Hips-hands — Hips-hands

Arms do not pull with muscular strength. They serve as connectors, like ropes, between the load and the hips and legs.

From left *hanmi*, with hips square, hands at waist, elbows down, knees bent,

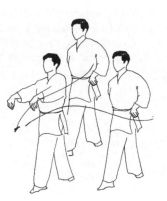

1. Shift hips forward thrusting out arms as if pushing an oar.
2. Shift hips back, drawing arms back to waist.

To test stability, *uke* may:

- Attempt to lift hands, or push up along axis of arm,
- Push straight back from shoulders.
- Push forward from hips or small of back.
- Hips remain at about the same height, which can be checked with two partners holding a *jo*.

Variations

1. *Uke* holds *nage*'s wrists as strongly as possible.
2. *Nage* attempts to move *uke* by pulling with arms or
3. Relaxing arms and moving hips with *funekogi-undo*.

    Observe the effect on *uke* regardless of his size and strength.

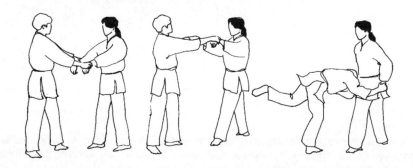

Another version of *funekogi* appears in *Ryote-tori kokyu-nage zempo-nage*, a variant of *Ryote-mochi kokyu-nage zempo-nage tenkan* on page 223.

1. Leaving wrists in place, *nage* step as far to the rear as possible on the left foot, taking up slack, then
2. Turn *tenkan* to *uke*'s left side taking *uke* off balance.
   Notice that the most powerful hold can be set up for a flying *zempo-nage*.

The actual "boat rowing" exercise can be seen in the opening scenes of Bruce Lee's *Enter the Dragon* as a young girl sculls across Tokyo harbor. Even without a traditional oriental boat, you can experience a similar feeling with Western oars or a rowing machine and more.

Apply *funekogi-undo* to mowing the lawn, or repeatedly opening heavy filing cabinet drawers to get the feeling of the back-and-forth motion of hips and legs, connecting with (rather than pulling with) the arms.

Udemawashi-Undo

"Arm-Dropping Exercise"

An exercise in raising the arm and then dropping it in alignment with gravity, using relaxation, mass and acceleration in the most effective way possible. This simple movement is the basis of many Aikido throws. It produces the "up" that makes an effective "down" in techniques such as *kokyu-nage* and *ikkyo*.

With feet shoulder-width apart (*shizentai* stance), *nage* will:

1. Raise arm to the highest point possible without straightening, stiffening or locking the elbow.
2. Allow the arm to drop, of its own weight, to the lowest point.
3. *Uke* test by attempting to lift straight up on the arm.

The same technique of dropping with gravity underlies sword techniques and other tools from hammers to hoes ("Gardens" on page 251). These fall of their own weight. They are not forced up or down. To do so is tiring and inefficient.

Variations

- Drop hand directly down as if the hand were sliding hand down a vertical staff.
- Working alone, raise and drop arm with a weight. After enough repetitions to tire the muscle, what is the most efficient way to raise the arm?
- In pairs, *nage* drops hand on *uke*'s outstretched wrist. (Drop arm only; do not push or attempt to muscle or force *uke*'s arm out of the way.)
  Compare *uke*'s resulting "down" to the degree of *nage*'s starting "up."
- As combination, if you drop arm while stepping to side and add an *udefuri-choyaku* (spin) in the middle you have *Kokyu-Nage Basic*.

Udefuri-Undo

ADS: Basic Exercise #15 ("Arm Swinging Exercise"), pp. 134-136; ZC: pp. 239-240.

In class, *udefuri-undo* is usually continuous with *udefuri-choyaku-undo* (below).

Nage stands with feet shoulder-width apart, with head, eyes, and chest straight ahead. *Uke* calls the count. Count is 1-2, 1-2, 1-2, 1-2 . . . until *uke* or instructor signals the end of the series by calling a 3-4. Notice that the torso does not turn until the final Step 4.

1. On "One," swing arms to the left, wrapping around body.
2. On "Two," swing arms to the right, wrapping around body.
3. On "Three," swing arms to left as on "One."
4. On "Four," swing arms right as you step forward with left foot.

   Uke may test for stability at this point, or *nage* may continue into *Udefuri Choyaku Undo* on count of "One."

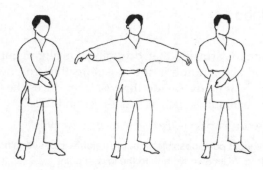

Udefuri-Choyaku Undo

ADS: Basic Exercise # 15 ("Spinning Exercise") pp. 135,136.

Remember spinning like a top when you were a child? This is the same.

This exercise develops balance, Center/One-Point, and relaxation. Keep foot motion as natural as possible, not leaping but stepping and turning naturally and comfortably. To end the motion, relax or drop into it, so there is no wobble or stumble at the end. Movement begins from the Center/One-Point, although rapid changes in direction can start from the little finger which acts like a small starter motor. Arms are not held out, they spin out due to centrifugal force; they should be so relaxed that you can feel tingling in the fingers. Extend *ki*, that is, have a goal. Pick points on two walls to serve as reference points. Continue from Step 4 of "Arm Swinging Exercise."

With arms wrapped to R side of body, LF forward,

1. Rotate hips 180 degrees to L. Arms spin out (they are not forced out) rising to shoulder height, then wrapping to L side of body. Draw lead foot back to close up stance into *hanmi*.
2. Reverse direction returning to original position with arms wrapped to R side of body. Draw leading foot back to close up stance into *hanmi*.

   The count is "1-2, 1-2, 1-2, 1-2 . . ." until the end of the series is signaled by "3-4."

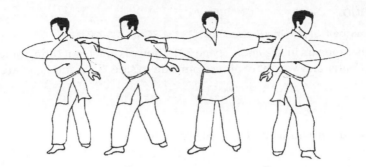

Variations

- Two spins.
- Three or more spins.

You may think this a frivilous exercise with no real value except perhaps "practice in accustoming oneself to functioning while dizzy." In fact, it teaches coordination, focus, relaxation, and good posture all in one — no small feat.

When ended with an *ude-mawashi* (page 91), it becomes *Kokyu-Nage Basic* (page 213), *Shomen-uchi ikkyo tenkan* (page 219) and many other "real throwing techniques."

It is also very "real" on its own.

When I first started practicing the martial arts (in January 1951 in Ashiya, Kyushu, Japan) I was told to practice a certain exercise called Udefuri-Choyaku Undo, explained as a defense against a tackle. For days, we practiced this one exercise for two or more hours at a time. After four days of this, I thought "Why am I here? I am not learning anything practicing just one exercise." When I returned to class on Friday, I resolved that if the teacher had me practice it again, I would quit. Fortunately he did not, until the last 15 minutes of class, when he had me doing the same old exercise. "Well," I thought, "I can do it, it's the end of the class."

The next evening I was standing in the barracks talking to several people when one of them yelled a warning. I turned around just in time to see a guy come screaming toward me in the tackle position. I turned automatically and the guy went flying. A couple of people held him down and one went to call the medics — he'd probably been drinking and flipped out. Later, one of the guys asked me how I threw him. I didn't know, I did not realize what I had done or how I had done it. I just made a move and . . .

Then the mental light came on. Practice, practice, practice. That is what it's all about. Through practice I did a throwing technique without even thinking about it. Actually it wasn't even a technique. It was "just an exercise."

—William Thorndike, Jr.

Sayu-Undo

ADS: Basic Exercise #13 ("Left-Right Exercise"), pp. 132-134; ZC: pp. 238-239.

This exercise appears in *ude-oroshi* (page 221). Body is erect, not tilting or leaning but dropping Center and weight of arms from side to side. Eyes and head are forward.

Static

With feet shoulder width apart, at center position,

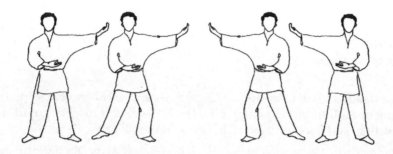

1. Swing left arm up to shoulder height and right arm to approximately waist height.
2. Bending left knee, shift to left side. Weight is underside, left arm settles with weight underside and right hand is at Center/One-Point.
3. Shift weight to center position as arms rise up to the right to a comfortable point.
4. Bending right knee, shift to right side, drop weight underside. Right arm settles with weight underside and left hand is at Center/One-Point.

In motion,

1. To move to left, cross outside (right) foot behind leading (left) foot while swinging arms up and to the left side.
2. Drop arms and Center/One-Point with weight underside, settling onto left foot.
3. To move to right, cross outside (left) foot behind leading (right) foot while swinging arms up and to the right side.

Uke may test either version of *sayu-undo* by:

- Testing for Unbendable Arm.
- Pushing on the shoulder from the side, eyes front vs. eyes forward.
- Attempting to lift up on the lower hand.
- Attempting to lift up on either leg.

Tenkan-Undo

ADS: Basic Exercise #10 ("Turning Exercise"), pp. 130-131; KIA: pp. 140-149; TOT: Tai no henko ichi/ni , pp. 36-39; ZC: pp. 235-236.

A *tenkan* is a "turning," a simple maneuver that is one of the most powerful and moves in Aikido. Its purpose and its power is to transform and redirect a blast of fast, incoming linear energy into circular motion. *Nage* stands safe at the center, turning calmly within the eye of the hurricane.

In left *hanmi* (left foot and left hand forward)

1. Extend left hand, palm down.
2. Curl fingers back towards palm, then step or slide forward with the left foot, pivoting 180 degrees. Draw the left foot back as necessary. Left foot is still forward and right foot back (still in left *hanmi* although direction is reversed).
3. Extend right hand, palm down then step or slide forward with the right foot, pivoting 180 degrees to original direction. Draw the left foot back as necessary.

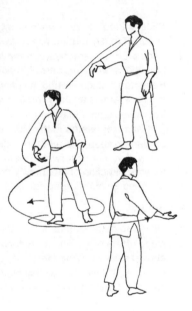

Note that Yoshinkan style does this very differently[1] swinging the leg back directly from the hip and turning 95 degrees rather than 180. Why 95?

Yoshinkan considers 95 degrees to be the smallest angle necessary to unbalance an opponent.

Variations

Once the motion is learned, *uke* can practice by:

- Pivoting around his own extended hand (alternating right and left hands) or around a staff.
- Turning in place.
- Turning every few steps while walking.
- Turn *tenkan* with a teacup of water. You may find it surprisingly stable.

  -What are the motions that keep it from splashing?

  -What are the motions that cause difficulties?

  -Compare with those required to turn *tenkan* with a balloon; with a ball and *lacrosse* stick.

---

1. See Gozo Shioda's *Total Aikido* for details of the Yoshinkan turn.

Ushiro-Tori Undo

ADS: Basic Exercise #16 ("Rear-Attack Exercise") pp. 136-137; ZC: pp. 241-242.

This exercise deals with rear attacks, specifically bear hugs and grabs to the shoulders. Facing forward in left *hanmi*,

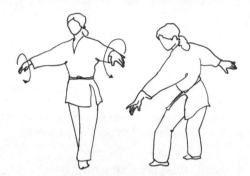

1. Slide left foot forward while swinging arms up in semi-circle leading with little fingers and simultaneously turning wrists inward, thumbs down.
2. Sliding LF further forward, bend left knee. Rotating hips, swing forward (L) arm to right until pointing forward, rear arm (R) pointing back.

    Back arm swings around in line with the front arm. When done as a throw from a bearhug, the back arm is actually the throwing arm; *uke* slides off the front arm.

    You will extend and bend forward from and in alignment with the extension of the back leg. The attacker rotates to the side, then slides forward and off.

    Be sure to keep hips and torso aligned with the plane of the throw. If you bend forward (that is, at an angle to the forward direction of the throw), your own hips will keep *uke* attached by blocking his forward movement.

Variation

1. *Uke* grab *nage* around shoulders.
2. *Nage* rotate wrists and arms forward (as in the exercise above) and walks forward.

    Uke will be drawn irresistibly along. By attacking *nage*, *uke* has sacrificed his own One-Point.

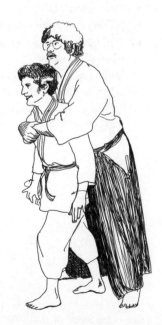

Ushiro Tekubi-Tori-Undo

ADS: Basic Exercise #17 ("Rear Wrist-Attack Exercise"), pp. 137-138; ZC: pp. 242-243.

Here the turning wrist motion of original *tekubi-kosa-tori* exercise appears again modeling a "wrist grab from behind" and the technique for dealing with it. Step 1 below also appears in *zempo* techniques.

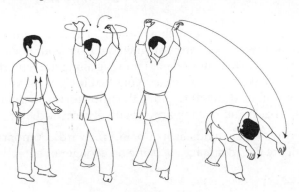

1. Step forward with left foot while curving fingertips inward, directing hands toward Center.
2. Swing arms up to forehead level and turn fingers palm down. (The image many people mention is that of a Praying Mantis.)
3. Bend body and drop arms tracing a large circle to ground over bent left knee.
4. Step forward with right foot as in Step 1.
5. Bend body and drop arms over bent right knee as in Step 2. With a partner, this will become a forward throw (*zenpo*).

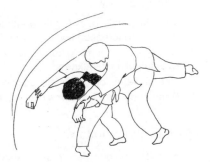

Variations

Uke may test as follows:

- Lifting up on *nage*'s wrists to see if shoulders rise or balance can be broken.
- Testing for Unbendable Arm.
- Pushing down on wrists when they are raised (a version of Unbendable Arm).
- Pushing forward from small of back.

  The "stooping" test prepares for and teaches stability in the final motion of this exercise and its *zanshin* version.

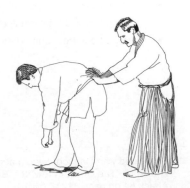

The following demonstration shows the power of this simple movement.

In pairs, with *uke* holding *nage*'s wrists from behind and pressing down firmly, *nage* compare the effort required in attempting to:

- Raise arms by bringing them out to the sides and up, or . . .
- Raise arms by doing the exercise (bringing fingers up center).

Some styles put heavy emphasis on "elbow power." The basic principle is that you are mechanically weaker when your arms are held out from your body. You are stronger when they are brought in to your Center or moving along the centerline of your body. The above exercise makes this very clear. Note that if *uke* pulls your arms back well past your hips, it will be difficult to move the arms forward. Therefore, step back, moving your hips back, and making arms relatively forward.

In the actual throw, *nage* extends arms up and forward. Compare with dropping elbows and compare the advantages of being on a longer or shorter end of the literal lever arm.

Ushiro Koshin-Zanshin

ADS: Basic Exercise #18 ("Backwards with Immovable-Mind Exercise") p. 138.

This exercise is essentially the same as *ushiro tekubi-tori undo* except that it involves stepping backward (*zan-shin*).[1] It deals with a two-handed grab from the front with incoming energy.

1. Step diagonally back (off-line) with left foot while curving fingertips forward and up. Swing arms up to forehead level and turn fingers palm down.
2. Sweep right foot back, bend body from center, and drop arms tracing a large circle to ground over kneeling right knee.
3. Repeat, stepping diagonally back with right foot as in Step 1.
4. Bend body and drop arms over kneeling left knee as in Step 2.

Uke may test as follows:

- Lifting up on wrists to see if shoulders rise or balance can be broken.
- Testing for Unbendable Arm.
- Pushing down on wrists when raised (a version of Unbendable Arm).
- Pushing forward from small of back during Step 1 or Step 2.
- Pushing back from shoulders during Step 1 or Step 2.

---

1. Combined with *funekogi-undo* (page 90) to set a static *uke* in motion, it makes up the technique known as "The Ghost Throw" (or "Swan Lake" in Ki Society *taigi*). See Projection #24 against Attack #4 on page 312 of ADS.

Ikkyo-Undo

ADS: Basic Exercise #5 ("First-Teaching Exercise"), p. 125; ZC: pp. 232-233

Ikkyo-undo is the high-flying reverse of *funekogi-undo*. It appears to be a block and in part it is, but it is more a means of aligning with *uke*'s energy, sensing and matching speed and direction of an incoming strike while rendering it harmless. In contrast to *funekogi-undo*, the Ki Society pattern for *ikkyo* is:

Hips-hands Hands-hips

Imagine that your thumbs are switches that allow your hips to move.

This is the exercise that brought me into Aikido from Karate. We were taught to directly block the most ferocious overhead blows with forearms and so spent years with sore, injured arms. "Isn't there a better way?" we always asked. Yes. Here it is.

With *nage* in *hanmi*,

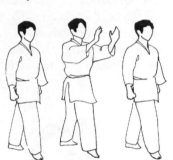

1. Hips shift forward.
2. Arms swing forward and up, fingers extended, stopping at forehead level.
3. Hips shift back.
4. Arms drop to sides, hands softly closed.
   Uke can test, with *nage* static or in motion by:
   - Pushing forward from the small of the back.
   - Pushing into and perpendicular to the chest.
   - Testing for Unbendable Arm (with *nage* standing still).
   - Feeling for tension in shoulders and upper back.

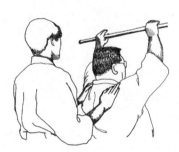

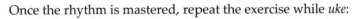

Once the rhythm is mastered, repeat the exercise while *uke*:

- Strikes *shomen-uchi* (see page 172) with hand.
- Strikes *shomen-uchi* with a plastic bat.

A plastic toy baseball bat is equivalent to the traditional bundle of split bamboo. It's noisy when *ikkyo* is incorrect, but causes no harm (and no splinters) and *ikkyo* improves like magic. Don't just go through the motions; with sensitivity to *nage*'s experience and skill, actually try to hit *nage* in the head with a correct *shomen-uchi*.

Rhythm and Timing

Musician Susan Chandler[1] uses this exercise to teach the rhythm and timing of *ikkyo*. Doing the *ikkyo-undo* as above,

1. Have *uke* count one/two with your movement; *one* at the top of the upward swing, and *two* when your arms rest again at your sides.
2. *Nage* focus attention at the moment of the count in the *ikkyo-undo* movement. *Uke* tests by:
   - Placing a hand in front of *nage*'s arm before it swings up and trying to stop its movement.
   - Placing a hand under *nage*'s arm after it has reached the top of the swing and trying to stop the arm from moving downward.
3. *Nage* repeat the exercise, this time focusing in between the counts on the movement of arms in time, not just on their point of arrival. *Uke* test as above.

Ikkyo and Attitude

Like so many things, *ikkyo* responds to internal attitude. When doing *ikkyo* in response to a strike, there is an initial tendency towards the "Oh No!" response. Arms do not swing up, they push up. They do not reach out to greet the attack, they fend off, a far less effective approach. Repeat the above while *nage* says or thinks the following. Which produces a more effective *ikkyo*?

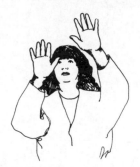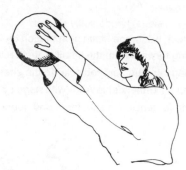

- "Oh no!" or "Oh-oh!" or
- "Stay away!" or
- "No no no!" versus "Yes yes yes!" or
- "Hi there!" or "Thank you!"

   The above shows the effect of internal orientation. Reaching out to catch a ball also produces proper configuration of hands and arms.

Spinning Ikkyo Undo

This motion appears in many throws.

1. Do *ikkyo* exercise as above but on raising arms,
2. Spin 180 degrees.
3. Drop arms.

   Practice on a mat seam or between two markers to ensure complete 180 degree turns.

---

1. For commentary, see "Essay: On Aikido and Music" on page 81.

Zengo-Undo

ADS: Basic Exercise #7 ("Forward-Backwards Exercise"), p. 126.

Zengo-undo involves a series of turns, reversing direction[1]. When applied to Aikido techniques, it models a response to attacks from two or more attackers coming from opposite directions. Internally, it models the demands of two different jobs or chores that threaten to divide time and attention.

Turn completely, directing *ki*, mind, and attention, strongly forward while remaining balanced and centered. Pattern as in *ikkyo* is:

Hips-hands-Hands-hips

As in *ikkyo-undo* it is as if the thumbs are the switch that "give the hips permission" to shift. In left *hanmi*, hands lightly closed and arms hanging naturally at sides,

1. At count of "One," shift hips forward, then swing arms up, open hands, extend fingers.
2. At count of "Two," drop arms back down to sides, closing hands softly; shift hips back. On balls of feet, pivot 180 degrees as weight shifts toward back foot.
3. At count of "Three," repeat Step 1, shifting hips forward, then swing arms up, opening hands and extending fingers.
4. At count of "Four," repeat Step 2, swinging arms back down to sides, closing hands into soft fists; shift hips back. On balls of feet, pivot 180 degrees.

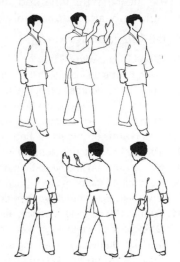

Variations

Uke count aloud, calling "Stop!" at any point.

To test,

- Push straight back on chest.
- Push straight forward at upper or lower back.
- Check for Unbendable Arm.
- Attempt to lift *nage* from ankle.

---

1. See *Shall We Dance?* on page 263 for how a dance instructor might teach it.

Happo-Undo

ADS: Basic Exercise #9 ("Eight-Directions Exercise"), pp. 127-130; ZC: pp. 234-235.

Happo-undo is *ikkyo-undo* (page 99) or *zengo-undo* (page 101) done with a series of turns to model multiple attacks from "eight" different directions.

On the compass:	In a room:
1. North-South,	1. Front-back,
2. East-West,	2. L side-R side,
3. Southwest-Northeast,	3. Corner, corner,
4. Northwest-Southeast.	4. Corner, corner.

Footwork is always: LR-LR-LR-LR or RL-RL-RL-RL

As in *zengo-undo*, the point is to turn completely, to direct *ki*, mind, and attention strongly forward while remaining balanced and centered. The temptation is to leave your mind behind, to split your attention, to be overcome by second thoughts, regrets, the accumulated weaknesses of small failures. Continuing through a series of turns, *nage* may become increasingly unstable and fall backwards in response to a soft test to the chest, having left mind and balance behind. Start with *four* directions, continue to eight only after comfortable with the first four.

In left *hanmi* (LF forward),

1. Step forward with LF.
2. Swing arms up into *ikkyo* then down.
3. Turn R 180 degrees stepping into R *hanmi* (RF forward).
4. Swing arms up into *ikkyo* then down.
5. Turn left 90 degrees stepping into L *hanmi* (LF forward).
6. Swing arms up into *ikkyo* then down.
7. Turn R 180 degrees stepping into R *hanmi* (RF forward).
8. Swing arms up into *ikkyo* then down.
9. Turn left 45 degrees stepping into L *hanmi* (LF forward).
   Swing arms up into *ikkyo* then down.
10. Turn R 180 degrees stepping into R *hanmi* (RF forward).
    Swing arms up into *ikkyo* then down.
11. Turn left 90 degrees stepping into L *hanmi* (LF forward).
    Swing arms up into *ikkyo* then down.
12. Turn R 180 degrees stepping into R *hanmi* (RF forward).
    Swing arms up into *ikkyo*; hold position. *Uke* test.

Variations

Step through the exercise as follows:

- Feet only, to establish direction and rhythm. When comfortable with these,
- Add the hands. When feet and arms are working together,
- Start on the R foot (rather than the left).
- Start in odd directions to eliminate dependence on specific visual cues.
- Place a mark on the mat before beginning. Finish at that same spot.
- Repeat above with eyes closed.

Shikkyo

ADS: pp. 324-325; TOT: pp. 46-47; BA p. 26.

> Am I the only one who thinks a matfull of students in hakama doing *shikko* looks like a
> bunch of drunken penguins trying to learn ballroom dancing?
>
> —K.S.

Shikko allows movement from a kneeling position. Aikido techniques done kneeling
are known as *suwari-waza* and require a more vivid awareness of balance, position,
and energy than the same techniques done standing.[1]

Shikko is confusing to beginners because it is referred to as "knee-walking." But it isn't
done by walking or *sliding* knees forward (knee-skiies) but by *pivoting* side-to-side on
alternating knees as a triangle. In the diagram below, the heavy line represents the
front body side of the triangle formed by two knees and feet behind.

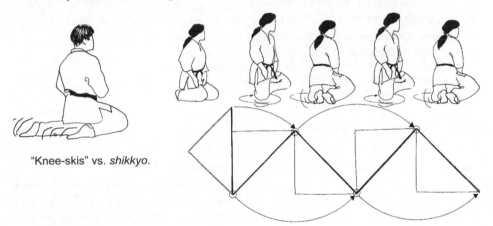

"Knee-skis" vs. *shikkyo*.

The side-to-side motion is very similar to that used in moving a chair by rotating it
around its legs (page 104). In *shikko*, knees create two points of the triangle base, toes
the third. Stay up on toes ("live toes") keeping *heels together* at all times.

Keep weight over shins and toes as much as possible, rather than knees. Avoid leaning
forward to avoid ramming your knees into the floor. From *seiza*,

1. Rise to L knee and bring RF forward.
2. Swing heel of LF to meet heel of RF.
3. Drop R knee to the floor.
4. Pivot on R knee, bringing LF forward.
5. Swing heel of RF to meet heel of LF.
6. Drop L knee to floor.
7. Swing heel of LF to meet heel of RF

---

1. *O-Sensei* scolded students for doing the techniques standing; techniques done kneeling (*suwari-waza*) are more difficult. Similarly, Yoshinkan Aikido with its emphasis on precise angles specifies 95 degrees for a *tenkan* turn because that is considered to be the minimum angle required to break balance. Training in what is more difficult will make easier approaches even easier.

Variations

See the difference "live toes" makes in maneuverability and balance. The two positions differ greatly in weight shift.

1. *Nage* assume a half-kneeling position with top of foot on mat.
2. *Uke* test by pressing directly forward at small of *uke*'s back.
3. *Nage* assume the same position but up on toes.
4. *Uke* test as above. Compare results.
   - Walk a chair across the room. How do you move it forward, backward, in a circle?
   - Many students think of the joined heels as "tied together by a bungee cord."

     Get a bungee cord and give it a try.
   - Do all throws on any test from *suwari-waza*.
   - Low shelves at the bookstore? Try shikkyo down the aisle.
   - *Shiatsu* practitioners work on floors, not on tables. Hands remain on the client at all times, in one continuous motion from start to finish, to eliminate the stress of anticipation or uncertainty for the patient. The means of moving about? *Shikko*. Experiment with moving around and over a prone partner.

While *shikkyo* is a critical skill for *suwari-waza* techniques, the hard fact remains that knee-caps were never designed to bear the weight of the body.

If you are not warned by the large numbers of elder Aikidoists with bad knees, please consider the findings of anthropologist Susan G. Sheridan who studied the bones of some 6,000 monks from the Byzantine monastery of St. Stephen c. 500 A.D. "The healthiest population I've ever studied," says Sheridan, "except in one respect — almost all the monks seem to have had arthritic knees."

The monks of St. Stephen's did a great deal of kneeling and knee-walking to the point that the insides of the kneecaps were rubbed smooth by impact with their thighbones. One monk wrote of descending 18 steps into a holy cave, with 100 genuflections on each step, a practice he did nightly across hard stone pavement[1].

You can wear knee pads, but they won't pad the *inside* of your kneecap.

Take care of your body. It's your only one.

---

1. Reported in *Discover* magazine, September 1997.

Wrist Exercises

The following exercises limber and strengthen the wrists while they also pattern movements used in wristlocks. Begin with the left wrist. A Common pattern is 2 sets of 5.

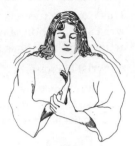

These are *wrist* exercises, not *shoulder* exercises. Movement starts from the tips of the fingers, not tips of shoulder! Because students commonly raise the shoulders first, then crank the wrist from there you will often hear instructions to:

"Relax the shoulders! Drop them 5 inches."

And students are shocked.

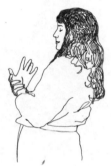

"Whaddya mean 'relax the shoulders'? They ARE relaxed!"
Sometimes it is impossible to tell the difference without outside help. *Ki* testing with a partner who serves as a bio-feedback sensor, quickly reveals the existence of tightness and tension by its side-effects. For example, see how easy it is to push over a *nage* with tense shoulders, weight upperside, and leaning back. Working in pairs, *uke* will:

- Push *nage* from side, directly into shoulder.
- Push *nage* directly from front or back.
- Lift elbow.

Nage may also practice with a mirror:

- Without raising shoulders,
- While consciously dropping them, or
- In combination with raising and tensing shoulders, arms and hands — then dropping them all together.

It is also useful to demonstrate how shoulders should feel by having the student place hands on the instructor's shoulders to feel muscle tension or lack of it while doing an exercise or a technique.

I use the "relax your shoulders" line quite frequently since students seem to like to put strength in their shoulders when practicing technique. Sometimes I put my hand on their shoulder when they perform and they can detect that they are becoming tense. Sometimes I have them put their hands on my shoulders and perform a technique with tense shoulders and then again with relaxed shoulders. They usually get the idea and stop using tension. Most of them had no idea that they were tense. Talk is cheap. A demonstration with feeling is much better.

—George Simcox, Ki Society

Ikkyo-Undo

ADS: Basic Exercise # 1, Ikkyo/Ikkajo ("First -teaching exercise"), p. 121; ZC: pp. 226-230; BA 44.

This exercise models the "first" Aikido technique which involves a bending of the wrist and rotation of wrist and arm forward of the body as a wristlock and throw. For actual *ikkyo* wristlock, see page 198; for technique, see page 217.

As wrist exercise,

1. Bring hands together with right palm covering knuckles and fingers of the left.
2. Raise left wrist to chest height, RH curling knuckles of the LH.
3. Drop hand and repeat.

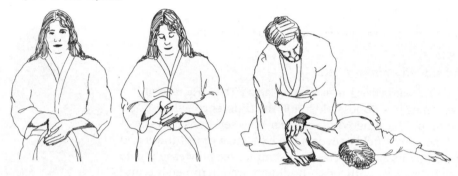

Nikyo-Undo

This exercise models a wristlock involving painful rotation and pressure on the bones of wrist and arm. It is not done in the Ki Society which uses *Ikkyo-Undo* above, in its place, but is common in other styles, provides a stretch that *ikkyo-undo* alone does not, and illustrates the mechanics behind the *nikyo* wristlock.

As wrist exercise,

1. Grasp back of LH with palm of RH. Thumb of RH is wrapped around the knife edge of the LH.
2. Rotate fingers towards chest while dropping the elbow.

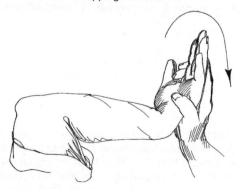

Nikyo as wristlock is described starting on page 201.

Sankyo-Undo

This exercise models the "third" Aikido technique which involves a painful inward rotation of wrist and arm as a wristlock and throw. Modified, it also appears (behind the body) as the Three-Palms-Up pin. Students tend to lean back from the waist while doing this exercise. Emphasize correct upright posture.

As wrist exercise,

1. Place thumb of RH on back of LH in line with index finger.
2. Wrap other fingers around the knife edge of right hand.
3. Extend arms until they form a circle, stretching the held hand.

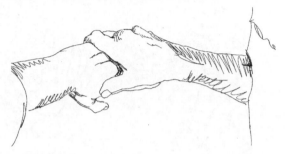

As *ki* exercise, extend arms into a circle. *Uke* tests by:

- Pressing into *nage*'s hands (towards chest).
- Pushing into hands and attempting to lift *nage*'s arms.
- Pushing into *nage*'s elbow toward center of circle or upward.

Nage experiment with the results of:

- Extending arms out from body.
- Pulling arms close into chest.
- Rotating thumbs up or down.

For *sankyo* technique, see page 203.

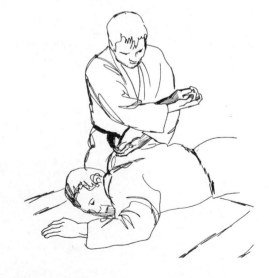

Kote-Gaeishi

ADS: Basic Exercise #2 ("Wrist-Bend"), p. 122; BA p. 45.

This models a throwing technique based on bending of the wrist. As exercise,

1. Grasp back of LH with palm of RH. Thumb of grasping hand is placed just below ring finger and other four fingers are wrapped around the "thigh of the thumb."
2. Bend wrist to 90-degrees and bring towards chest.
3. Drop the hand vertically down the center of the chest. For additional stretch, twist hand slightly outwards.

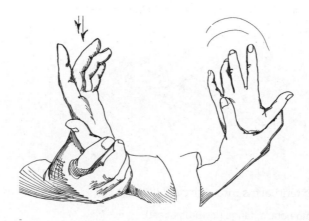

For *kote-gaeshi* as wristlock, see page 208. For throw from *kote-gaeshi*, see "Mune-Tsuki Kote-Gaeshi Tenkan" on page 220.

Leg Exercises

In all exercises below, move from Center/One-Point, not from shoulders. Do not bounce and do not overstretch. Overstretching activates the body's stretch inhibitors designed to protect the muscles from damage and which may actually leave your muscles shorter and tighter than they were to start with. Proper stretching will actually increase muscular strength, and prevent physical problems such as knee and back pain related to shortened muscles.

Many of these can be done with a partner. This approach offers the fun of working with a partner, but requires even more care. In many military-style schools, a student will stand on another student's back or knees, then wonder why the partner doesn't return. Be sensitive to your partner's capabilities. Be as careful and sensitive as if working with a child.

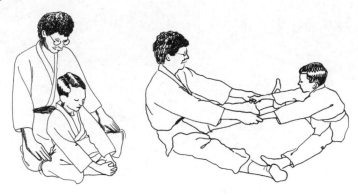

Limbering Knees and Legs

Standing with feet together, hands on knees,

- Rotate knees in a circle to limber and stretch. Combine with squats, quad and hamstring stretches after *muscles* are warm.

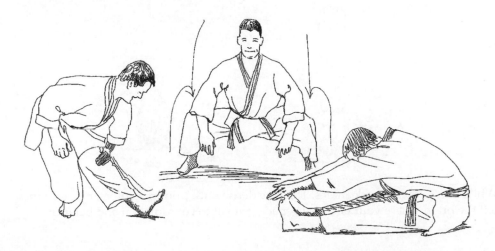

- With legs extended and toes up, bend forward from Center/One-Point (not shoulders). *Relax* into the stretch. If you cannot, you are stretching too far.
- With toes up and legs spread, bend forward from Center over left leg then over right leg, a combined hamstring / adductor stretch.

  Note that tight adductors can restrict toe-touching even more than the hamstrings themselves while giving rise to groin pain, pelvic pain, and even a common misdiagnosis of shin-splints.

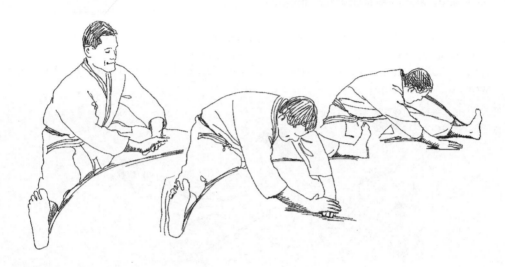

Sitting Cross-Legged and Bouncing Knees

With soles of feet together and drawn into hips, bounce knees gently several times then lean forward from Center/One-Point to stretch the hips.

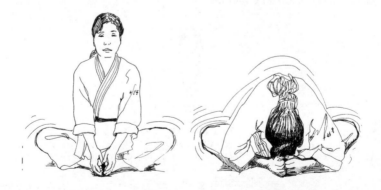

While you're there, work ankles. They are dense with priprioceptors, nerves which tell the brain where your body is in space, critical to coordination and balance.

Bending Back in *Seiza*

On most mats, this is the primary exercise for stretching all four quadriceps muscles, the abdominals and groin — a tall order. Flexibility in these muscles can avoid much knee pain and be critical to safe "round" rolling.

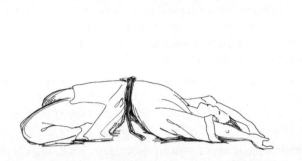
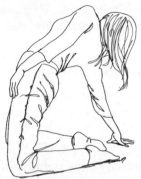

This exercise can be difficult for persons with lower back or knee pain because of the interplay between hip and knee (page 114) and between lumbar vertebrae and psoas muscles (see page 117.) You can separate this into its component parts. Lean back part way. Support the torso with one arm. Take care to extend hips *forward*.

Quads can be also be stretched "by hand" but those who don't understand the muscle attachments usually stretch only three of the four quadriceps muscles. To get them all, you must extend the hip.

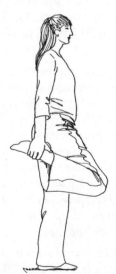

The position at left stretches the three vastus muscles only.

Flexing the hip removes the rectus femoris muscle from the equation.

To stretch all four quads, extend the hip by pushing the pelvis forward relative to the thigh. Torso must remain erect throughout.

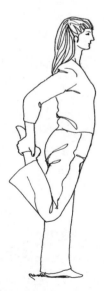

But why does this matter? And why do otherwise healthy knees hurt in kneeling or the layback exercise?

On Muscles and Pain and Effective Stretching

Aikido exercises work the body, muscles, and brain helping to prevent strain, pain, and resulting dysfunction and disability. Before skipping warm-up exercises "to get to the good stuff" (throws), consider another aspect of "self-defense."

Imagine finding yourself pinned down by a gang of masked attackers. One, armed with a razor-sharp knife, slices you open with surgical precision. It is a traumatic experience from which you may need months or years to fully recover because back surgery, neck, abdominal, and thoracic surgery is serious business. It is financially and physically draining. And often it isn't even necessary.

Muscles and connective tissue *alone* (no other pathology involved) can produce remarkably individual patterns of pain and dysfunction that appear in areas of the body far from the actual point of origin. Over 80 percent of the time, the spot where you hurt is not the source of the pain.

Neck muscles cause brutal pain in areas as diverse as head, teeth, arm, back, and chest yet the sufferer may notice no problem with the neck at all. Different pains may be known as "migraine," neuralgia" or "sinus" but originate in muscle and fascia.

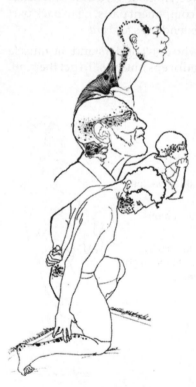

For example, the trapezius muscle of the upper back and posterior neck (shown top left) creates a classic "fish-hook" headache that travels up the neck, around the temple and to the back of the eye possibly combined with dizziness, nausea, and tooth pain. The pain is usually called "migraine" but it comes from muscle fibers of the lower neck / upper shoulder which may have been strained by cell phones, sword exercises, heavy bags, or poor footwear and poor posture .

The middle drawing shows pain patterns arising from the suboccipital muscles. The common head-forward position strains muscles of posterior neck and upper back (trapezius and more). It also requires an upward tilt of the head with constant strain and shortening of the suboccipital muscles. This posture (and the mysterious headaches that accompany it) is seen in persons who wear bifocals (and must hold the head in a fixed position in order to see), who watch TV with heads propped on elbows, and who sit slouched on the mat.

One of the oddest examples of referred pain is jaw and head pain from the soleus, a calf muscle which may be strained by kendo or high heels.

Large black dots are common sites of trigger points (TrPs). Stippling indicates areas of resulting pain.

This may seem impossible. Western medicine says that there is no nerve, pinched or otherwise, which runs from calf to cheek. But there *is* a connection.

Fascia ("fash-uh") is a our original nervous system. It is made up of enormously strong connective tissue (tensile strengths of 2,000 to 4,000 psi). It is the Force that surrounds and penetrates every cellular structure of the body. Superficial fascia surrounds the body like a shrink-wrap leotard; deeper fascia surrounds individual muscle fibers, muscles, and groups of muscles. However, for the most part, Western medicine ignores fascia except where its fibers blend together to form the local structures known as "ligaments," "tendons" or "adhesions."

Fascia stabilizes and supports, like guywires on a radio tower, the rigging on a ship, steel belting in radial tires. It is also piezoelectric, able to produce electrical charge under pressure. This integral body system, largely ignored by Western medicine for 500 years, appears to be the origin of the Eastern "meridians."

Ancient Chinese medical writers spoke of a "lining" of the body and organs, called the *Li*. Today this word is usually translated as "internal" and relegated to the philosophical opposite of "external" in Taoist dualistic thought. But during the Han dynasty (206 bc–ad 220), *Li* indicated a specific physical lining, what we would think of as "membrane." You can see these "membranes" separating the individual muscles in a cut of meat. The vegetable equivalent separates the segments of an orange, pomegranate, or other fruit.

The high correspondence between the lines of meridians and the lines of muscle blend the two schools of thought[1]. Rolfer Tom Myers has verified a continuous line of fascia running from the the tips of the toes to the eyebrows connecting muscles (and their pain signals) in series. But what does this have to do with Aikido class? A lot.

It explains why stretching the suboccipital muscles can improve hamstring flexibility. It exlains why treating tight calves relieves plantar fasciitis and why therapies such as *shiatsu / kiatsu* based on "lines" can be very effective. It also suggests why gentle stretching of a warm body is most efficient: both muscle and fascia lengthen when treated gently, but contract under sudden force which the body perceives as a threat.

Shortened muscles and fascia can be painful and dangerous.

Think of a phone cord that must stretch 10 feet. Tangles take up slack in the cord. If it must still stretch 10 feet, you will notice areas of fibers that are over-shortened and others that are overstretched. Strain on the connections may cause static.

The same problem occurs in muscle and fascia. Taut bands of overstretched fibers and areas of overshortened fibers are weaker than normal and can also be painful. Areas of shortened tangled fibers feel like pea- to walnut-sized hard nodules under the skin. They are characterized by adhesions, scar tissue, and spurious electrical signals and known as Trigger Points (TrPs) for their ability to trigger pain and other symptoms to far distant areas[2].

---

1. Myers studied with biochemist Ida Rolf, whose 1920 Ph.D. thesis formed the basis of what we long knew about fascia. Myers, a sailor, went on to detail a brilliantly logical fascial support system similar to the rigging on a sailboat. In his book *Anatomy Trains*, Myers uses the analogy of fascial train tracks, connecting bony landmarks and muscles in series.
2. In the various pain pattern diagrams in this manual, TrPs are indicated by black dots. Notice how rarely the TrP source corresponds to the area where the pain is actually felt.

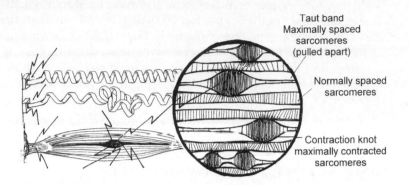

Taut band
Maximally spaced
sarcomeres
(pulled apart)

Normally spaced
sarcomeres

Contraction knot
maximally contracted
sarcomeres

Areas of shortened fibers accumulate waste products. Strain on attachments stimulate the Golgi tendon apparatus causing more tightening to protect the muscle. With sustained stress, attachment TrPs (in fascia) can provoke inflammation, fibrosis, and calcification.

Pressing out TrPs before stretching helps to return the muscle to its normal resting length especially if followed with a gentle stretch. However, standard stretching tends to lengthen the already overstretched fibers still more. The same exercises done after gentle resistance (post isometric stretching) helps return both shortened and overstretched fibers to normal.

Understanding muscles and TrPs can help your flexibility and general health. It may also help students appreciate the value of "pre-class" exercises and the rationale behind them. Here are just a few of the muscles that can cause problems if ignored.

Lower Body

Quads and Knee Pain

The "four-headed" quadriceps muscles are critical to correct knee function. All four quads extend the knee (kick the knee forward). All four refer unique patterns of pain and dysfunction. They are common causes of knee pain, grinding and crackling and/or improper tracking of the kneecap, weak thighs, aching or buckling hips and knees, tight hamstrings, and gait problems. They lurk behind "growing pains" in children and mysterious falls in daily life. [1]

Because of its attachment to the anterior pelvis, a tight rectus femoris (with help from tight adductors) rotates the pelvis forward (see page 154). Unfortunately, tight quads are rarely stretched fully. What are stretched are the three vastii muscles alone; rectus remains short. You stretch vastus muscles just by kneeling in *seiza*. Your knees will probably continue to hurt until the quads are fully stretched out. But no need to spend

---

1. The image of hopping about on one leg trying to pull on trousers is a comedy staple, but an unbendable knee that causes a fall won't be very funny.

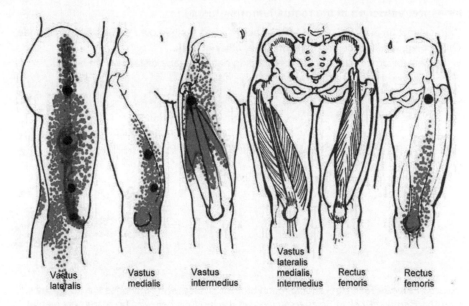

| Vastus lateralis | Vastus medialis | Vastus intermedius | Vastus lateralis, medialis, intermedius | Rectus femoris | Rectus femoris |

Black circles indicate common sites of trigger points. Solid areas show essential or most common pain; stippling indicates areas of less common or spillover pain.

months or years waiting for this to resolve. Work the trigger points[1] then stretch against gentle resistance.

Range-of-Motion (ROM) tests reveal shortening in specific muscles and can be used for effective stretching.

To measure restriction in vastus muscles,

1. Test lying on back. Flex thigh to 90 degrees relative to torso. Heel should be neutral, that is, do not point toe; keep foot at 90 degrees to shin.
2. Press heel gently towards buttock; heel should contact buttock.
3. When movement stops, measure distance between heel and buttock.

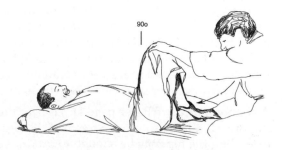

Vastus Test. Heel should reach buttock. Those who can't pass this test will find kneeling painful. They may also have pain on walking *up* hill, *up* stairs.

---

1. Davies, Claire (2004) details one approach. For ROM tests, see back of this manual.

To measure restriction in the rectus femoris muscle,

1. With subject on back at edge of table or bench, drop test leg over edge; bend other knee.
2. On test leg, tester place one hand on knee, other at ankle.
3. Bring heel towards buttock until knee starts to rise. Measure distance from buttock.

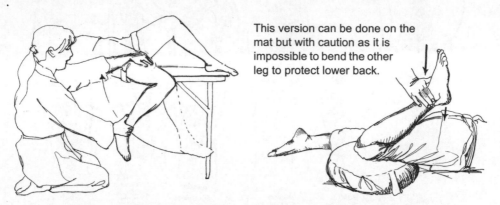

This version can be done on the mat but with caution as it is impossible to bend the other leg to protect lower back.

Rectus Femoris Test. Heel should reach buttock. Those who can't pass the test at left will find the *Bending Back in Seiza* exercise and the leg lock below to be extremely painful. They may also experience kneecap pain on walking *down* hill, *down* stairs.

At a seminar, I tested some 20 attendees with the Rectus Femoris Test. Those who passed were sent to one side, those who failed were sent to the other. On completion, all those who suffered knee pain were asked to raise their hands.

In the "fail" group, all hands were raised.

In the "pass" group, not one hand was raised.

On the mat, there may be other consequences.

Judo is designed to allow maximum force with minimum danger of injury. You are not allowed to attack the muscles, especially those of legs and knees. Leg locks like the one shown below are illegal precisely because they are so likely to injure someone with tight, inflexible muscles. Nevertheless, they are seen when Judoka or Aikidoka are "playing." They are seen in Gracie / Brazilian Jiu-Jutsu (BJJ) but uncommon, perhaps because of its Judo roots. They are more common in Russian Sambo, despite its Judo roots. They are *very* common in Mixed Martial Arts (MMA) whose "anything-goes" image of No Holds Barred competition is marketing hype. MMA has rules too; you are not allowed to gouge eyes or rip out lungs. You *can* take advantage of tight muscles so these holds are very common and very effective. Fexible players will almost always be less prone to injury than inflexible ones, regardless of style.

A common rectus TrP (see page 115) is near the attachment at the hip, the section of the muscle that is so rarely stretched. Because of this area of shortening, merely extending the hip may be enough to produce extreme discomfort. The lock will be even more painful if psoas is tight (common in *karateka* and kickboxers). Players with tight psoas may tap out even before the knee is flexed. The reverse is also true.

Wiley Nelson who has trained and coached in MMA demonstrated this leg lock on a class of trigger point therapists. He was shocked to find that he was unable to get *anyone* to tap out. Classmates worked on each other every day and muscles were relaxed and stretchy.

No discomfort, no pain.

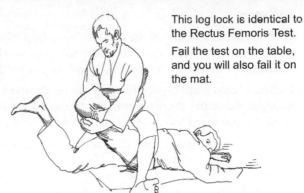

This log lock is identical to the Rectus Femoris Test.

Fail the test on the table, and you will also fail it on the mat.

Psoas and Sit-ups

The rectus test and the leg lock above also stretch the psoas and the iliacus muscles of the hip which join to form the iliopsoas. Fibers run through the pelvis connecting spine to the thigh. Psoas major and minor combined onnect to all the lumbar vertebrae and their disks, the reason why straight-leg situps can severely strain the lower back. The Yoshinkan *kamae* position of extended hip and knee is excellent for psoas but in inflexible beginners, it may cause problems until the muscle relaxes.

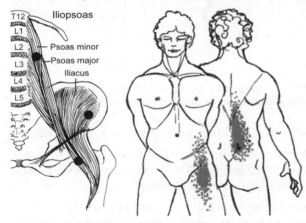

Psoas are shortened when hips are strongly jack-knifed as in desk work, driving, or sleeping in the fetal position. They are also strained by forcing hips to flex against tight hamstring or back muscles in attempting to touch toes. In kicking styles, repetitive front kicks[1] beyond the student's strength and endurance can cause chronic pain and distress.

Pain from lumbar attachments runs vertically up the back . The TrP at the lower attachment send pain down the thigh and up to groin and abdomen.

Psoas and iliacus muscles join to form iliopsoas. Notice attachments to lumbar vertebrae and disks.

Sufferers may attempt to relieve the lower back pain with back stretches, but notice that the source of the problem is in *front*. Psoas TrPs are best treated by a professional myofascial trigger point therapist[2] or a massage therapist trained in the technique. However, moist heat and gentle stretch, properly applied at hip and groin can provide great relief.

---

1. The 1000 kicks done for Anniversary Celebrations are a notorious source of injury.
2. Find a therapist at www.myofascialtherapy.org. See also "Resources,"

Adductors

In various stretch and exercise classes (including Aikido) hamstrings seem to get most of the attention. Oddly enough, adductor magnus (largest and most powerful of the adductors) can restrict "hamstring" stretches more than the hamstrings themselves.

Tight adductors are especially likely to be strained or injured in the *uke* caught in a strong *tenkan* turn. Adductors bring the legs together. In *tenkan*, they must pull the outside leg inward towards the circle for the next forward step.

Strain in these powerful muscles can be painful and disabling.

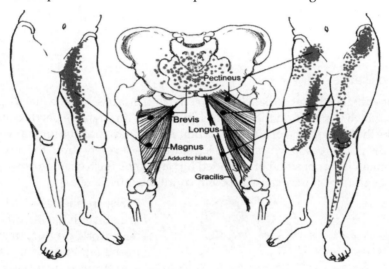

Pain patterns arising from adductors range from medial and anterior thigh, to the groin, pelvis, and knee and down the tibia to the medial ankle.

Pectineus, short but powerful, produces a local pain interpreted as a "groin pull."

Adductor longus and *brevis* acting together can cause hip pain that may extend down to the knee. Pain may continue down to the inside ankle. Because it follows the fascia along the shin, this pain is readily confused with shin-splints.

Gracilis is a slender "graceful" strap-like muscle that can cause a burning pain along the inside thigh extending down to the knee. It can also cause a jolt of pain into the pelvis, sometimes described as feeling "like a firecracker."

Adductor magnus refers pain up to the groin and down the inner thigh to the knee. In both males and females, a TrP near the attachment at the ischial tuberosities (the "sitz-bones") refers a deep burning pain inside the pelvis. In females, the combination of inner thigh and pelvic pain has been attributed to inflamed ovaries. When surgery reveals perfectly healthy organs, the pain has been labeled "psychosomatic" and the patient referred for psychiatric counseling.

Notice also the *adductor hiatus* (a "break" in the adductor magnus muscle). Through this opening pass the femoral artery, femoral vein, and femoral nerve. In some people the hiatus is relatively small; when the muscles are tight, it can become even smaller, strangling the neurovascular bundle so effectively that the victim may temporarily lose deep tendon reflexes and ability to walk.

Another symptom of tight adductors may be migraines. Many seem to begin with tight adductors and many can be halted by working adductors and calves. Migraine sufferers may protest. "But migraines are vascular!" Perhaps, but "vascular" does not stop at the neck. Avoid the pain (and that masked gang of knife-wielding attackers) by keeping adductors healthy and relaxed.

Two ROM tests for adductors.

Test 1 removes gracilis (which crosses the knee joint). Test 2 includes it.

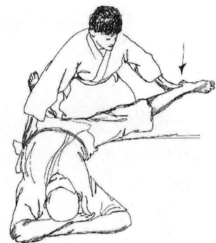

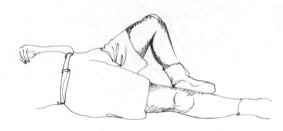

Adductor Test 1

1. Place heel of test leg on table next to knee of other leg.
2. Lower knee to table. Note how close to table it comes.
3. Sliding heel to crotch can be blocked by vastus medialis (see Vastus Test).
   If no restriction, knee comes to mat.

Adductor Test 2

1. Stabilize opposite hip bone so subject doesn't roll.
2. Raise opposite leg to 90 degrees then lower at 90 degrees out to side.
   If no restriction, leg can reach mat.

Like tight quadriceps, tight adductors may be utilized in pins. Again, you probably won't see this pin in Aikido, but it might appear when Judoka are "playing."

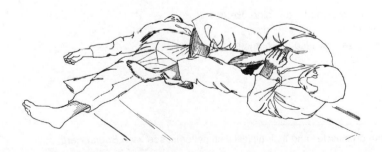

Quadratus Lumborum

Quadratus lumborum (QL) connects pelvis to rib cage. It is so critical to walking that if paralyzed, walking is impossible even with crutches. Few know of this muscle but many have experienced it at some point as severe back, glute, hip or groin pain[1].

When shortened, it can be strained by strong sudden twisting motions, whether *giri* from sword, golf club or bat, by carrying a weight on one side of the body, or simply by arising from chair, bed, or mat while simultaneously twisting the torso.

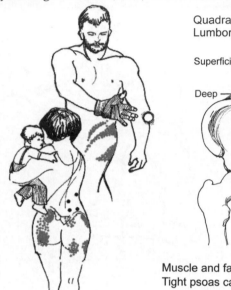

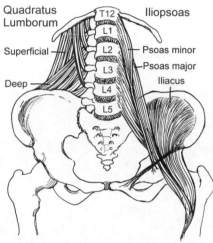

Muscle and fascia of the iliopsoas blend with that of QL.
Tight psoas can eventually cause QL problems.

The resulting pain can be hellish, is usually assumed to involve disk problems, and so can lead to unnecessary and unsuccessful back surgery with the many health issues that flow from that. The gentle twisting of the Three-Minute Ki Exercise for Health helps avoid these risks.

The Torso Twist stretches QL and pectoral muscles. With pelvis perpendicular to mat and leg extended as shown, yes, you *should* be able to drop shoulder flat to mat! If not, the exercise below will help loosen things up.

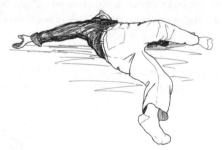

On back with arms at 90 degrees to torso,

1. Cross L leg over body to R side. Return.
2. Cross R leg over body to L side.
   This exercise may also be restricted by *abdominals*.

---

1. For more on muscles and their typical pain patterns, see *www.Round-Earth.com.*

Abdominals

Healthy, well-toned abdominals are critical to good posture and pain-free living.

Abdominals round the torso hence they are critical to safe rolling. Many schools emphasize abdominal exercises, rarely stretching out afterwards. In one "No Pain No Gain" school I visited, students were told that cramping and pain were the proper results and "If the muscles *don't* cramp up, you're not doing it right."

Wrong. The instructor who inflicts such abuse on students is setting them up for disaster. Unfortunately, tight or strained abdominals cause a wider range of pain and dysfunction than any other muscle group. Consequences may range from merely inconvenient to the brutally painful[1]. Symptoms vary widely, but can include:

- Pain in back, hip, chest, gastric region / solar plexus, groin, pelvis, bladder, testicles. Colic, indigestion, "gas pains," belching, diarrhea, nausea and/or vomiting. Urgent (non-productive) urination.
- Symptoms that mimic: Appendicitis, diverticulosis; ulcers, hernia, renal colic, heart or gallbladder disease.

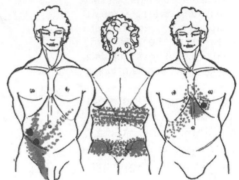

Some of many pain patterns arising from abs.

L and R: lateral abs; Center: rectus abdominis.

Many people can produce the back pain simply by leaning slightly backwards, stretching rectus.

Can't do a sit-up? Then *don't*. Those who strain to do so with weak abs will substitute with psoas. (You can tell this has happened when the lower back is arched rather than rounded.)

Out-of-shape beginners should start abdominal exercises gently. A good start, safer than a sit-up, is the sit-*back*.

Sit-Back Exercise

On floor, with knees bent and feet held in place by a weight or a partner,

1. Curl the torso, tuck chin to chest, and slowly lower torso to mat.
2. From back, roll to side and return to sitting position.
   Eccentric contraction (*lengthening* a muscle under load, rather than *shortening* it) strengthens muscle more efficiently. Many who can't sit up can sit back. This can be done as a partnered exercise, each helping the other to return to the sitting position.

The Shrimping Exercise comes from Judo groundwork. It is more dynamic than sit-backs and trains a useful skill while still avoiding the back strain of full sit-ups.

---

1. Symptoms must be carefully checked as they are so similar to those of serious diseases; however, symptoms of muscles are often mistaken for serious diseases. For example, appendectomies are the most common emergency abdominal surgeries in the U. S. Appendicitis is so dangerous that it is better to err on the side of safety; in theory, surgeons accept a false diagnosis rate of 20 percent rather than risk death due to a missed diagnosis. In clinical practice, the *reported rate* of false positives among women has been as high as 42 percent. Both psoas and abdominal muscles can produce symptoms mistaken for appendicitis when pain is on the right side (Raman, S. S. 2008).

Shrimping Exercise

This develops abdominal strength critical to safe rolling. *Round* the back rather than merely flexing at the hips. The first works abdominals, the second psoas.

On back, knees flexed and arms up,

1. Roll to L side, simultaneously curl torso, push arms to thighs, and straighten legs to push hips towards head.
2. Return to starting position; flex knees and raise arms.
3. Roll to R side; curl torso, push arms to thighs, push and straighten legs above.
4. Continue down the mat shifting from side to side. You will progress the length of your lower legs. The motion can be reversed by arching back and pulling with hamstrings.

Tight or weak abdominals are a classic cause of visceral and back pain. Always stretch out abdominals after crunches or other exercises.

The "Cobra" pose from yoga is a good choice

Cobra Exercise

1. Lying prone, raise straight up on arms tilting head back. Keeping hips on ground stretches psoas and rectus femoris.
2. Turn torso side to side looking over shoulders to stretch obliques.

To add a quad stretch,

1. Have partner press heels *gently* towards buttocks.
2. The one stretching should resist the stretch with about 10 percent of strength, then relax into partner's push.
3. Repeat.

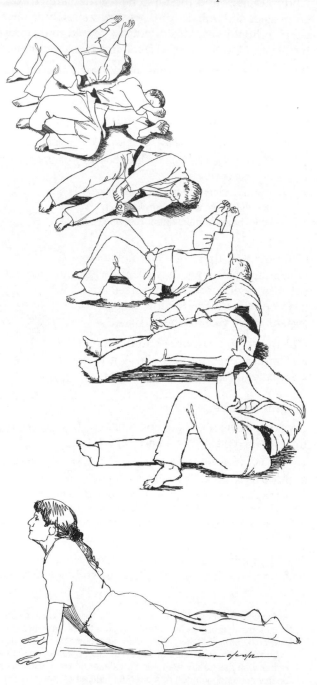

Upper Body Stretches

Trapezius

Because trapezius helps raise the arms, it is strained by sword work and in daily life by hunching shoulders to hold cell phones, straps, bags, and more.

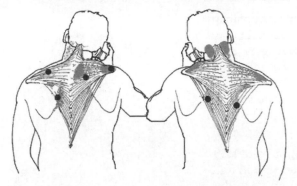

Trapezius pain to upper back, base of skull. It also extends into temple and back of eye (see diagram of the trapezius headache on page 112).

Aching or burning pain may range across the upper back, between the shoulder blades, to the point of the shoulders or up to the base of the skull. Severe head pain with nausea and visual disturbances may be called *migraine*, but very often the headache begins with the upper fibers of trapezius.

When things get tense, stretch out!

Trapezius Stretch 1

1. Hold on to a pillar, a post, or a doorknob,
1. Round back, drop head forward, and
2. Lean back.

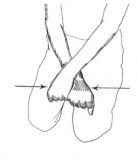

Trapezius Stretch 2

1. Extend arms to front crossing wrists at little-finger sides.
2. Make fists and press them against each other.
3. Partner press head down gently as you turn head side to side.

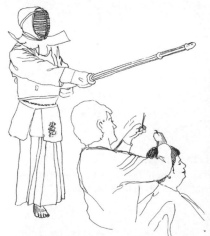

When weightlifters and martial artists suffer head and neck pain, it is likely to be seen as muscle strain and, with luck, treated effectively.

Female hairstylists with the same problems tend to be diagnosed with "fibromyalgia" and dosed with pain killers and anti-depressants. Male colleagues are likely to be diagnosed with "a pinched nerve." The entire group invariably suffers trapezius strain, as do others who spend their days holding their arms up or doing overhead work such as wiring or carpentry.

Pain also arises when trapezius muscle fibers are overstretched by shortened pectoral muscles.

Balance is key!

Pectorals

Chest (pectoral) muscles can tighten in the course of daily activities such as keyboarding (music or computer). Aikido can add to the problem via sword and staff work, or centered arm positions (such as the *kamae* stance of Yoshinkan). Short, tight pectorals have their own pain patterns. They also rotate the shoulders forward and overstretch the opposing trapezius muscle of the back. (See trapezius pain on page 123.)

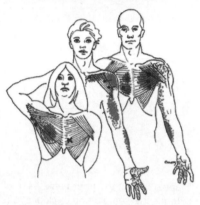

Pectoralis major can cause numbness or pain in chest, shoulders, and arms. houlder pain may be interpreted as bursitis. In men, chest pain extending down the left arm may be mistaken for angina pectoris, the warning sign of a heart attack. Women may be given repeated mammograms. Pain should be checked out by your doctor, but if nothing is found, check muscles.

Pectoralis minor (see diagram on page 157) connects ribs to shoulder blades. Blood and nerve supply to the arm should dive under this muscle and come out the other side with nerve impulses and blood supply intact. This doesn't always happen. If pectoralis minor is tight, you may suffer odd symptoms such as waking at night to find your arms still "asleep." The problem can be relieved by

Pain from pectoralis major (right and left), and from subclavius (center). A TrP just below the 5th rib at X can cause frightening heart arythmias.

stretching your shoulder back (thus stretching the muscle that is compressing the artery). *Subclavius* compresses the same artery and also sends pain down the arm.

Prevent problems with shortened chest muscles with the doorway stretch.

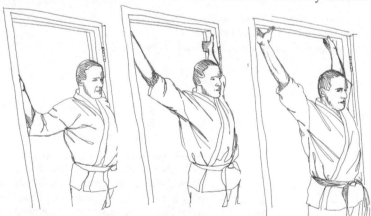

1. Stand with arms on either side of the doorway and lean through it.
2. Shift arms between high, middle, and lower positions to stretch the three different groups of pectoralis muscle fibers. Another stretch is the Paired Chest and Hip Exercise.

Paired Chest and Hip Exercise

This exercise provides a stretch through the arms, chest, abs, psoas, and the fun of doing it with a partner. Standing back to back, hip to hip, arms hooked,

1. First partner bends forward balancing partner 2 on hips and back.
2. Second partner bends forward balancing Partner 1 on hips and back.

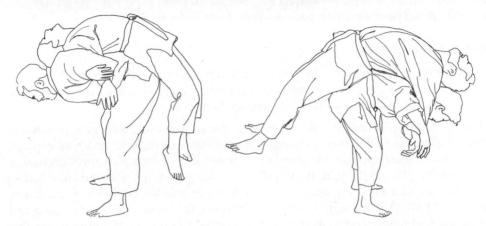

Per muscles, notice that one partner shown here had flexible psoas and quads. The other had tight psoas (hip does not extend) and tight quads (shin kicks forward rather than dropping down under gravity). He also had knee pain.

Per mechanics, notice that a partner's weight seems almost negligible as long as it is over hips and legs.

Pills and Perils

I have sat at table with muscle-weary Aikido friends who were passing around the bottle of "Vitamin I" with the beer and the whisky. It came with the implication that the greater the number of tablets washed down with the beer, the greater the pain and suffering, *ergo* the greater the dedication as a Martial Artist soldiering bravely on. If you are doing this, please stop and compare the level of pain and disability between sore muscles versus liver or kidney transplants.

NSAIDS (Non-Steroidal Anti-Inflammatories) have earned an important place in pain control but they are not innocuous; they are powerful drugs with debilitating side effects such as liver damage and a rising number of kidney failures (even in young people) per year. All reduce platelet count and clotting time which in turn lead to capillary breakage and increased bleeding in both body and brain.

- **Ibuprofen** (sold as Advil and Motrin) blocks new bone growth and in large doses or on an empty stomach can cause stomach bleeding and ulceration.
- **Naproxen** (sold as Aleve, Anaprox, Naprelan, and Naprosyn) has been shown to increase risk of heart attack or stroke by 50 percent among healthy elderly patients.
- **Acetaminophen** (sold as Tylenol and others) is changed by alcohol into liver-damaging chemicals, even when used at recommended dosages. As few as 8 extra-strength

caplets over a period of 24 hours can cause severe liver damage if taken with alcohol or for the after-alcohol hangover. It is best to simply avoid the combination entirely.

- **Aspirin** increases risk of gastrointestinal bleeding at *all* levels of alcohol consumption.

Use these medications for their very real benefits when needed — but read labels and use with caution. Even if prescribed by a physician (who is perhaps very busy and overscheduled) don't turn off your own good self-defense sense.

Self Defense

Self-defense is far more than Hollywood scenarios. Read a chapter or two of *Financial Management for Dummies* and you'll wonder why you're wasting time learning to defend against overhead strikes and punches to mid-section.

Why? Because self-defense is also defending against pain and injury, against medical interventions and bills (now a leading cause of financial disaster and bankruptcy). Sometimes it's just good ongoing care and maintenance of your body through motion and healthy play on the mat. It's PhysEd class for grownups with our tight office-bound muscles and aching joints. You may never encounter a mugger on the street, but if you haven't raised arms overhead in 30 years, then *ikkyo-undo,* and turning and spinning and rolling and limbering will be wonderful exercise. In the long run, this may be the most practical physical self-defense of all.

A fine example appears on page 194. For many years this young woman suffered from intractable muscle spasms which were finally discovered to be from spina bifida occulta. When muscle relaxants did not help, she was faced with the agonizing choice of continuing pain or having her tendons cut and spending the rest of her life in a wheelchair. By some lucky chance, she visited an Aikido dojo with a friend and was urged to join in by the instructor.

"I can't!" she protested. He, an amputee, snorted.

"You can!" he said. And got her onto the mat.

Over time, the stretching and motions of Aikido relieved the painful spasms in a way that muscle relaxants had never been able to do. Now, the only sign of her disability is the one shoe she wears on the mat. When last I heard from her, she was a *nidan* with her own school.

Play, stretch, strengthen, relax, and yes, you can stretch away the pain.

Aikido is a great way to do that.

Aikido is also a terrific way to learn to defend against the most constant attack we face in daily life: gravity and falls.

CHAPTER 4

Rolling, Falling, and Flying

Ukemi is the most practical, real-world self-defense that we teach. Few of us get into fights regularly, but all of us (in Kansas!) have to deal with ice, or stairs or curbs — we will fall and falling is dangerous. People die every day from falling down. Good idea to learn how to do it with some safety, eh?

—Stan Haehl, Kansas Ki Society

Whoa! Gravity is a harsh mistress.

—The Tick

Did you start Aikido for self-defense? And do you think of rolling practice as a waste of practice time, or at best a "warm-up"?

In Real Life it is the skill with the most real and immediate application On The Street, because On The Street, we trip over curbs, slip on ice, and stumble over our own feet. We land in emergency rooms where the most common injuries are broken wrists and broken collarbones due to falls.

Safe falling is one of the most challenging and important skills in martial arts. Critical to Judo, Ju-jutsu and Aikido, it is rarely taught in Karate. In competition, many moves are forbidden because of the danger of falling. This situation was gleefully exploited by the Gracies for years until the rest of the world caught on to what they were doing — purposefully taking opponents untrained in falling or mat work down to the mat.

In Real Life, falls are a far greater daily danger than street attacks. Consider the data on accidental deaths. Despite the lurid headlines, more people in the U.S. die each year from falls than die from drowning, fire, choking, and firearms accidents combined. Motor vehicle crashes (horizontal falls) beat all others. Someday you will fall.

We have driver education classes, seat belts, child car seats, swimming and water safety lessons, smoke and carbon monoxide alarms, and gun safety classes.

But who is taught to fall safely?

U. S. Accidental Deaths by Cause and Rate / 100,000:	No. of Deaths[a]
Motor vehicles (14.9)	44,700
Poisoning (solid, liquid) (8.5)	25,300
Falls (7.1)	21,200
Suffocation / Choking (1.4)	4,100
Drowning (1.3)	3,800
Fires, Flames, & Smoke (0.9)	2,800
Firearms (0.2)	680

a. National Safety Council, *Accident Facts*, 2006 data on 120,000 accidental deaths.

Judo and Aikido teach balance under extreme conditions and how to fall should you lose that. Defense against finding oneself hurtling toward a hard and painful surface is real self-defense, useful on a regular basis.

The art of receiving an attack (by people or planets) and falling safely is *ukemi*.

In performances of carefully rehearsed "movie-do" the rolls and falls by stuntmen, protecting themselves from real harm, are the most real part of the performance. In the entertainment art known as "WWF" there is little actual wrestling. The apparent opponents and referee all work together as a team; competition is largely illusion. But the risk of injury is very real and so the *ukemi* is very real.

In real life, the most common injuries "On The Street" are from trying to break a fall and breaking a wrist instead. In the U.S. most accidents happen at home on ladders, stairs, slippery floors, in bathtubs, or any and all possible combinations of factors. In the U.K., thousands of injuries severe enough to require hospital admission were caused by tea cosies, vegetables, and sofas; false teeth were responsible for 933 and toilet-roll holders for 329. There were 5,945 "Trouser Incidents" as compared to 1,207 chainsaw injuries[1]. In 1999, over 10,000 were hospitalized by socks.

Closer to home, one of our students was thrown by socks and his Sunday newspaper.

> I answered the door in socks and our friend handed me the newspaper as she came in. The Sunday issue weighs several pounds and as I turned, the paper in its plastic sack hanging off one hand took me slightly off balance, my socks slipped on the tile, and I fell backwards down the stairs to the den. The den is concrete slab with carpet over it, but the automatic back roll (the only form of *ukemi* I'm reasonably good at) made it a non-event even though I was recovering from a detached retina and falls are on the Major No-No list. I sustained no injury, not even bruise or soreness, and don't remember any sudden impact, just a soft landing and half a roll. I'm a "Noh Kyu" and have only been practicing a few months, but the back roll *ukemi* has already come in handy — and was completely automatic.
>
> —Michael Bartman, Ki Society

Ability to fall safely is one of the most valuable self-defense techniques there is.

But how is such a thing possible? How and why does it work?

Dr. Wendy Gunther explains.

---

1. Department of Trade and Industry data (1999 and 2001). At the Royal Society for the Prevention of Accidents spokeswoman Jan Eason admits: "It seems odd there are so many more accidents involving trousers than chainsaws but everyone has trousers and hardly anyone has chainsaws." Because of patient confidentiality, the department cannot reveal the details behind the accidents. It is, therefore, impossible to know precisely how 750 people happened to be seriously injured by household sponges, but chances are it had to do with falls. See also page 114.

Essay: The Physics of Ukemi

"Falling down" is equivalent to being hit, slugged, punched, or shot at by the ground moving at the acceleration of gravity. Whether you are hit by ground or by bullet, the wounding energy is proportional to:

mass (m) multiplied by velocity (v) squared

divided by the time (*t*) it takes for the wounding surface to contact you,

and also divided by the area (*a*) of the wounding surface.

In symbols, this is expressed as:

Wounding energy = mv^2 / ta **(EQ 12)**

Hence wounding energy decreases if we can increase time and area.

Increasing Time. If I take a bullet and touch it slowly to your skin, you aren't wounded because the marked reduction in velocity means a marked increase in *t*. During falls, you slow down the contact by rolling into it or slapping the mat with your arm like a spring. Even fractions of seconds of increase in *t* significantly reduce wounding energy.

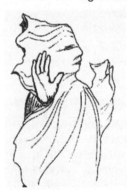

Increasing Area. Suppose I take the same bullet and hammer it into a huge flat sheet of lead and fire it at you (in a vacuum where there's no air friction) with the same velocity (*v*) as a bullet leaving the muzzle of a gun.

The bullet will wrap itself as a flattened surface over your skin (with an area of say 720 square inches). You are extremely unlikely to be wounded simply because of the increase in area (*a*). Wounding energy is extremely low[1].

In contrast, if the area through which the kinetic energy is being transferred is reduced to the size of your chin, say 2 square inches, wounding energy is high.

To recap:

The greater the mass and velocity of the oncoming object, the more dangerous the situation.

The larger the area and time of contact, the safer the situation.

We usually can't change our mass or velocity, but we can increase time and the surface area of contact with the oncoming mass, mat, sidewalk, or planet.

The means of doing so are the skills of *ukemi*.

—Dr. Wendy Gunther.

---

1. Pads and helmets work to reduce the wounding energy in the same way, by spreading the force over a larger area and by increasing time required for the force to reach you. Baseballs, punches, and planets all move much more slowly through plastic foam than through air.

On *ukemi*, see ADS: pp. 139-142; TOT: pp. 48-49; BA pp. 36-39.

On Learning to Roll — A Course of Action

To start the lesson, your instructor will . . . ski a short distance down the mountain, just to the point where it gets very steep, and swoosh to a graceful stop, making it look absurdly easy. It IS absurdly easy for [him], because underneath his outfit he's wearing an antigravity device. All the expert skiers wear them. You don't actually believe that "ski jumpers" can leap off those ridiculously high ramps and just float to the ground unassisted without breaking into walnut-sized pieces, do you?

—Dave Barry

My wife is often the only woman in class and feels a bit humiliated when she can't roll in front of all the guys. Backward rolls are fine, at least pretty good. But on forward rolls, she hurts herself more when she falls on her shoulders and neck rather then going over. For me, it's frustrating because I don't know how to help her. And for her, she's getting more and more afraid.

—L. J.

Rolling is one of the most important skills in Aikido, yet informal surveys of students and instructors strongly suggest that a big reason for student dropout is problems with rolling. Many students are lost due to fear of rolling and being pushed too hard too soon. Many quit due to pain or injuries from rolls. Consider then,

- How can teaching of rolling skills be made safer and more effective?
- How can we protect students until they are able to protect themselves?
- How can a student most effectively practice and develop rolling skills?

Ueshiba's students, the original Aikido students, report that techniques were done *kneeling (suwari waza);* they were reprimanded if caught doing techniques *standing.*

Tatami (the traditional Japanese straw mats) are very hard. A bad standing fall will hurt. Techniques done from the floor have far less potential to injure. By necessity, they also teach the importance of balance and center. You *must* move hip with arm in order to be effective. This sensible approach allowed students to learn to roll safely, eventually progressing to standing techniques and standing falls. However, these were students who were culturally accustomed to kneeling.

In the U.S., the process was reversed. American knees, accusomed to sitting in chairs, were less flexible. When the choice became Standing Aikido or No Aikido, classes were necessarily taught standing. As a result, in most schools, *kneeling* versions of techniques are considered to be the advanced versions of the *standing* techniques. Standing *up* is a separate issue from falling *down to the* mat.

Standard procedure at many dojos is to demonstrate a beautiful roll with some basic instruction on placement of head, hands, and feet. "Here is a forward roll, a backward roll, a breakfall. Please practice." How well this works is reflected by the dropout rate due to injured shoulders and aching heads plus other considerations.

For example, in the story above, a new student starts with stage fright causing general stiffness. There's no time to concentrate on the backrolls that she can do just fine or at least pretty well, because she needs to be doing something else that hurts more with every roll so that every subsequent roll whether done wrong or done right, becomes more and more painful. Talk about negative reinforcement!

Consider starting students with rocking-chair back rolls (*koho-tento-undo*) followed by full back rolls. Begin forward rolls after backrolls are mastered and comfortable. If a beginner has never done rolls before, it may be counterproductive to start them off with forward rolls. There's no lack of other things to do, too little reason to push this particular skill plus too much danger of injury and bad experience without careful and caring supervision.

Many instructors try to encourage frustrated students by revealing that they themselves took more than a year or two to learn to roll well. This may be helpful *or not*.

- For students who are merely frustrated and who need to understand that any new skill takes time, it can be a useful reminder.
- For students who are frustrated — and hurt and injured — you have just promised them a year or two of continuing pain, headaches, bruised or separated shoulders, failure and embarassment. The more apprehensive the student, the more tense.
- For students who are frustrated, injured, apprehensive and tense, the more panic, injuries and pain, and the once enthusiastic new student disappears.

There is no need to hold back students who are familiar with rolls, pick them up quickly, or are ready for new challenges. Less confident or less skilled students should not be expected to progress at the same rate or made to feel inferior if they don't. This is not boot camp and it is not a contest.

Certain classes, groups, or techniques can be limited to a certain proficiency in *ukemi*[1]. Meanwhile, it should be OK to stay with something that feels safe and accomplishable for awhile. If that something is back rolls, then back rolls it is.

Ukemi skills should be taught carefully and methodically, not just "absorbed" through random experience. Consider the following progression.

1. **Rocking-Chair Rolls**. This simple rocking backwards and forwards roll (*koho-tento-undo*, page 135) teaches rounding and relaxation through movements that are already familiar to everyone. It allows the beginner to join in practice or someone with injured shoulder to continue practicing. *Koho-tento-undo* offers plenty of interesting dynamics for exploration. Once simple rocking-chair rolls are mastered, and the feelings and sensations associated with them are comfortable and familiar, move on to . . .
2. **Full Back Rolls**. Full back rolls (page 136) require attention to head position to avoid straining the neck, but they completely avoid the problem of crashing forward onto head, neck, or shoulder joint. In Ki Society, even beginning students quickly learn to segue into full back rolls because of *taigi*. Allowing the physics and inertia of *koho-tento-undo* to return *uke* to attack position may take too long to meet the time requirements. The solution is to continue over backwards into a true back roll. *Taigi* helps improve rolling because the focus is on needing to get back up and attack again rather than on the rolling itself, a useful distraction.

---

1. *Taigi* are paired *kata* practiced by the Ki Society to emphasize rhythm and flow. At the Merrifield dojo, *taigi* class was originally listed as an Advanced Class and limited to persons considered to have acquired adequate rolling skills. This encouraged both rolling practice and *taigi* practice (presence there automatically declared one to be an Advanced Student). When the rolling requirement was dropped, interest in both rolling practice and *taigi* class faded.

3. **Small Forward Rolls with a Partner.** Small forward rolls (page 145) can be presented as an exercise at first; not as actual *ukemi*, that is, as *uke* the student can "walk out" until rolls are usable; partners should allow them to do so. Practice with partner ensures proper position and opportunity to work on patterning, to develop body memory and awareness of what a successful roll should feel like and how the body should behave. Note that proper positioning can depend heavily on body type. See "Male and Female Rolls" on page 141.

4. **Individual Small Rolls.** When student is familiar with position and purpose, rolls can be done by the student alone. Combine with rolling exercises and games.

5. **Standing Rolls.** Front and back. By now the student should feel comfortable enough with the process to realize that the mechanics are the same, regardless of starting height.

6. **Breakfalls.** Breakfalls are rarely the first thing taught. However, forward and backward rolls need not be perfect before starting breakfalls. Furthermore, the extension required for roll-outs (a beginning form of breakfalls), may clarify the problem that a student may be having with proper position for other rolls. For example, it is impossible to do a proper rollout if the student is "pancaking."

Students often feel that they must *do* something to roll. All that is needed is to set up the inbalance.

In all these exercises, the student should feel for the point of balance and unbalance, of stability and instability.

On opening night of Ringling Brothers, Barnum and Bailey Circus, a wonderful clown came out with a large newspaper, dragging a park bench. Throughout his attempts to merely sit down on the bench (without getting his hands, feet, or head stuck) he took some of the most wonderful *ukemi* I have ever seen.

As the park bench "threw" him about, he took backward *ukemi* (as the bench tipped while he was sitting on its back), forward *ukemi*, and some *major* breakfalls. He simply threw himself forward, flipping, and landing on the ground (no mats).

To the untrained eye, I know it looked phenomenal.

To my semi-trained eye, I saw some wonderful *ukemi*, sometimes with the hand reaching back to "spot" the ground, occasionally with slapping, and one or two that might be described as "falling leaf *ukemi*."

If you think we have it tough learning *ukemi*, try doing it in size 40 clown shoes!

—Scott Crawford, Yoshinkan

The story of me and aikido is basically. "Hey... this aikido stuff looks fun.

Hey, you get to throw people... and not only do they not get hurt, they're not even angry? And you don't get hurt either! Sign me up!"

—Paul Gowder, Ki Society

Preparation

Mats and Padding

I once taught a class where the only available space was thin industrial carpet over concrete, no pads, no mats. Students were nearly all retirement age, except for one very overweight young man and one very athletic young man. I purposely restricted class practice to back rolls; no front rolls unless students came to the *dojo* and its mat for safe practice and individual attention. One day when I was absent, my assistant seized the opportunity to correct what he saw as a blatant omission of a critical skill: Front rolls. On concrete. I returned to find the entire class damaged and unable to continue, with shoulder injuries, neck injuries, bruises, broken veins and hematomas.

Obviously students should not start forward rolls on concrete. Safe learning requires proper equipment, but the most critical item is good sense by both student and instructor. We are accustomed to turning over control to a teacher, but part of self-defense is knowing just how far this transfer of personal responsibility should go. Learning is a balance between challenging what you don't know you're capable of versus knowing what you're *not* capable of quite yet. A young man in superb physical condition may be completely unaware of the potential fragility of other bodies. A long-time skier may be unable to remember not knowing how to ski. Many a friend has taken a novice skiier straight to the top of the expert slope. "It's OK! It's *easy!*" This may be true for the "friend," but not for the beginner. Both teacher and student must be aware of limitations. What the student risks should be up to the student. That said, reduce risk with good equipment.

- **Mats**. The flip side of beginning rolls on concrete is beginning rolls on a too soft surface which interferes with forward momentum and rhythm. The student sinks to a halt and "pancakes" (falls flat sideways) right about the time that hips begin to go vertical and weight is concentrated down into the pad. On the other hand, a very soft mat, a crash pad, eases beginning breakfalls.
- **Crash Pads**. It's one thing to roll into a breakfall (a "roll-out"). Quite another to flip into a breakfall from a standing position. During the course of the learning process, a standard mat will punish new students severely (especially when they are tentative or tense). A crash pad makes the process much easier.

  Much easier than on the regular mat. I have a tendency to try to support myself on my arm, which is nowhere near strong enough. When it inevitably collapses, I fall on my shoulder and it hurts, and makes me less interested in doing it again. Knowing that I was landing on the equivalent of a feather bed let me do the little jump that is necessary to get you over the top before landing. A bit more practice like that and I may have the pattern of movement ingrained enough that I'll do it right on the regular mat too. — Michael Bartman
- **Pads**. Beginners may bump hip bones at lower back (the "knobbies") or hit shoulders (especially females) yet I've never known anyone to suggest pads to get them through this stage. Motorcycle and skating pads protect from impact while allowing freedom of movement.

Risk Issues

Specific physiological issues greatly increase the risk of falling. Because of promises of "no physical strength required" Aikido tends to attract students who are less fit, or who have already been damaged in more extreme arts. But students who are injured attempting to learn to roll are students who tend to leave, never to return. Avoid both problems with awareness of underlying issues such as:

- **Poor fitness**. Abdominal strength is especially critical (see page 85).
- **Tight inflexible muscles**. See quadriceps (page 114 and page 153).
- **Heavy hips and thighs**. An issue of body shape (see page 138).
- **Dizziness**. It can come from tight muscles (see page 154).

Curling the torso , critical for safe rolling, requires abdominal strength. The student who can't curl at the very start of the roll must play catch-up for the rest of the roll. Roma Patrykus *Sensei* notes that non-athletic women in particular tend to lack abdominal strength. Men, athletic or not, tend to feel that they should do at least an occasional "crunch."

Tall men of average physical condition often have difficulty, perhaps because of a longer waist and longer abdominal space to control. In general, students unable to do even one bent-leg curl / sit-up[1] should not be thrown into rolling exercises until they have developed basic abdominal strength.

The person most at risk is the Tall Heavy Man. Often seen as unbreakable, he is made of the same tissue and may have no stronger bones or muscles than the smaller classmate.

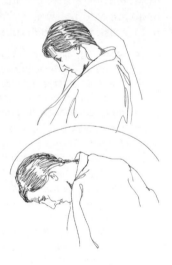

His high Center means that he is easily unbalanced. His greater mass makes bad falls exponentially more severe than for the smaller lighter students. To survive a fall, he needs *more* technique and *more* skill. A beginner simply doesn't have that.

Tight muscles can also inhibit the tucking and rounding critical for safe rolling. To protect the head and to round the neck and upper back, we usually think of tucking the chin. But that thought tends to stop at the chin and neck may be merely bent rather than rounded. Thinking of rolling and tucking the *forehead* is "rounder."

To round the neck,

1. Tuck chin into lateral (shoulder side) of your collarbone and look over shoulder.
2. Now think of rounding your forehead into your chest.
3. Notice any pull or strain which reveals tight muscles in need of attention.

---

1. Bent-leg situps require more abdominal effort.

Back Rolls

Back rolls are easiest to learn and least frightening to beginners. The motions are already familiar from lying down in bed or on a rug from a sitting position.

Backwards and Forwards

ADS #19, *Koho-tento-undo, "Rolling Backwards and Forwards"*

This is a simple rolling back and forth (*koho-tento-undo*) like a rocking chair. Sitting cross-legged with hands on thighs,

1. On count of One, roll backwards by rounding the lower back. Motion begins by rounding the lower back and dropping chin to chest. Focus on your belt knot.

   Do *not* begin by flinging back the head, an unsafe position. Be a ball, not a brick.

2. On count of Two, roll forward to original position. Focus on a point across the room.

   Hands remain on knees or thighs; they do not touch the mat.

   Tempted to use hands? Clap them.

   Respect the natural rhythm of the roll. Do not try to force yourself up by flinging the legs forward or arching the back (which means concave or flat instead of round).

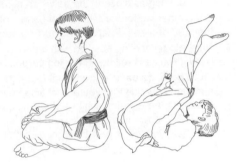

Variations:

- What motions roll you backward most effectively?
- What motions absorb excess energy?
- What motions return you to your original upright position with the least effort from you? Try rolling backward while:

  - Extending legs up rather than overhead.

  - Keeping legs extended.

  - Keeping legs tucked.

  - Tracing an arc in the air with your toe.

For smoother rolling, imagine . . .

- A goldfish bowl in your pelvis filled with water or liquid, white light. Roll and stand in such a way that you do not splash the water or disturb the fish.
- A rubber band stretching from your Center/One-Point to the opposite wall that allows you to roll back but helps you to come forward again.

What happens:

- If the near leg is not tucked?
- If the angle of the forward leg is greater than 90 degrees?
- If you place attention on things behind you while rolling, especially while coming up? Compare with extending your attention forward.

From here we will progress into full back rolls.

To prepare,

1. Roll back,
2. Touch toe to mat,
3. Experiment with the most comfortable position of head and neck. Notice that it will not be directly down the back of your head or over the nape of your neck.

   Finding the place where your head *is not* will ease transition to full back rolls.

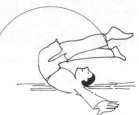

Backwards and Forwards to a Kneel

Roll back as in previous exercise, but on coming forward,

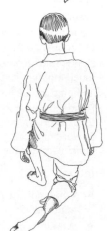

1. Tuck one leg as close to the pelvis as possible.
2. Bring other leg forward, bent at an angle of up to (but not greater than) 90 degrees. Push off with tucked back leg (not hands).
3. Rise into a kneeling position with back leg at an oblique angle to the body. (You can't roll back with leg perpendicular to the body).

   From here, it's easy to drop back to another backward roll or to rise and stand. Notice that you do not fling yourself backward. Drop Center/One-Point first, while curling into a ball. The motion is exactly like sitting down in a chair. You do not fling yourself backward into the chair, you lower your hips, *then* shift back.

Small Full Back Rolls

A complete back roll continues the motion of the beginning backward-forward roll. Dropping down from a kneel gives additional momentum.

To do a complete back roll,

1. Start from the kneeling position, left foot forward and left knee up, right knee and leg on the mat at an oblique angle to the body.
2. Look at your left knee. You will be "throwing" this left knee over your left shoulder.
3. Now look right, rock back and sit down beyond the mat leg while throwing your left leg over your left shoulder. Look at your right armpit. As hips go overhead, continue the motion by pushing off with left arm.
4. As you complete the roll, bring your left leg forward to the original starting position.

Variation

- Repeat small back rolls in series, two in a row, three in a row . . .
- Continue into non-stop back rolls around the mat.
- Alternate right and left sides to avoid the habit of rolling on just one side.
- Combine with *koho-tento-undo*, rising to one knee.

Back and Stand

This roll is similar to the previous back roll but ends standing. Rolling as above,

1. Tuck near leg as close to the pelvis as possible.
   Your body must pass *over* this leg in order to rise; you can't rise if the leg is in the way.
2. Roll back and up with leg still tucked and rise. Note that:
3. "Forward foot" refers to the forward foot of your starting *hanmi* position. If right *hanmi*, that will be the right foot; if left *hanmi*, it will be the left.
   Knees never touch the ground (i.e., get on your feet immediately by "kicking" the forward foot towards the ceiling.
   Arms are used only at the end of roll to push yourself to the upright position. Try to do it with no arms at all.

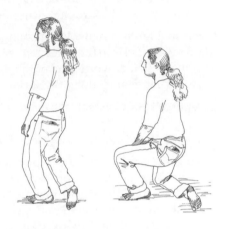

Rising one-legged from this roll is a good practice in coordination and balance. It builds thigh strength *and* helps clear the the hakama thus avoiding the dreaded "hakama toe."

Standing Back Rolls

Standing backward rolls are done like small backward rolls from the kneeling position except: place top of foot on mat, drop to the kneeling position and roll from there. Rather than angling the "sitting" leg, some styles, such as Yoshinkan, tuck the buttocks as close as possible to the heels. Try both options.

Forward Rolls

The Aikido roll (unlike the tumbling roll taught in schools) does not go straight down neck and back, but slightly sideways down the back of the arm (triceps), across the scaupla and mid-back to opposite hip. Head is tucked *away* from the rolling arm. This roll protects the nape of the neck and the spine so well that, properly done, it makes no difference whether you are rolling on a mat or on concrete as long as you are round.

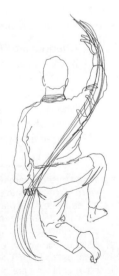

But few new students start out round. Demonstrate a roll and they see and copy the hand on the mat, the forward motion, the head going down towards the mat and then "pancake" — fall sideways collapsing into puddle of mat-hugging confusion.

Pancaking occurs when hips fail to rise above head and torso. Body falls or rolls to the side, rather than rolling down the line of arm and hip. This may be due to trying to support the entire roll with arms, or, the startling sensation of finding oneself upside down and apparently about ready to fall directly down, crashing headfirst into the mat. Panic!

It is not enough to keep Unbendable Arm while standing and concentrating on the far wall. Unbendable Arm requires learning to *relax*, to be calm, and to focus but the real problem is learning to *apply* those skills. "Advanced Students" are merely those who've learned to "Do the Exercise!" and put it back together again. Most people can do Unbendable Arm on walking into the dojo, but lose it completely in their first rolls or techniques. Rather than emphasizing "Unbendable Arm," consider emphasizing "Unbendable Arms In A Circle." Have student actually grasp right and left hands.

On the other hand, do not expect to support the full weight of the body on one arm, even an Unbendable one. Leave forward foot on the mat, supporting weight, until the last possible moment, until you are actually rolling.

Instructors should be very clear on exactly where the head is supposed to be, what the student should be looking at (belt, back leg, anything but the mat). Students should review this "pre-flight checklist" before every roll until it is automatic.

Even small rolls can involve crashing down on head or shoulder. The whole point of the forward roll is to translate vertical momentum (falling) into horizontal movement (rolling). In other words, never think of falling into the mat. Instead, imagine rolling forward, skimming along the surface of the mat.

Despite all your best efforts, however, safe rolling may come down to body type.

Forward Rolls, Balance and Body Type

As a group, the ones who separate shoulders and break collarbones tend to be women. This may be accepted with the notion that women are Naturally Less Fit than men. Yet female athletes who play soccer three times a week, with aerobics at lunch, who can run rings around males who are merely males and not male athletes, may spend years of their Judo or Aikido careers with chronic shoulder injuries.

Fitness and muscle development can be issues but so can different bone structure and weight distribution compared to men. Oddly, gender differences tend to be dismissed as "sexist[1]" or hotly denied — by both male and female martial artists. Nevertheless, the world of competitive and Olympic sports suggests a very different picture.

- **Children are "ITs."** Skeletal shape and proportions are essentially the same for girls and boys. The ones who excel in gymnastics are essentially balanced — like an apple — until puberty, around age 12 or 13, when bones, muscle, and body fat begin to change.
- **Olympic contenders in "Women's Gymnastics" are not women**. They are little girls who compete as long as their bodies are essentially the same as those of little boys[2]. When they begin to be shaped like *women* changes in weight distribution, balance and angular momentum cause disorienting changes in the dynamics of their rotating bodies.

---

1. When this topic arose on the Aikido-L Internet mailing list, several men (both student and instructor) were incredulous *that it was even possible to hit a shoulder while rolling*. At least one woman agreed with them but admitted to having a narrow-hipped boyish figure. Noting physical differences between the sexes tends to be denounced as *sexist*. Attributing a pattern of female injuries to female incompetence or poor conditioning is not. Go figure.
2. Strict division of style along gender lines means you will see no little-boy equivalent of little-girl gymnastics in the Olympics. Men's Gymnastics emphasizes strength and power that boys won't have until they are grown, hence there are no serious male competitors under about 20.

Their competitive gymnastics careers are usually over by the time they are 14 to 16 years old. This also applies to figure skaters; Olympic gold medalist Michelle Kwan shocked the skating world when she competed successfully at the advanced age of 22, but in order to do so she had to change her entire program.

- **All Bodies change**. Roma Patrykus observes that adults who have the most difficulties in Judo and Aikido are not the ones who *never* studied. It's the men who played Judo as *children*. They wired all the moves into muscle memory — then stopped. When they return as adults, the skills they learned in the body of a *boy* no longer work in the body of a *man*. And they get hurt.

For women in martial arts the problem seems to be:

- **Male bodies are the martial arts norm**. In Judo and Aikido the proportion of male to female arts students tends to run about 6:1 and greater. Women roll as they have been taught although with experience, they learn to make the necessary adjustments in mid-air[1]. With time, upper-level females learn to initiate the roll best suited to their body type. Unfortunately, the chance of most females having an upper-level female instructor is fairly low and few others are aware of the differences.

- **The Master taught it this way**. The Master may have been a short Japanese man who started Judo as a child. Until recently, most Japanese men were about 5' 4"[2], women shorter, in a culture remarkable for its physical *uniformity* and where Judo was standard Physical Education in school. Uniform body type is characteristic of all restricted cultures from the Alps to backwoods Kentucky but the urban American "melting-pot" has bodies with wide variations in height and proportion.

- **Either / Or Thinking**. "I'm a male / female so this doesn't apply to me!" In adults it isn't necessarily an issue of "male / female" but of variations along the body-build spectrum. There is a continuum of human body configurations, of height, width and proportion. It's the body build and fitness that counts.

Roma Patrykus and Fred Strathman are sixth *dan* instructors in Tomiki Aikido, with extensive Judo backgrounds. This husband and wife team report arguing for years about the "proper way to roll" until they realized that their different rolling styles were due to their different bodies. Their classes are the best I have ever seen for acknowledging and dealing with varying body mechanics[3]. The following material on body type and rolling is based on their investigations. See if it works for you.

---

1. "A mid-air Athletic Event," says Roma Patrykus
2. Minimum height for the Japanese Army was 5' 2". Aikido founder Moriehei Ueshiba couldn't qualify until he spent a night hanging by his feet to stretch out his spine.
3. Their classes in Karl Geiss Tomiki Aikido are in College Park, MD.

The Body Type Continuum

Between the Extreme Male and Extreme Female there is a continuum of weight and proportion.

- **Children**. Especially those good at gymnastics who have not yet differentiated sexually.
- **The Extreme Female**. Narrow shoulders and broad heavy hips (a *pear* shape, a.k.a "Hips of the Goddess"). Weight and Center of Gravity are low. A man with a powerful "basketball butt" and enormous muscular thighs[1] is closer to this than to extreme male.

The Extreme Male. Narrow hips and wide shoulders (broccoli-oidal). Weight and Center of Gravity are high. Idealized in body builders and Marvel Comics. Rare in athletes (other than swimmers) for whom a bulky upper body is an unnecessary or unbalanced load. The current (comic book) ideal woman with broad shoulders, huge breasts and snake hips is closer to the extreme male than to female.

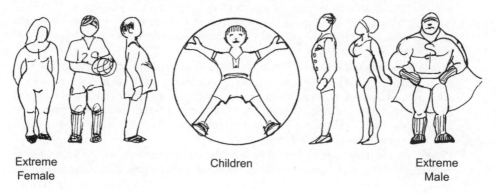

Extreme
Female

Children

Extreme
Male

Exercises and Experiments

One-Point or Center or Hara is traditionally said to be two inches below the naval. But it varies from person to person. If you still don't believe these differences are real, then there's nothing to do but see — and test — for yourself. Here are some exercises that demonstrate the differences in body type, body mechanics, and finding (or changing the location of) Center.

Chair Lift

This classic party trick is based on the different distributions of weight and center of gravity between different bodies. The classic prop is a simple straight-backed chair so subject need not bend over.

1. Stand with heels against the wall and lift chair by back.
2. Observe which bodies can lift the chair — or not.

---

1. This would describe a sprinter in track or soccer, or a basketball player whose powerful legs are everything for running and jumping but upper body weight is a relatively useless load.

    For a beautiful and illuminating study of the continuum of adult human bodies, see *Athlete* by Howard Schatz. Notice distribution of weight and muscle, the widely differing centers. Notice that you can *predict* the sport at which the subject excels based on body build.

As variation, stand with heels against the wall and try to touch your toes. See "The Ma-ai of Balance and Flexibility" on page 189. The physics behind this impossible feat is the same physics behind many seemingly impossible throws.

Weighting

An exercise in *changing* body mechanics. Highly recommended for instructors.

1. With weight belt and / or vest and 5-10 pound weights,
2. Observe the differences in rolling and basic technique with:
   - Weight belt at lower hips, mid-hip, waist.
   - Weight loaded around chest, shoulders.

     Warning! Differences may be extreme! Consider wearing a padded motorcycle jacket (with padded shoulders) until you adapt to the differences.

Leaning and Reaching

Another example requires only a belt and *uke*.

With *uke* holding *nage*'s belt and braced for weight support,

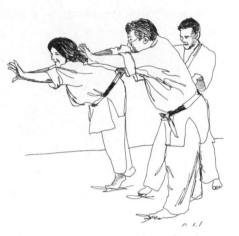

1. *Nage* see how far it is possible to reach forward before losing balance.
   Uke is not there to hold *nage* up but for safety and to allow nage the opportunity to push to the edge of balance and hold it there long enough for observers to see what is happening.
   - Observe which bodies can lean or reach the furthest and when foot leaves mat.
   - Repeat this experiment with weight belt/ vest (see "Weighting," above).

Male and Female Rolls

See which positions work best for your own body type. Starting position is on one knee, one leg extended to side and fingers pointed inward. Ending is a rollout with slap for ease of illustration.

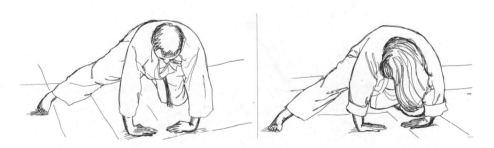

What works for "Male"

1. Reach out, shifting weight forward of belt towards shoulders.

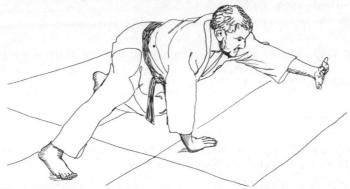

2. As weight shifts forward, tuck for the roll by reaching straight *between* the legs.

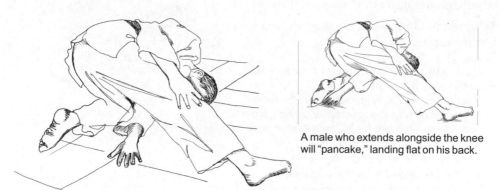

A male who extends alongside the knee will "pancake," landing flat on his back.

Notice the feeling of instability. Stefan, who posed for this picture, found it extremely difficult to hold the position long enough for me to shoot it. Exactly as it should be!

3. Roll, ending slightly to one side.

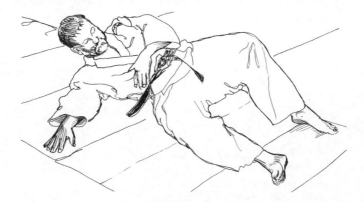

What works for "Female"

From starting position,

1. Tuck forehead, but do *not* reach *forward*. Instead . . .

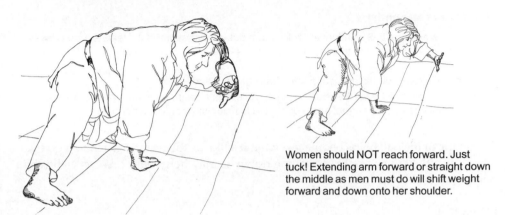

Women should NOT reach forward. Just tuck! Extending arm forward or straight down the middle as men must do will shift weight forward and down onto her shoulder.

2. Extend arm at an *oblique* angle, down one side alongside knee . . .

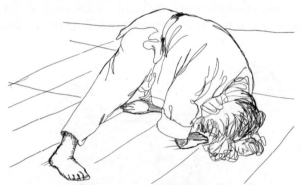

3. Notice the tipping point where you go from being on balance to off balance. Slowly move past that tipping point and release your body into the roll.

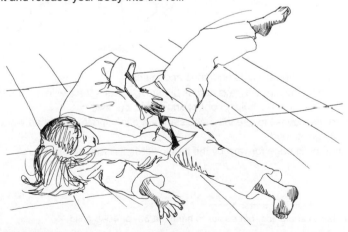

Beachball Rolls

Students are often told to "imagine rolling over a big beach ball." So try using a real ball. Aikidoist Scott Crawford (Yoshinkan) reports that the PhysioBall (about 3 feet/ a meter in diameter) is a wonderful tool for teaching forward rolls to kids[1].

With partner as spotter,

1. Child lies over the ball with forward rolling arm out in front as normal. Head is turned away from the rolling hand and tucked as much as possible around the ball and away from the rolling arm.
2. Hold child from side by legs, supporting back of neck and head.
3. Slowly roll the ball forward by pushing the child's legs forward until balance is broken and gravity takes over. Be careful not to dump the kid sideways onto his/her back.

The shape of the ball helps people feel what it's like to "be round" when you go over. Also, since they're basically just laying down, it may help them relax as well while helping to build body memory.

Horse Rolls

If you don't have a big enough ball or are working with full-grown adults, the following exercise helps ease the student into the position, the process and the unfamiliar sensation of being upside down in a slow and carefully controlled way. In groups of three,

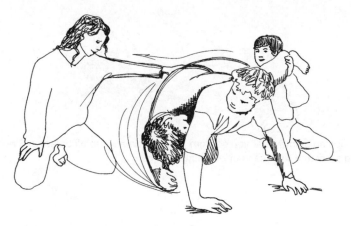

1. One *uke* ("the horse") gets on hands and knees.
2. *Nage* (the rolling student) lays across the first partner's back with the intent of sliding forward and off. This provides height control and speed control.
3. Second *uke* checks to see that nage's arms are in a circle, that head, shoulder, and back are correctly positioned.
4. *Uke* then pulls *nage* forward by the belt towards the mat and into a roll.

---

1. Applicable to adults too, but easier to handle a 30- or 40-lb child.

Nage will,

1. Slide forward over "horse" placing hand of right Unbendable Arm on mat. (Or join hands forming arms into a large circle).
2. Tuck and turn neck and head away from the rolling arm (to the left) sliding towards the mat.
3. Feel for the tipping point where balance is lost and body begins to move with gravity.

   A student tried this roll at her dojo but was unenthusiastic when I asked her how it went. "I hurt my neck again," she sighed. How? Why? Because her instructor's version was: "Take terrified student, have her dive over kneeling *uke*" — rather than moving slowly and gradually. *The explicit purpose of this exercise is slow, gentle practice in feeling roundness and correct hand, arm, and head position.*

Variations:

> Try the above exercise at home with a helper, rolling off a pile of sofa cushions or the edge of a low bed or couch, forward onto another cushion for safety.

Upside-Down Rolls

Much fear of rolling is the fear of being upside down. Children or small adults may have a parent or partner who is tall enough or strong enough to simply hold them upside down by their ankles, slightly back of vertical, then lower them carefully and under complete control, to the mat.

As in Horse Rolls, the second partner checks for proper position of arms, head and neck. *Nage* curls into a roll as *uke* lowers *nage* to the mat.

Do this carefully and under control. The point is to develop confidence in positions required for rolling, to help mind / body understand that it will not break or die merely if upside down for a few seconds.

Small Individual Forward Rolls

With the foregoing preparation, students should be ready to practice forward rolls individually, noting any rough spots. A hard thump at the small of the back or hip means the back is not round enough. Thinking of touching knee to nose or looking at the belt while rolling helps to maintain roundness. Are you rolling down the arm, or landing splat onto the shoulder? Note and adjust.

> Imagine "pumpkins falling off the back of a truck." Some will land hard and go splat while others will skitter along turning smoothly.
>
> —Philip Akin, Aikido Yoshinkan Canada

But what happened to the injured and frustrated lady on page 130?

> Brad, a new student and Judo black belt, asked politely, "Have you tried these yet?" and does this tiny little Judo roll where you put your shoulder on the ground and one leg forward and roll.There was silence. "Umm, do that again?!" she said.
> She tried it, lived through it, and then Bob Sensei laughed and made her do 50 of them. She wasn't even in pain the next day!
>
> —L. J.

The 6-Count Rolling Exercise

This exercise is a series of forward and backward rolls performed in a specific sequence to a strict count. It provides rolling practice, but also offers useful *distraction*: striving to keep in sequence and rhythm leaves little time and attention to spare anguishing over an individual roll while improving skill and flow. A new student who was having trouble with individual rolls described this as:

"Awesome! No time to stop and think, especially of all the reasons why I can't do this. I'm too busy trying to remember the pattern, and keep the rhythm. And I'm rolling!"

Instructor calls the count and the class rolls in unison.

1. Rock back into Rocking-Chair "roll" (*koho-tento-undo*).
2. Rock forward rising to one knee and continuing into . . .
3. Forward roll then back into . . .
4. Back roll. On coming up . . .
5. Rock back (*koho-tento-undo*) . . . then
6. Rock forward to return to starting position.

Cross-Rolls

Cross-rolls (*zempo-kaiten waza*) are forward rolls begun with left knee up and right arm on mat. In the Ki Society, the first test requires three of these small rolls done in series while maintaining the same arm/leg relationships.

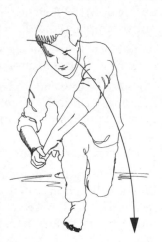

Years ago Tohei noticed that beginners did cross-rolls naturally. He adapted the test to accommodate this roll. But beginners usually adapt so quickly to moving arm with leg that going back to the cross roll seems awkward. Nevertheless, one must learn to roll from either position. To eliminate confusion between right and left, start your practice with a sock on the "rolling" foot.

Standing Forward Rolls

Standing forward rolls are done in the same way as small forward rolls except that you must first drop down to kneeling position. Keep your forward foot on the ground until you are actually rolling over your shoulder.

These should be done only after the student is comfortable with small rolls and has demonstrated a good round circle. They should grow gradually.

Diving rolls cover the greatest distance. Although it seems contrary to every instinct, you must extend out for maximum distance then assume the correct rolling position rolling in air before you contact the mat. How you think of the roll also matters.

Not a falling rock, but a landing airplane.
Not falling into the mat, but skimming over it, just passing through.

With these images in mind, aim for a specific point, extend and go there.

I dreaded rolling for years. With chronic migraine and neck problems, I was always trying to protect my head and neck, not yet realizing that what I was doing did not protect but only made me stiff and tense, perpetuating the cycle.

One year while assistant-teaching, the county Adult Recreation Department class was mis-scheduled and replaced with children's Aikido classes. I dreaded them. They were like the "Toon Town" scene in *Roger Rabbit* with children too young and too many. But what can you do when a small child goes through the motions of a throw? — except let out a shriek and go diving across a mat crowded by little people who would be squashed flat if I hit them. Suddenly I was more concerned about extending out and over and through to that particular open spot right *over there* than I was about my head. And suddenly the rolls were smooth and soft and magical.

An amazing lesson. If concentrating on the roll or on me, it falls flat. If projecting out, concentrating on a larger circle, a larger goal, it works. Beautifully.

—C.M.S.

Rolling in the Air

You will often see an experienced *uke* tilt the head back then fling it forward to start a roll. The weight of the head adds energy to the roll where energy is lacking and helps keep *uke* safe[1]. *Uke* is rolling long before the first touch of the mat. Eventually arms are not needed at all and become less for weight-bearing, more for simply feeling and sensing the exact location of the mat — sometimes in surprising ways.

An Aikidoist from New England Aikikai told me that she attended a seminar at Montreal one winter. It was bitter cold but well-attended, so in short order the room was steaming and wet like a sauna. When they opened the door for air, cold dry air met supersaturated hot air. Presto! Fog! — of the ground-hugging variety. Those who were thrown were landing blind, and those throwing would watch their partners disappear into the mist and re-emerge meters away.

—Janet Rosen, Aikikai

Jo Rolls

Combine *jo* practice with rolling practice. Good throwing practice for nage and a wonderful aid to helping *uke* learn to roll. Here's why.

One doesn't "fall" when rolling, one provides forward, circular energy and *then* rolls. Many folks dive into the mat, never letting their hips raise up in the air to form the "rolling circle." Instead they dive forward *into* the mat. This puts part of their circle below the surface of the mat and creates a problem.

Once I had a student who just didn't grasp the idea of rolling so I had him grasp the end of a *jo* then I described a large, vertical circle in the air. His hand was taken upward, outward and matward. His body followed and he did one heck of a good roll. As he bounced up he said, "Is that all??"

I think he had built up in his mind that it was a very complicated, multi-muscle direction thing and he could not organize all the parts at one time. When he found that was not true he was just fine. This can be illustrated by tying a ribbon on to the end of a *jo*. If the tip of the *jo* moves in a circle, the ribbon does too.

—George Simcox, Ki Society

---

1. There can be problems with the head-flinging technique. See page 154.

Breakfalls

Rolling extends and continues energy enabling *uke* to land safely on his feet ready for the next attack. A throw with enough energy and forward momentum can be thought of as "help in getting back up." But sometimes it simply isn't possible or safe to roll. Breakfalls absorb and neutralize energy by placing as much surface area as possible in contact with the ground at one time. No one point hits the mat. It is a full-body *splat* — full arm, full side, and flatfoot — that spreads energy over a wide area rather than concentrating it all on the point of a shoulder, heel, chin. Some pointers:

- **Do not cross legs with contact**. Ankles may bump, bruise, or chip. Men may suffer other painful results as the upper leg comes crashing down.
- **Practice repeated breakfalls on forgiving surfaces only**. Limit extensive breakfalls to crash pads, sprung floors, or other yielding surfaces. Breakfalls reduce the *potential* for severe injury. They do not not necessarily *eliminate* injury entirely. Some take great pride in how far they can repeatedly breakfall onto concrete and still walk away; others believe anything less than 300 breakfalls a night to be less than Serious Practice. Injury may not be visible as broken bones but it may still exist as repetitive microtrauma and possibly brain damage. It takes far less force to tear neurons than to tear blood vessels.
- **Stay properly fed and watered**. Dehydration and nutritional deficiencies set you up for internal injury. Vitamin C deficiency and anemia allow capillary breakage and bruising. If your gums bleed when you brush your teeth ("pink toothbrush"), you may risk internal bleeding (brain or body) from every hard brush with the mat.

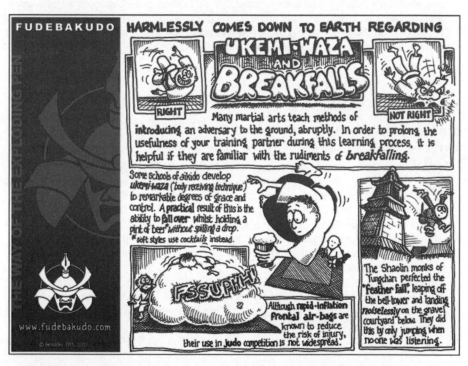

—Reproduced by kind permission of David Whitehead. See www.fudebakudo.com.

Rolling Side to Side

This very beginning exercise enables the new student to practice the feel of a breakfall and correct positioning of body, arms, and legs in the safest manner possible. In a slightly more advanced version ("fish-flops") hips and legs are lifted off the mat in the course of the movement. Because the body moves across the mat, this exercise can be used as a game or relay race for children or adults.

1. Lie on back with chin tucked to chest
2. Roll to the right, striking mat smartly with flat of right arm and right palm.
3. Roll to the left, striking mat smartly with flat of left arm and left palm..

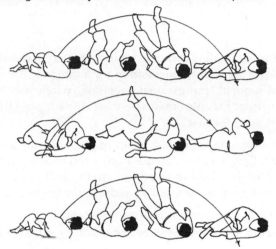

Arm-Pull

A good beginning exercise for breakfalls. It allows *uke* to learn at his own pace, the "unfurling" action as you turn in the air is natural, and you pretty much land in the "correct" landing position.This exercise provides an actual fall but still allows a low-stress and relatively low energy check for body position and timing. Aim to land more on your side than on your back. In a more dynamic fall, landing flat on your back will knock the wind out of you.With *nage* on hands and knees,

1. *Uke* reaches under nage's body to his opposite arm.
2. *Uke* pulls arm towards him, flipping *nage* into a breakfall. Another exercise from the same beginning position is to unfurl not sideways but "over your head," sort of a mid-air front roll and land. It's a bit more advanced, but more what you should be doing in a front breakfall (instead of rolling out to the side).

—Jun Akiyama

Rollout

A "roll-out" begins with a standard forward roll, but ends in breakfall position. This introduces the feel of breakfall in motion, and helps develop good positioning.

Breakfall Over Partner

This step adds height but adds it safely. In groups of three with a crash-pad,

1. One partner with belt, is on hands and knees.
2. Student slides hand palm-up under kneeling partner's *obi* for stability.
3. Instructor or other partner applies *kote-gaeshi* flipping student onto crash pad.

Breakfall With Jo

"Gaining height" for breakfall is contrary to almost every natural instinct. But, it's good physics. It allows *uke* to get into position for a safe fall. You will see this demonstrated again and again in "professional wrestling" where *nage* helps *uke* vault off his back or thighs in order to come down safely into the supposedly devastating (but mostly just noisy) slam to the mat[1].

In a breakfall from a *kote-gaeshi* (a wrist technique which may involve diving over *nage*'s arm) you are falling 3-4 feet. Practice from a roll means you've practiced only from a few inches of height. This exercise allows individual practice from *any* height, controlled by the position of the student's hands on the lower end of the *jo*.

- Use a T-shirt or *gi* to protect the mat from the edge of the jo.
- Use a crashpad to cushion falls that will be higher than the student has been accustomed to taking.

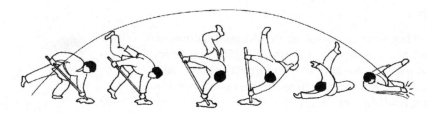

Ukemi from Ikkyo

A slightly different technique is possible for *ikkyo* techniques in which you are diving forward to the mat, secured by one arm. *Ukemi* for this technique is a sort of modified forward breakfall[2].

In *ikkyo*, it is common to see *uke* flopping down to the mat with full weight on the kneecaps just prior to transferring weight to the wrist at the end of a nearly vertical arm. This may work on the mat but would have devastating results on street or sidewalk: a shattered kneecap, a broken wrist. Instead,

---

1. See "Exposed! Pro-Wrestling's Greatest Secrets (Don Wiener, 1998)" on page 262 of this manual.
2. See also BA p. 40-41.

On falling forward,

1. Drop to knee and shin (not just kneecap) of inside leg.
2. Fully extend the outside leg. The extended leg provides a counterbalance which prevents your *full* weight from transferring to hand and forearm. As weight transfers forward,
3. Place entire forearm (not just the wrist) on the mat and extended forward. Arm is Unbendable and slides forward with body.

   Grasping the cuff of the *gi* before taking the fall prevents mat burns.

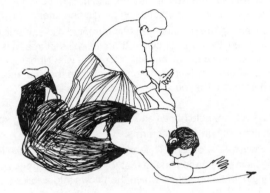

The following version is limited to persons whose bellies do not extend significantly beyond their thighs. Hence, it is unsuitable for pregnant women or for men of similar configuration. On falling forward,

1. Extend the outside arm with knife edge of hand towards mat (thumb up). Simultaneously,
2. Kick heels up and back as if trying to kick yourself in the fanny.

   This aligns the entire lower body so that impact is spread across the extended forearm, torso, and thighs. Kneecaps are tucked safely out of the way.

   I like *ikkyo* because it offers the most control over an untrained *uke* who doesn't have to know how to take a flying *ukemi* for me to get *uke* safely to the ground and pinned.

   —Peter W. Boylan

Rolling Exercises and Games

Games are not just for children, and they are valuable not just for fun but because the student's focus is diverted elsewhere. Often, the best beginning exercises are those that provide some sort of distraction. Reframe the fear of falling into love of flying via a shift in attention. In the Six-count Rolling Exercise (page 146), it's the next roll in the series. In Rolling Tag and Maximum/Minimum it's the contest. In 50 Rolls it's sheer exhaustion versus critical conservation of energy.

- **Rolling Tag**. Kids love this and although some instructors think it unseemly for adult dignity (or their own), adults have a great time too. As in any other game of tag, choose someone to be "It" and chase the others, but only with rolls or knee walking (*shikkyo*).
- **Minimum/Maximum**. Who can cover the length of the mat in the fewest rolls? Who can fit the largest number of small rolls along the length of the mat? (Tip: Try cross-rolls!)
- **50 Rolls**. Roll back and forth in alternating directions without pause. Key to success (or survival) is to not stand up between rolls. Instead, rise partway then turn and fall. Use the

momentum to bring you back up so that you can fall again. Vary by working as *uke* with two partners practicing *zempo* throws. *Uke* rolls back and forth between the two.

- **Forward Rolling Nonstop**. There is a tendency to separate motions and undertakings into individual parts. This exercise emphasizes continuous rolling. Do not stop between rolls, just keep rolling. Not Roll, stand, and ponder but Roooolllllllll2lllllllll3lllllllll. Combine with Obstacle Course.

- **Obstacle Course**. An exercise in revealing and changing mindset. Once students learn to roll, place an obstacle in the way. It may be: a *jo* held out by the instructor, a rag on the mat, a body or series of bodies laid flat or on hands and knees.

  Also useful for observing the peculiar games your mind plays, panic at the supposed impediment even when it is lower or closer than the roll requires. It is a *perceived* barrier, not a real one. The exercise is: roll anyway. Combine with Nonstop Rolls in a circle around the mat. Scatter more laundry or bodies around the mat, use the in-between spaces for target practice. Do you notice any difference in the rolls? How do you overcome that?

- **Rolling in Pairs**. Partners hold hands and roll in tandem, matching speed (and direction). They must, of course, roll on opposite arms.

- **Rolling With a Sword (Yokomen)**. This exercise provides practice in overcoming dependency on placing the hands on the mat to roll. The oblique *yokomen* strike provides the downward beginning momentum which then flows into a roll.

- **Parking Lot Rolls**. For the experienced upper belt who has forgotten how terrifying rolls are to beginners: practice rolls (carefully!) on concrete or asphalt in jeans and T-shirt. Useful as a demo to the performer and to the observer that "this stuff really works ("On The Street" and on concrete) and is not just a function of mats or magic clothes. Especially for circular rolls, once the techniques and dynamics of rolling have been mastered it doesn't really matter whether the "wheel" of your body rolls over a mat or over asphalt.

- **Water Rolls**. Eliminate mats, pads, and hard ground by rolling into water at the beach or the edge of a pool. Notice the sensation of cool water moving up your neck, back and hips. Notice the path it takes. You can't roll across the surface of course, but you can get the feeling of hips going over head.

I did breakfalls in the surf the other day. Got the kids a little too excited though. They didn't want us to stop. NB: Eliminate the slap. — Tarik J. Ghbeish

Had fun with a friend from class this weekend. He practiced throws that would need breakfalls on land. I got to take them as flip/dive forward or back in the water.

I am so at home in the water and it was cool not to think about how I was landing. Did lose the diagonal feel but it worked without a thought. — N. B. R.

For more variations, nuances, and good solid information, see Bruce Bookman's DVDs on *ukemi* and advanced *ukemi*.

For application of falling and rolling in actual throws and techniques, see "Nage and Uke — Partners in the Dance" on page 177.

Injuries

Bones

Collarbones and Shoulder Injuries

> I thought I could do a couple of rolls. As I went over, I was still a bit hesitant, and so I didn't keep my arm round enough to roll on it, which resulted in, that tell-tale crunch! pop! I got up quickly, frantic, saying to my *sensei*, "I broke it again. No! No! I broke it again!"
> *Sensei*, thinking I was overreacting, said soothingly, "No you didn't. Lift your arm above your head." I did so with ease.
> Sensei: "If it were broken you wouldn't be able to do that."
> Me, still frantic and wanting nothing more than to turn back time: "No, I felt it pop! It's broken! I bleeping broke it again!"
> *Sensei*: "Shoulders pop and make weird sounds all the time. You're OK."
> —A student just back after 6 weeks off the mat with a broken collarbone, and yes, a second break.

Ability to raise the arm in a suspected collarbone break depends on the nature of the break. Unless the bone is broken completely through, offset, and/or poking through the skin, athletic persons can have a broken clavicle and remarkable range of motion because of stabilization by the surrounding muscles. Arm-raising can compress the fracture rather than pulling the pieces (painfully) apart.

Instructors and their students owe it to themselves to understand possible injuries and consequences. However, in general, don't be diagnosing OK-ness or treatment without the training and experience that requires.

Obviously there's another issue here: just back from a major injury is not the time to dive right back into the action that caused the first injury.

Pelvic Distortions

One of the most insidious and unrecognized injuries in falling is pelvic distortion.

The pelvis is not a rigid block of bone, it is three separate bones joined by shock-absorbing fibrocartilage (see illustration on page 120). These joints were long considered immovable, a notion coming from centuries of studies on cadavers. There is very good reason why these pickled remains are referred to as "stiffs" but in live folk, the situation is different[1].

The joints move allowing the pelvis to torque, twist, and tilt in normal daily life in response to muscle tension[2]. They also move when the pelvis suffers impact from planets and other moving bodies. As a three-part structure, it is impossible for any one piece to be misaligned without distorting the other two which in turn distorts the

---

1. As for skull sutures, pelvic joints can be immobile but this condition is considered by many to be pathological. A locked sacroiliac joint has been linked to chronic spasm of the hamstrings.
2. Tight adductors, gluteal muscles, hamstrings, piriformis and rectus femoris (one of the quadriceps) are particularly likely to shift the pelvis.

spine. One bad fall can cause pain and dysfunction for years because when the pelvis is wrong, everything above it is going to be wrong.

Something is definitely wrong whenthe crests of the hip bones or the dimples at lower back are at different heights, or one side of the pubic bone is higher than the other.

A good chiropractor or osteopath[1] is an important part of your sports bag. Putting the pieces back where they belong will relieve pain and dysfunction in a way that muscle relaxants, pain relievers, and other pills and potions can never do.

"Knobbies" and Knee Pain

Pain from repeated blows to the "knobbies" of the lower back[2] is commonly known as "the knobbies." It may be suffered after too many breakfalls by skinny people who lack padding or by well-padded people falling onto too-hard surfaces.

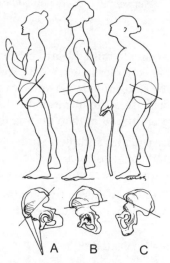

The knobbies can also develop from ordinary rolls on good mats; if the pelvis is rotated forward it can be almost impossible to round the back fully. This can occur due to tight rectus femoris and adductor muscles. Anterior pelvic rotation produces sway-back (often mistaken for "big butt"), can cause abdominal contents to shift forward ("big gut") and can also be responsible for knee pain in *seiza*.

A quick test for anterior pelvic rotation is to lie flat on a firm surface. Soft tissue blends. Bone does not. If there is a tunnel under the waist, where you can slide a hand (or arm) with ease, you may have found the source of your "knobbies" (and maybe even knee pain; see page 114).

The pelvis rotates forward (A) due to pull by the rectus femoris, tensor fascia lata, sartorius, and adductor muscles.

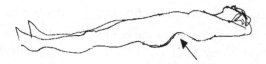

Dizziness

Sometimes dizziness is simply a matter of getting used to the disorienting feeling of being upside down or spinning through the air. But sometimes dizziness comes directly from the sternocleidomastoid (SCM) muscle of the neck.

---

1. American osteopaths have largely lost the manipulative skills for which they were once renowned. Look for D.O.M. licensing, a separate degree program of training in manipulative skills. Cranio-sacral therapists are trained in some osteopathic techniques. Find a therapist near you at Upledger.com but look for the ones with three or more classes especially those who have done visceral work. Cranio-sacral therapy 101 is not enough.
2. These are the dimples at adjacent to the sacro-iliac joint of the lower back. They are actually anatomical high points, the "posterior superior iliac spines."

SCM is the big ropy muscle that runs from behind your ear (from the mastoid process, the rounded bump) to the joint between collarbones and sternum at the base of your throat. This paired muscle pulls the head forward and down, and prevents the head from falling backward. Both actions are involved in tucking the head for rolling. Thus it may be strained by tucking, as well as by headlocks, and by "neck-a-nage[1]."

SCM receives nerve motor fibers from the spinal accessory nerve and fibers from the vagus nerve which wanders about the body to the viscera and heart. A tight SCM, clamping down on its own nerve supply, can cause an amazing range of symptoms: nausea, motion sickness, bad balance, headache, even tinnitus and teary eyes. These are commonly mistaken for inner-ear problems, migraine, sinus headache, trigeminal neuralgia and more. Yet despite having one of the most extensive patterns of pain and dysfunction, SCM is one of the easiest muscles to self-treat. Students who have suffered years of chronic dizziness may improve remarkably in minutes.

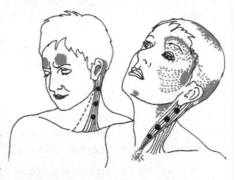

Sternal and clavicular SCM pain patterns.

The SCM is easily tested simply by gently grasping the body of the muscle. A relaxed, pliable SCM will perceive the squeeze as pressure, but not pain. A tense, hard muscle will be painful, and may even produce the referred pain patterns shown here.

To treat the sternocleidomastoid,

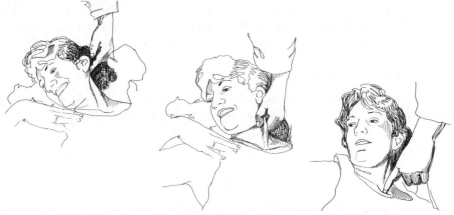

1. Look for a tender spot at the mastoid process, the bump behind the ear.
   Apply gentle pressure until perception of "pain" or "tenderness" decreases to "pressure" only. Repeat down the muscle to the point where you can actually grasp the muscle between thumb and index finger. Do not press or squeeze anything that pulses.
2. Using thumb and the *side* of finger as shown, grasp muscle and squeeze gently.

---

1. For details, see http://round-earth.com/HeadPainIntro.html

3. Continue to sternum, feeling around the inside of the notch for tender points.
4. Repeat for clavicular division of the muscle which attaches to the upper side of the clavicle.

Be sure to grasp the *muscle*, not just the skin. In healthy athletic persons, this muscle will be much larger and deeper than you think. It should be as pliable as any other healthy muscle, but in some — especially in those with dizziness problems, it is often rock hard.

Warning!
The mastoid process is the large rounded bump behind the ear. Below the ear and the angle of the jaw is a small spur of bone, the *styloid process*. It is relatively fragile. Do NOT press in this area!

Headaches and Neck Pain

Headaches and neckaches were a big part of my experience in learning to roll. The exercises presented here should ease the process of purely mechanical bumps and thumps. However, headaches may occur due to muscle strain in unexpected places.

Trapezius headache is illustrated on page 112. Avoiding this headache is a good reason to relax your shoulders—in sword work, with cell phones, bags, or purses. The TrP shown sends pain up the neck and around the temple. Other trapezius TrPs send pain to the back, to the base of the skull, and out to the acromioclavicular joint. Trapezius may also fire off the temporalis and masseter muscles producing a deep aching pain in the molar teeth.

Sternocleidomastoid (SCM) is commonly strained in the course of tucking and the pain that results is mistaken for "sinus." See discussion on dizziness (page 155).

Posterior neck muscles are strained in the course of attempting to walk out of a roll in a stooped position but holding head forward—like a bowling ball on the end of a stick— rather than allowing it to drop down naturally. This strains the trapezius, the suboccipitals, and other muscles which contribute to headaches.

Shoulder / Arm Pain and Tingly Fingers

Aikidoists commonly strain scalene muscles through repeated forceful tucking of the head for rolling. "Neck-a-nage" throws are also dangerous (see page 214).

> So dangerous is this move considered to be to the necks of large, heavily muscled, and extremely physically fit men, that its use in a professional football game results in an automatic 15-yard penalty.
>
> —P. F. Kozey

Dangerous how? Injury to the neck with many possible neurovascular consequences. An experienced instructor (notorious for his emphasis on "controlling *uke*'s head") once gave me a herniated disk. The more common injury of strained neck muscles, particularly the scalenes, is no picnic either.

Problems begin when scalenes tighten compressing blood vessels and the nerves of the brachial plexus which supplies branches to chest and upper back. Problems are exacerbated by a tight pectoralis minor muscle, which the brachial plexus must squeeze under on its way to supply the arm and fingers.

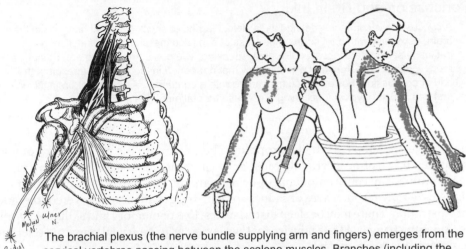

The brachial plexus (the nerve bundle supplying arm and fingers) emerges from the cervical vertebrae passing between the scalene muscles. Branches (including the median nerve responsible for Carpal Tunnel Syndrome) must then tunnel under the pectoralis minor muscle of the shoulder with the axillary artery. Pain patterns for scalenes and entrapped nerves extend from chest to back to arm to fingers. Pain from pectoralis minor alone tends to run down the inside of the arm as far as the 4th and 5th fingers; it is heavily involved in Thoracic Outlet Syndrome.

These anatomical relationships are often responsible for symptoms of Carpal Tunnel Syndrome and Thoracic Outlet Syndrome — the reason why carpal tunnel surgery is so often unhelpful[1].

Symptoms range from tingling of thumb and index fingers to brutal pain in shoulder, upper back, down arms to fingers, with fingerlike projections of pain in chest (where it may be mistaken for a heart attack). Victims may receive a diagnosis of Carpal Tunnel Syndrome (CTS) or Thoracic Outlet Syndrome (TOS). They may be be referred for radical surgery which involves removal of one or two of the three scalene muscles and removal of the first and possibly part of the second rib. The surgery is remarkable for painful side effects and often poor relief rates[2]. It is a high price to pay for being sloppy with someone else's neck or with your own.

---

1. Scalenes are also strained by bad posture, chest breathing, playing the violin, and swimming the crawl. There are at least half a dozen reasons for carpal tunnel syndrome (tingling or numbness in the thumb and forefinger). Scalenes and pectoralis minor muscles are the most likely and of all the possibilities, the carpal tunnel itself is dead last.

2. For more information on scalenes (and pain patterns arising from other neck muscles) see: www.round-earth.com/HeadPainIntro.html. For self-treatment, see Davies (2004). For medical background, see Travell & Simons (1999).

Concussion and Brain Injury

A *concussion* is commonly defined as "a violent jarring or shock." When it happens to the brain, especially with brief or prolonged loss of consciousness or bodily function, a patient is said to be *concussed*. Properly speaking, you don't arrive at the emergency room with a concussion; that was the blow that happened in the past. As a result of the earlier concussion, however, you may arrive with a *contusion* — bruising of brain tissue that can impair physical functioning and cause mental/emotional problems.

—Dr. Wendy Gunther

Injuring your brain is much like dropping a hammer onto the motherboard of your computer. It will almost certainly cause some amount of damage. Even a very minor head trauma may cause emotional upheavals and mood swings for a week or more. These may range from waves of sadness or hair-trigger anger to a lowered tolerance for frustration. There may be sleep disturbances, loss of memory and skills, ADD, and personality changes. Head injuries that we consider to be trivial may cause serious symptoms for years onward.

The human computer is a truly wonderful computer in that it is self-healing, but it does not heal in the ways that people often think it should. For example, it is not helpful to push getting back on the mat after a head injury. Trying to "work through" the pain, nausea, or dizziness is no more sensible than trying to repair your laptop computer by hitting the motherboard again with more hammers. Doing so is dangerous to the point of equipment dysfunction, or to the point of fatal error.

Always treat head injuries gently and properly. But what is proper treatment?

Concussions are traditionally classified based on confusion, amnesia, and loss of consciousness. However, consciousness is controlled by the brain stem; one can suffer severe injury to other parts of the brain yet remain fully conscious. And return to activity must not depend on schedules, tests or game dates but on healing.

Now that symptoms of healing (or lack of it) are tested and tracked by computerized testing systems, traditional guidelines for concussion have been thrown into serious doubt. Testing of cognitive functions reveals that healing generally takes longer than was previously believed. The athlete who returns to play too soon risks second-impact syndrome. This is a rapid, fatal swelling of the brain that may occur if there is another head injury (even a minor one) before the symptoms of the previous concussion have fully resolved.

Treatment for concussion is drug-free rest and observation[1]. What does this mean?

---

1. Much of the information here was provided by Dr. Wendy Gunth, triple board-certified forensic pathologist. As Dr. Gunther says, "Don't end up on my slab!"

1. **Drug-Free Rest and Repair.**
   - **No NSAIDs**. This means: No aspirin, no ibuprofen, no Motrin, no Tylenol, no Advil. These destroy blood platelets required for clotting and destroy Vitamin C encouraging even more bleeding via capillary breakage. If surgery is required, neither you nor the surgeon will benefit from poor clotting time and increased bleeding in the brain.

     Once blood platelets are destroyed, it takes 2 weeks for the body to regenerate a new set. (You'll be up to about half the normal level in one week). Patients scheduled for surgery are restricted from aspirin for 2 weeks. Advil and Tylenol reduce platelets to a level replaceable in 6-8 hours but even this is too much to risk with a head injury.

   - **No alcohol**. Alcohol alone reduces clotting and promotes bleeding. And, if surgery is required, it may also have toxic interactions with the anaesthesia.

     Alcohol may also cause vomiting, extremely dangerous during unconsciousness. You may choke to death on your own vomit. Or you may breathe (aspirate) the vomit into your lungs resulting in the worst and most painful case of pneumonia you've ever had. This involves burning of lung tissue by stomach acid (pH 2) plus introduction of enzymes and bacteria that are great in the stomach, very bad in the lungs. For all these reasons, never attempt practice (or any other physical activity!) while drunk.

   - **No diet sodas, no Aspartame (NutraSweet), no MSG**. Glutamates occur naturally in the brain and normally are carefully controlled. When controls are overwhelmed by accident or design, free glutamates actively destroy brain cells for hours or days after the initial trauma. In patients with severe head injuries, levels high enough to destroy neurons were detected in cerebrospinal fluid within 24 hours of the injury. Levels continued to rise up to 72 hours later[1]. Once levels of neurotoxic glutamates have risen, it may take a week or more for them to come back down to harmless levels.

     The food industry provides the same free glutamates in processed foods. MSG is manufactured by breakdown of protein into its component amino acids, one of which is glutamic acid. MSG is often disguised under other names such as *hydrolyzed protein* from any source. Glutamates are especially high in broth and soups — the very foods fed to the ill and injured. Read labels with an eagle eye to avoid adding injury to injury.

   - **No heavy meals**. If surgery is required, an empty stomach is safest under anaesthesia.

   - **No intense activity**. Inflammation will subside and minor bleeding will be reabsorbed over time. But if there has been any serious bleeding, a clot can form which takes more time to be reabsorbed. A clot jarred loose before it can be reabsorbed travels through the vascular system as an embolism. It may lodge in an artery of the brain as a thrombus causing cerebral thrombosis or "stroke." Or, there may be hemorrhage of damaged or incompletely healed blood vessels. Strangely, blood is toxic to neurons.

     Take a break from practice and rest. Really rest. Please don't decide that because you're skipping the breakfall class, that you'll go to the gym and lift weights or do aerobics instead. If you're injured, you may not feel up to it anyway. Problems arise when people think they must "work through" the pain, nausea, fatigue. Please just *rest*.

2. **Observation. What exactly are you observing?**
   - **PERL (Pupils Equal & Reactive to Light)**. Pupils of unequal sizes or pupils that do not change in response to light after a head injury can indicate a dangerous rise of pressure in the brain due to internal bleeding / swelling. Emergency surgery may be necessary.

   - **Confusion, disorientation, and sleep patterns**. Do not allow a person with a head injury to spend the night alone, nor to sleep through the night. Awaken the patient every couple hours to verify that he has not slipped into a coma. Use a flashlight to verify that

---

1. Baker and others (1993); Zhang H and others (2001).

pupils are reactive and normal. Marked disorientation or inability to awaken is a signal for immediate emergency medical attention including X-ray to check for bleeding.

Victims may feel queasy and dizzy. The heart may be racing, mouth may be dry. There may be physical discomfort, emotional instability, and depression. If sleepiness, headaches, or vision changes occur (whether weeks or months later) head to the ER.

Another interesting symptom: If, when blowing your nose, fluid squirts out of a tear duct and onto your glasses, you have also broken some of the delicate internal nasal bones that normally separate tears and nasal secretions. If you hit hard enough to damage those, there is almost certainly damage to the soft tissues of the brain, possibly including the delicate olfactory nerves which provide sense of smell.

Martial arts do not necessarily expose you to a higher risk of head injury than other sports. Football, basketball, and skating are far more risky. Nevertheless,

- Avoid potentially damaging activities that are under your control such as repetitive microtrauma from constant breakfalls. There are students who think that 300 breakfalls a night is just Serious Practice and who later pay the price.
- When you practice, avoid practicing in ways that increase the likelihood of head injury; use brain-saving equipment such as crash pads and sprung floors.
- Realize that you cannot "toughen up" your brain by doing more of what hurt it in the first place. If you try, realize that in Real Life there will be terrible consequences. Your brain is who and what you are, how you form relationships, how you make a living. Protect it.

For more information on head injury and healing the damage see:
www.round-earth.com/Neurofeedback-Info.html

I never liked *ukemi* practice and even saw it as an annoying side-trip taking valuable class time from the "real" techniques.

That was so as long as I was afraid. Later it was flying. Years later, when I slipped and fell in an ice storm, it probably saved my life. I went airborne, then despite tucking and slapping, hit the high curb. I ended with a basal skull fracture and a very severe concussion. At 10 pm that night the emergency room was packed to the walls. It was standing room only, overflowing with broken arms, legs, wrists, heads, every possible combination of hurt from falls.

How many of those people had ever been mugged "On The Street"?

I would guess somewhere around zero to none, yet on that day, almost every one had been mugged, hit, shot at *"By* the Street."

Now I tell new students that *ukemi* is the *real* self-defense portion of our program and that the throwing techniques are just for fun. That isn't quite true of course.

Despite the many accidental injuries and deaths due to falls, there are also *purposeful* injuries and deaths.

There are terrible places and terrible situations.

That is another thing entirely and it is why we have Aikido techniques.

CHAPTER 5   *Grabs and Strikes*

Real life attacks range from tentative testing of the waters, immediate intent to harm (strikes and punches) to restraint (to prevent the subject from drawing a weapon or harming another). In Aikido, all of these may be practiced singly or in combination.

In beginning classes, *uke* normally attacks to the forward foot, shoulder, or ribs. In general, it would be foolish to extend past the forward side and arm to attack *nage*'s rear side or arm. As the Aikidoist becomes more experienced, stance becomes far less rigid but the underlying rationale remains.

Whether attacking or defending, arm moves with leg (see "Standing, Stepping and Stance" on page 44). Since Aikido assumes a right-handed attacker, *nage* usually does techniques on the left side first. Also note combinations. For example,

- *Kata-tori* is a grab to the lapel,
- *Shomen-uchi* is an overhead strike.
- *Kata-tori shomen-uchi* is a combination grab with strike.

Grabs are easy to break and so many martial arts do just that. In Aikido, grabs are *not* broken — they will even be secured in place and used to provide the starting point of techniques. Grabs tell you where *uke* is and limits his options while breaking the hold can mean a new and different attack. And, while *uke* may be thinking "Ha! I've got you!" from *nage*'s point of view, *uke* has just tied up or given away one or both or all of his weapons[1].

Basic Practice

Practice below is for the beginning student working as *uke* with a more experienced *nage*. Variations will provide *nage* with additional practice in response to attack. At home, the new student can also work with a "Closet *Uke*" (see page 232) or even an arm chair.

To drill with a partner,

1. Experienced student as *nage* calls out names of attacks.
2. New student as *uke* provides the requested stance, grab, or attack.
3. Reverse roles.

---

1. Hence Aikido described as The Art of 'I've Got You, I've Got You . . . Oh Nooooo!'"

Variation

As *uke* provides the requested grab or attack, *nage* notes the direction of motion, and continues the energy and motion of the attack. *Nage* can also test effectiveness of the hold by raising/lowering hand or moving it from side to side. Also apply the *hitori-waza / aiki-taiso* exercises from Chapter 4. For example, for *katate-tori,*

- For inward motion, rotate attacker's wrist inward with t*ekubi-kosa-undo* (page 88), start of many *irimi* techniques. Notice *uke*'s shoulder.
- For outward motion, duck under *uke*'s arm (start of *sankyo*, page 203).
- For incoming motion or static attack, turn *tenkan*. Notice what makes the easiest and most effective *tenkan*, and the difference between relaxing the held arm and trying to force your way through it.
- Deflection ("wax on, wax off"). See how little effort deflects by a few degrees.
- For two handed grabs, *funekogi-undo* to start the motion, then continue motion into another exercise such as *tenkan*.
- "Standard Response." As punch or grab comes in,

  1. Sweep your opposite arm down *uke*'s attacking arm stopping at the wrist.
  2. Step back, then draw back forward foot, ending in *hanmi*.

  Observe the difference between a) brushing down incoming hand then stepping back and b) stepping back and then brushing down the incoming hand.

Focus on attacks, their names, and the exercises. Do not continue on to a throw.

Be aware of real-life differences between attacks on men and attacks on women.

Men tend to attack *men* with punches and blows, in usually face-to-face, territorial, pummeling, dominance sort of behavior. Restaurateurs and bartenders report that a common attack is what we would call a John Wayne right/left hook, perhaps because it is so common in movies that many think it is the way to fight.

Men tend to attack *women* with chokes. The most common *street* attack on women is from behind, typically with *ushiro kube-shime*, the "mugger's hold" (page 169) of one arm in a stranglehold around the target's neck, the other grasping one hand. A choke from the front is especially common in domestic violence. I have heard botched attempts at choke techniques dismissed as follows: "Oh, well, it's not like anybody would actually attack like that anyway[1]." Actually they do.

For women, practice in groundwork and choke-hold techniques may be critical to training and safety.

---

1. A new student sputtered when she heard this. Contrary to popular belief, street attacks by strangers against women are rare. Attacks by abusive husbands or partners are common and they commonly involve choke holds. Her estranged husband had attacked her on four separate occasions, each time with a chokehold. "But of course!" she said. "So easy when he is big and you are small. It isn't as blatant or obvious afterwards as shooting or stabbing or breaking an arm but it offers total control as you will do anything to get air." Each time, however (and with no training) she was able to turn the attack into a hip throw knocking him cold on the hardwood floor. She then resolved to buy a gun to protect herself. On the way to the store, she realized that she *had* protected herself — and started Aikido instead.

Front Grabs

Judo grip or "aiki grip" or "soft grip" to a wrist starts by grabbing first with the little finger then each finger in order up to the index. This, as opposed to starting the grip with the index finger and bringing each finger into play down to the little finger. It's like holding a sword, the reverse grip of milking a cow.

—Dennis Hooker, Aikido Schools of Ueshiba

For key to books referenced here, see "Preface" on page viii.

Hand and foot positions are indicated as follows. LH=Left Hand, RH=Right Hand, LF=Left Foot, RF=Right Foot.

Katate-Tori

ADS: Attack #1 ("Single-hand attack" [to same-side wrist]); TOT: Katate-mochi, pp. 58-60.

Katate-tori is the basic beginning attack in Beginning Aikido.

Uke:	RH and RF forward, grab *nage's* LH; fingers toward *nage* like gripping a tennis racquet, not toward self.
Nage:	LH and LF forward, palm down

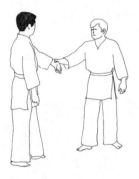

- Observe the ways that a one-handed same-side grab can be entirely different, for example, pulling in or pushing out.
- Using different motions above, *nage* practice setting up the beginning motions for:

  Sankyo, rotating *uke's* arm *in* relative to *uke's* body (see page 203).

  Shiho-nage, rotating *uke's* arm out relative to *uke's* body (see page 207).

  Tenchi-nage, leading *uke's* arm out and down behind his body (see page 225).

- *Technique*: "Katate-Tori Kokyu-Nage Tenkan Ude-Oroshi" on page 221.

Katate Kosa-Tori / Kosa-Tori

ADS: Attack #2 ("Single-hand cross attack"); TOT: Katate-ayamochi, p. 107, for nikyo.

This "cross-handed" attack is the start of *Kokyu-nage Basic*. If "overhead" (a strike instead of a grab, with slight change in angle) it becomes *shomen-uchi* (page 172).

Uke:	RH and RF forward, grabbing *nage's* RH. Fingers are pointed toward *nage* (as if you are gripping a tennis racquet) not towards self.
Nage:	LH and LF forward, palm up, palm down, or with hand vertical (thumb up and pinky finger down).

For palm up, rotate *uke*'s wrist inward across his body by rotating your hand thumb down. Observe behavior of shoulder and its natural lead-in to *irimi* techniques.

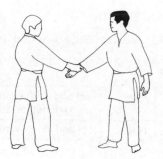

- As for "Katate-Tori" on page 163, practice setting up the beginning motions for *sankyo* (page 203), *shiho-nage* (page 207), and Nikyo 2 (page 202).
- *Technique*: See "Kokyu-Nage" on page 212 and "Katate-Kosa-Tori Kokyu-Nage Irimi Tobikomi (Kokyu-Nage Basic)" on page 213.

Katate-Tori Ryote-Mochi / Morote-Tori

ADS: Attack #3 ("Attack to single hand with both hands holding")

Uke:	RF forward, both hands grabbing *nage*'s LH.
	R (outside) hand is above L (inside) hand on *nage*'s arm; this protects *uke* by keeping *nage*'s elbow from bending out for a strike.
Nage:	LH and LF forward, palm up or down.

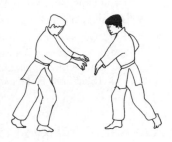

- *Tekubi-tori.* Combined with *tenkan* and *ude-mawashi*, generates a spin used in several *en-undo* techniques.
- As for "Katate-Tori" on page 163, practice setting up the beginning motions for *sankyo* and *shiho-nage*.
- *Technique*: See "Ryote-Mochi Kokyu-Nage Zempo-Nage Tenkan" on page 223. See also "Katate-Kosa-Tori Kokyu-Nage Irimi Tobikomi (Kokyu-Nage Basic)" on page 213. From Katate-tori ryote-mochi, the technique would become "*Katate-tori ryote-mochi kokyu-nage irimi tobikomi.*"

Katate-Tori Ryote-Tori / Ryote-Tori

ADS: Attack #4 ("Both [single] hands grabbed by both [*uke*'s] hands"); TOT: ryote-mochi, p. 164.

Uke:	RF forward, holding both of *nage*'s wrists.
Nage:	LF forward, palms down.

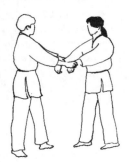

- *Tekubi-kosa: rotate uke's* wrists by rotating yours.

  Observe how difficult or impossible it is for *uke* to halt this motion and what can be done with it, including conversions to *tenkan*, *irimi*, and *shiho-nage* movements. Reaching under one hand with the other, grasp knife-edge of *uke*'s hand. (See *"Kote-Gaeshi 3" on page 211).*
- *Funekogi* shifts a static *uke* into motion.
- Technique: "Katate-Tori Ryote-Mochi Kokyu-Nage Tenchi-Nage" on page 225.

Kata-Tori / Kata-Mune-Tori

ADS: Attack #5 ("Lapel-" or "shoulder-attack"); TOT: Kata-mochi, p. 63.

Uke:	RF forward, seizing L lapel of *nage*'s *gi*.
Nage:	LF and L shoulder forward.

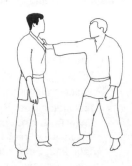

- *Tenkan.* This is often combined with *shomen* or *yokomen* strik (ADS attack #17). Notice how easy it is to turn *tenkan* if you do not freeze up and get stuck in your own clothes.
- Try stepping back into a no-hands *funekogi*.
- For incoming motion, practice "Standard Response" (page 162) three or four hundred times, brushing down on incoming arm, stepping back, and drawing up the forward foot. (Step back first if *uke* is already holding.)

Ryo-Kata-Tori / Ryo-Munetori

ADS: Attack #6 ("Grab to both lapels/shoulders"); TOT: Kata-mochi, p. 63.

Uke:	RF forward, seizing *both* lapels of *nage*'s *gi*.
Nage:	LF forward, hips squared.

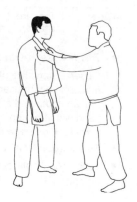

- *Tenkan.* Notice that this still works just as it did for the one-handed lapel grab.
- Experiment with a no-hands *funekogi*.
- As for *kata-tori*, for incoming motion, practice the "Standard Response" (page 162) reaching over the near arm to brush away the outside arm with an *ude-furi* motion, or to deflect the outside arm into an *irimi* motion.

Back Grabs

Ushiro ('behind") in a technique name indicates an attack from the rear.

When *nage* was armed with two swords, the safest place to be was behind them, a situation vividly portrayed in the opening scenes of *The 47 Ronin*. The point of *ushiro-tekubi-tori* ("wrist attack from behind") is to pull *nage*'s arms to the rear, rendering the target supposedly helpless while the attacker remains safely behind, shielded by *nage*'s own body. You may remember the name and the configuration of arms pulled back and seen from above as:

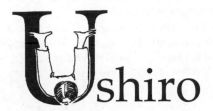

Ushiro-Tekubi-Tori / Ushiro Ryote-Tori

ADS: Attack #7, "Rear-Wrist-Attack"; TOT: Ushiro Ryote-Mochi, pp. 65-66.

Uke:	Behind *nage,* pulling both wrists down and back.
Nage:	*Shizentai*

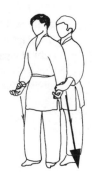

- *Ushiro tekubi-kosa* and *ushiro tekubi tori*. Raise arms to sides, then compare with doing the exercise by raising hands up center.
- Technique: "Ushiro-Tori Tekubi-Tori Ura-Gaeshi" on page 224.
- Practice flowing into position for *sankyo, shiho-nage, ikkyo, kote-gaeshi,* etc.
- As an exercise in balance and stability plus a good stretch, combine with the "Paired Chest and Hip Exercise" on page 125.

Ushiro-Hiji-Tori

ADS: Attack #8, "Rear-Elbow-Attack"; TOT: Ryohiji-mochi, p. 68.

Uke:	Behind *nage,* holding both elbows back.
Nage:	Shizentai

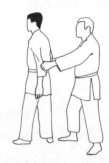

- *Ushiro tekubi-kosa, ude-furi, funekogi,* and *tenkan.*
- With *ushiro tekubi-kosa,* flow into the position for *sankyo.* With *tenkan,* flow into position for *kote-gaeshi.*
- As variation, compare with the standard schoolyard attack of one arm behind and forced upwards along the spine. It seemed like the Ultimate Attack at the time, but see what happens now if *nage* turns tenkan in the direction of *nage*'s elbow.

Ushiro Kata-Tori

ADS: Attack #9, "Rear-Shoulder-Attack"; TOT: Ushiro ryokata-mochi, p. 67.

Uke:	Behind *nage,* holding both shoulders of *gi.*
Nage:	Shizentai

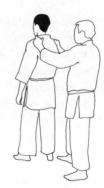

- *Ude-furi choyaku, funekogi, tenkan* and bowing. The *zempo-nage* on page 43 can also be applied to a standing bow.
- *Uke*'s intent is to unbalance *nage* to the rear by moving shoulders behind hips. What happens if *nage* moves his own hips backward? Compare difficulty between tilting a standard chair backward and attempting to do the same thing to a chair on casters.

Ushiro Kubl-Shime

ADS: Attack #10/#16, "Rear-Neck-Attack"; TOT: pp. 188-189

This is commonly known as "The Mugger's Grab" and is the most common street attack on women[1].

Uke:	Behind *nage*, R arm around nage's neck, LH grabbing *nage*'s L wrist.
Nage:	*Shizentai*

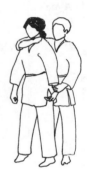

- *Ushiro-tekubi-tori* (page 97): As L wrist rises (preparing for *sankyo*, *zempo-nage*), combine with *sankyo* and see what happens to *uke*'s neck grab.
- Press the arm holding your neck *into* your chest. Observe the difference between this and attempting to pull it away.
- What are the positions of neck and head where you will choke yourself against *uke*'s arm? What are the positions which will give you breathing room? Note that the best option is *not* pressing your neck into *uke*'s forearm in an attempt to "get away."
- Observe also, how little control *uke* has over your hips.

Ushiro-Tori

ADS: Attack #11/12, "Rear-Attack"

Uke:	Behind *nage*, a bear hug with both arms around *nage*'s shoulders or waist so that arms are pinned.
Nage:	*Shizentai*

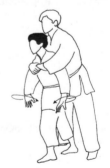

- *Ushiro-tori-undo* (page 96). Observe what happens to *uke*'s stability when you rotate or do not rotate thumbs down or raise arms.
- On moving into throwing position, observe what happens to *uke* (and how successful the eventual throw would be) if you bend forward from the waist versus rotating and bending from sideways with knee, hips, shoulders, and arms in the same plane. The throw is actually from the rear arm out the forward finger. Experiment with feeling the connection between the two.

---

1. According to studies by IMPACT Self-Defense.

Names and Numbers

The venerable *Aikido and the Dynamic Sphere* (ADS) by Westbrook and Ratti, is almost The Standard Aikido Textbook. Its numbering system for attacks and techniques is a neat solution to the problem of different terminology between styles. However, it can be difficult to decipher, especially for beginners. The following chart is organized by attack number and name, keyed to the "Immobilization" (Imm.) or "Projection" (Proj.) and referenced to the ADS page number on which the combination appears. See ADS pp. 56-57 for attacks, then practice them by offering the different energy and options which set up different techniques.

Attack	Attack Name	Defense Name	Defense	ADS Page
#1	Katate-tori	Nikyo	Imm. #2	180
		Sankyo	Imm. #3	192
		Kokyu-nage	Proj. #1	227
		Ude-oroshi	Proj. #2	244
		Kaiten-nage	Proj. #3	252/332
		Tenchi-nage	Proj. #9	272
		Sumi-otoshi	Proj. #10	278
		Shiho-nage	Imm. #6	330
#2	Katate-kosa-tori	Sankyo	Imm. #3	193
		Kokyu-nage	Proj. #1	230
#3	Katate-tori-ryote-mochi	Ikkyo	Imm. #1	168
		Nikyo	Imm. #2	182
		Kote-gaeshi	Imm. #7	219
		Kokyu-nage	Proj. #1	232
		Sumi-otoshi	Proj. #10	280
#4	Ryote-mochi	Shiho-nage	Imm. #6	209
		Kokyu-nage	Proj. #1	236
		Koshi-nage	Proj. #4	257
		Tenchi-nage	Proj. #9	274
		Ghost-throw	Proj. #23	332

#5	Kata-tori	Ikkyo	Imm. #1	169
		Sankyo	Imm. #3	194
		Yonkyo	Imm. #4	200
		Shiho-nage	Imm. #6	210
		Ude-oroshi	Proj. #2	246
		Aiki-otoshi	Proj. #5	260
		Ude-kiri	Proj. #7	269/332
		Tenchi-nage	Proj. #9	276
		Sumi-otoshi	Proj. #10	281
#6	Ryo-kata-tori	Kokyu-nage	Proj. #1	237
		Ude-oroshi	Proj. #2	247
#7	Ushiro tekubi-tori	Ikkyo	Imm. #1	170
		Nikyo	Imm. #2	184
		Shiho-nage	Imm. #6	211
		Kokyu-nage	Proj. #1	238
		Ude-oroshi	Proj. #2	248
		Koshi-nage	Proj. #4	259
#8	Ushiro-hiji-tori	Kote-gaeshi	Imm. #7	220
		Kokyu-nage	Proj. #1	239
#9	Ushiro-katate-tori	Yonkyo	Imm. #4	201
		Kokyu-nage	Proj. #1	240
		Ude-oroshi	Proj. #2	249
		Aiki-otoshi	Proj. #5	264
#10	Ushiro-kubi-shime	Ojigi-nage	Proj. #15	294
#11/12	Ushiro-tori	Zempo-nage	Proj. #13	292
#13	Shomen-uchi	Zempo-nage	Proj. #13	286
#14	Yokomen-uchi	Koshi-nage	Proj. #4	260
#15	Mune-tsuki	Kaiten-nage	Proj. #3	254

Strikes

Beginning Aikido deals with three basic strikes. Two (*shomen-uchi* and *yokomen-uchi*) are derived from the Japanese sword tradition.

Shomen-Uchi

ADS: Attack #13, "Front-Strike"; TOT: pp. 50-51.

To differentiate this $traight-up-and-down $trike from *yokomen,* think of it as:

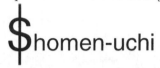

$homen-uchi

Uke:	LF forward, raise RH overhead, then drop strike straight down to *nage*'s head while stepping forward onto RF.
Nage:	LH and LF forward.

Initial set-up and stance vary between styles and schools. At the Virginia Ki Society, *shomen-uchi* is essentially a *katate-kosa-tori* ("cross-hand-attack" page 164), targeting head rather than wrist.

Uke starts in a stance opposite to where he will end. This allows a step into the strike, often explained as "attack the *back* foot" or "Attack *nage*'s forward RF foot with your RH hand," that is:

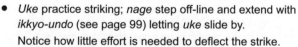

- *Uke starts* on LF simply to move into the attack, just like throwing a ball.
- Step forward onto RF, striking down with your RH.

  This configuration allowed two persons to pass, back to back, if the fight was not entered into. The aim was to expose as little of yourself to the opponent as possible.
  —*George Simcox, Ki Society*

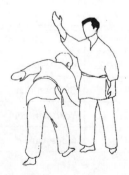

- *Uke* practice striking; *nage* step off-line and extend with *ikkyo-undo* (see page 99) letting *uke* slide by.
  Notice how little effort is needed to deflect the strike.
- Techniques: "Shomen-Uchi Ikkyo Irimi" on page 217.
  "Shomen-Uchi Ikkyo Tenkan" on page 219.

Yokomen-Uchi

ADS: Attack #14, "Side-head-strike"; TOT: p. 53.

To differentiate *yokomen* and *$homen-uchi,* observe the diagonal stroke of the *Y* in:

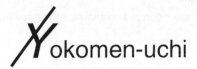

Yokomen-uchi is an "oblique" cut to the "head." Raise the arm and/or weapon straight up just as for *shomen,* but cut down diagonally while rotating the hips.

As in *shomen-uchi,* raising the sword overhead then dropping it down allows you to blend with gravity and hips for maximum power.

Uke:	LF forward, RH overhead, striking diagonally to *nage*'s neck while turning hips and stepping into R *hanmi*.
Nage:	LH and LF forward.

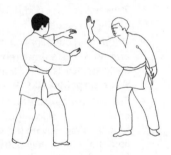

- *Uke* observe power generated by starting the strike from side; from overhead.
- As *uke* strikes *yokomen, nage* observe the path of the arm. This is the path of travel, the vectors, that you must blend with.
- *Ikkyo. Nage* practice "blocking" — actually feeling, flowing with, redirecting — the strike. How softly can you do this? By aligning and blending, how invisible can you become to *uke*?
- Techniques: "Yokomen-Uchi Shiho-Nage Irimi" on page 215 and "Yokomen-Uchi Shiho-Nage Tenkan" on page 216.

Mune-Tsuki

ADS: Attack #15, "Middle-punch"; TOT: *Shomen-tsuki*, p. 56

Uke:	L *hanmi*, draw back RH in fist; stepping into R *hanmi*, punch forward to the solar plexus or belt knot. *Practice*: Do the same punch to punching bag or *makiwara* to check form and effectiveness.
Nage:	LH and LF forward.

In traditional Eastern styles, *mune-tsuki* ("middle-punch") or "punch to chest" tends to be an uppercut punch to the solar plexus.

Students often hesitate to offer a real punch for fear of injuring their partners (see page 182) or simply because they have no idea how to punch. Either option deprives the partner of practice with real punches, real energy, and real commitment behind them. This is important because although Aikido doesn't emphasize punches, other martial arts do.

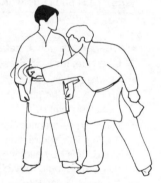

- *Tenkan:* As "fisty dodge-ball," observe that it doesn't matter how hard *uke* hits — if you aren't there.

- *Ude-furi*: In combination with *tenkan*, sweep same-side arm down *uke*'s arm preparatory for *kote-gaeshi,* especially for a curled wrist with uppercut. (See "Finding the Wrist" on page 210.)

- *For beginning uke:* Aim for the knot of *nage*'s belt. This provides a specific target especially for the *uke* who "punches" by waving his arm in a vaguely forward direction often completely outside *nage*'s body, often due to fear of harming nage.

  Aiming at the knot gives partners the opportunity to know that the block or *tenkan* was effective or ineffective, while protecting *nage* from harm.

  Meanwhile, practice with a pillow, punching bag, *makiwara*, to learn the actual dynamics behind effective punching.For the *nage* working with a beginning *uke* who may not realize that he's not really punching, work on *ma-ai,* backing up across the mat to force forward movement and commitment.

- For beginning *nage*: *Uke* start slowly with a punching *motion*, gradually increase force and speed to a fast and powerful "real" punch.

Other Techniques

Kicks

Kicks are rarely used in Aikido, but are common in other styles and appear in various Ki Society *Taigi* (notably *Taigi* #7.) They are always of interest to new incoming karate students, but avoid them unless an instructor is present. If unbalancing *uke* is too successful, the consequences from a kick are far worse than from a punch and karate students rarely have experience in falling. Kicks include:

- *Choku-Geri* ("straight-kick" or front snap kick),
- *Mawashi-Geri* ("round-kick" or roundhouse kick),
- *Yoko-Geri* ("side-kick")

Atemi

Atemi is a "strike" or blow, which in Aikido is used to distract, startle, or in general, to disrupt an attacker's focus and rhythm. Ideally, it is not usually intended to smash or injure; it operates more on the level of distraction or psychological warfare. It may take the form of a punch, a kick, or even more subtle motions: a palm whizzing by the face, a *Stooge-ido* poke towards the eyes which startles, surprises, unbalances.

An attacker may be fully prepared to take on the most ferocious blows, but a soft unexpected flick to the tip of the nose diverts brain cells to dealing with the problem of *"What was that?!?"*

Some insist that there are no punches in Aikido[1] but this is not the case.

> In Ki Society's Taigi 13, the third technique is *"yokomen-uchi kokyu-nage atemi"* and is done with a *ki-ai* on the *atemi*. Taigi 19, *Mune-Tsuki*, has only one technique that does *not* include *atemi*. My favorite is called simply *mune-tsuki kokyu-nage shomen-uchi;* the *shomen-uchi* is the response to the attack. There are others that are in the test requirements, such as the *katate-tori tenchi-nage* that used to be in our 5th kyu test.
>
> —Brian Kelley, Ki Society

> A fairly high ranked student of Chiba Sensei once told me that he doesn't teach *atemi* to beginners, not because it isn't important, but because everyone thinks they know how to hit people. If you include *atemi* when teaching new students, they tend to focus on what they think is familiar to them, and end up pounding on each other instead of learning good body mechanics.
>
> —J. Toman

---

1. A quote attributed to a high-ranking and notoriously combative USAF-West (Aikikai) Sensei: "He said there were no strikes in Aikido — so I hit him again."

Breathing

> The principles of breathing and also using your opponent's breathing to your own advantage are contained in all martial art practices that I have encountered in 45 years of practice. Control of your own breath should be included at fundamental levels of study. It is built into all kata and some teachers don't make a big deal out of it at basic levels, but I believe it is very important. Using your own breath and then your opponent's breath as strategy is part of all techniques. As we become more sensitive to timing and rhythm we will find that breathing ties everything together.
>
> —Chuck Clark, Jiyushinkai Aikibudo

Breathing is the most obvious of self-defense techniques. (Stop and you die quickly). It is possible to disrupt an opponent's attack through disruption of his breathing. Attacking or closing *ma-ai* when the opponent is breathing out is not so much an issue of "being weak when exhaling" as it is an issue of being interrupted before a startled opponent has completely inhaled the oxygen needed for further physical effort.

Practice breath awareness with DVDs of familiar movies. Speak the lines with the actors. Watch and listen for the intake of breath and notice what happens to the power of your speech if you fail to follow their breathing.

Ki-ai is a powerful exhalation, a shout or cry "with *ki*" intended to concentrate and focus mind and body. It is fundamental to karate and to other styles including IMPACT Self Defense training (heavily based on karate). Nowadays *ki-ai* seems rarely taught in Aikido although it was clearly important to Ueshiba.

For *nage*, a spirited *ki-ai* is invigorating if only because it requires *breathing* rather than holding the breath. For the attacker, an unexpected *ki-ai* can also be more — for man or beast. And if you're ever attacked by a moose . . . .

A Norwegian politician was hunting rabbits when charged by a moose protecting her calf. Rather than trying to fend off a half-ton of angry mother moose with a rabbit gun, he decided to use his best weapon — his voice[1].

> "I unleashed a tremendous shout . . . The moose instantly collapsed onto the ground, a meter from me."

As corroborated by witnesses, the stunned moose lay there for several seconds before staggering to its feet and wobbling quietly away.

In the same year, the sudden frenzy and collapse of an Okapi, a rare antelope, was attributed to a rehearsal of Wagner's opera "Tannhauser" in a park some 300 yards from the Copenhagen zoo, perhaps similar to epilepsy induced in humans by certain frequencies and rhythms of sound. A shocking sensory overload may be the mundane explanation of many seemingly mystical "no-touch throws."

Nothing more, but nothing less.

---

1. Associated Press, Jan. 2., 1997.

Nage and *Uke* — Partners in the Dance

Before starting throwing techniques, it is important to understand the relationships in the partnered practice that is Aikido,

- *Uke* offers the raw material of the attack then "receives" the technique.
- *Nage* "throws" or performs a technique appropriate to *uke*'s attack.

New students are often disturbed by the notion of cooperation and teamwork between *nage* and *uke* which seems to make it "faked" or "staged" or "phony." Aikido is indeed cooperative, but it isn't just *uke* who's cooperating. *Nage* cooperates even more by following, aligning with, and blending with *uke*'s attack.

In the performance art known as "Pro-Wrestling" you will see excellent gymnastics and superb *ukemi*. No one is supposed to get hurt, but it works only because of careful cooperation[1] between the players.

For example, in the breakfall technique known as a "Body Slam," *uke* vaults off *nage*'s thighs or shoulders to gain height. *Nage* helps by delaying any downward force until *uke* has head properly tucked and is fully horizontal in order to obtain the greatest possible degree of surface area in contact with the mat. In the "Flying Body Break," the "attacker" leaps from the ropes to land on his quarry. Or so it seems. In reality, the "victim" is the "catcher" or "spotter" there to help the "attacker" land safely. Each is protected by his *ukemi* skills and by his partner. Yes, it's comic book, yes, it's staged — but the physics are real, the risk of devastating injury is real, and the *ukemi* is real. The cooperation between *nage* and *uke* is real and keeps both parties safe so that they can come back and play another day. In Aikido practice we must do no less.

How to Be Nage

- See *uke* as your partner and teacher (page 177),
- Match speed and direction of the attack (page 178),
- Continue the motion (page 178),
- Don't muscle the technique (page 179),
- When *uke* counters, stop and ask for correct energy (page 179), and
- Respect *uke*'s ability to take a fall — and let go (page 180).

See Uke as Partner and Teacher

Uke is *not* your enemy. *Uke* is a partner who has loaned you a physical body for a time so that you may learn Aikido skills. Treat that gift with gratitude and respect. In Aikido and *ki* exercises, *uke* serves as the biofeedback monitor that makes the exercises real. Are you off-balance or not? Is your technique effective or not?

You can dance through the motions forever on your own. Only *uke* can tell you if they are truly effective.

---

1. See *Exposed! Pro-Wrestling's Greatest Secrets*, page 262.

Match Speed and Direction of the Attack

> My eyes, his eyes. My feet, his feet. For the enemy, that agreement is the one thing they can't handle. It doesn't have to be long but it does have to be total. Opposition they can handle, but when instead of presenting them with more opposition, you present them with agreement, it's absolutely devastating. And it's the soul of the art.
>
> —Terry Dobson

In matching *uke*'s speed and direction, staying just barely out of reach, *nage* actually blends, vanishes, disappears into the attack. This matching and blending is a form of camouflage, a weapon in and of itself. Blend into the attacker's power and direction and he will feel only himself and be unable to counter. It is extremely disconcerting to attack, to be aware that something astonishing is happening, but to feel nothing.

Notice that a tense tight grip by *nage* adds new and different directions of force. Notice that trying to speed through the technique faster than the attack is itself an attack. There should be only one attacker.

Learning to blend in Aikido is very much like a two-year-old learning to pet a cat. It is the same balance and sensitivity required to drive a manual transmission, to pull a weed complete with root, to "stick to *uke* like white on rice," to turn touch into music.

> As pianist and piano teacher, it's interesting to note that while we're pressing down what is basically a block of wood against a string, some have a good 'touch' while others just play. It's the touch, the blending with the block of wood that makes all the difference.
>
> —Margarete Brandenburg, Kokon Ryu Renmei Aikido

Continue the Motion

Continuing the motion continues the preceding principle of matching speed and direction. Many martial arts styles respond to an incoming punch or kick with an opposing block of greater force or inertia. In Aikido, an arm may appear to be blocking a strike but is not. It is more a *feeler* to sense the speed and position of the oncoming attack. The apparent block may deflect the incoming energy, but the purpose is never to block it with opposing force.

Cattle herders needing to slow or stop a stampede did not gallop headlong into an oncoming wall of longhorns (page 70). They matched speed and direction with the leaders, deflecting and turning the mass into a large roiling circle. Similarly, when the Highway Patrol wants to slow or stop high-speed traffic, they do not block oncoming cars by driving at greater force and inertia into oncoming traffic. Neither do they throw up a stationary roadblock to bring vehicles to a sudden slamming stop. Instead, they employ a rolling roadblock. Troopers driving in each lane of the roadway match the speed and direction of traffic, then gradually decrease speed as necessary.

In Aikido, the attacker's incoming energy is your raw material for unbalancing *uke* and allowing a throw to happen. What if you don't get a real attack? What if you only get uncommitted strikes and punches and there is no motion or energy to continue?

New students often simply don't know how to punch or strike, or may fear causing harm and aim so far off line that it provides no threat and no energy to work with.

If *uke* is punching or striking offline, not moving at all makes it clear what is happening. If *uke* is unfamiliar with the whole concept of striking, it also helps to provide a specific target. Have *uke* aim for the knot in your belt, a specific target that is also padded should they fear connecting and harming you.

Nage can also compel a committed attack by repositioning. For example, if *uke* is stopping short with a punch or a strike, keep backing up across the mat just out of range. For *nage*, it is useful practice of *ma-ai*, and will eventually produce a genuine committed forward motion. If *uke* doesn't realize what he's doing, this will help to clarify the situation. It is far more effective than complaining that "there's no energy there."

For a weak overhead strike (*shomen-uchi*) I step back and place my hands so that they would catch the strike with palms up if it were to be in the correct place. The miss is obvious and *uke* usually doesn't need any more correction. If they do I have them practice striking into my hands (usually held at waist level) a time or two and then, without telling *uke*, fail to step back and execute the throw instead. Works about 90 percent of the time.

—George Simcox, Ki Society

I have a mentor in the psychotherapy field, Stephen Gilligan, a psychologist in San Diego and an experienced Aikidoka. One of the many things he has written that stays with me is the way *uke* and *nage* relate:
Heart to heart.
Mind to mind.
Center to center.
As Steve says, in psychotherapy, if you do that, the rest is easy.

—Leonard Bohanon

Don't Muscle the Techniques

If they try to muscle me, I just lean on them until they get tired.

— Big Dave, Aikikai

Purely physical strength is limited by the physical body. There will always be someone bigger and stronger, if not now, then tomorrow or 20 years from now. Aikido allows you to use *uke*'s strength, rather than exhausting your own. Aikido gives you a tremendous advantage over a larger, heavier, stronger opponent *provided you avoid a weight and strength contest*. To use his size, strength and energy, you must blend; align with it, stay with it, go in the direction that it is going.

The more you struggle and strain, the less likely you are doing Aikido. The more you feel you have done nothing, the more likely you have done the technique correctly.

When Uke Counters . . .

1. Stop and ask for the correct energy or
2. Use the counter-attack energy.

When an *uke* does not understand his real role, every technique seems to work about twice. Partners counter to avoid being thrown are frustrating and confusing for the beginning *nage*. For example, *tenkan* techniques are designed to deal with incoming energy. If *uke* pulls back, the *tenkan* technique won't work. *Uke* is setting himself up for an *irimi*, but of course a beginner won't know that.

Both partners must understand the energy the technique is intended to deal with. If *uke* is providing the wrong attack for the technique being practiced, tell him so. Do not, however, be too quick to blame failure of technique on *uke* "giving the wrong energy." Be sure that you are doing the technique correctly and then if the energy is incorrect, correct it. If there is any doubt, ask *Sensei* for help. At higher levels (and respecting *uke*'s ability) match the technique to the energy and attack presented.

Two things will happen.

1. The technique will work.
2. The aggrieved *uke* (completely unprepared for being thrown across the mat when he thought he was countering so very well) will protest:

   "But that's not the technique we're supposed to be doing!"

   The answer is: "Why don't we try it again with [the correct energy]."

   A useful lesson for both partners.

There is a tale told of nearly every master.

"Amazing!" cries the student. "Please do that one again!"

The master agrees and the student attacks again.But the result is an entirely different technique. Then another. And another.

"Why don't you do the same technique as before?" cries the frustrated student.

"Because you haven't given the same attack as before," says the Master.

Respect Uke's Ability to Fall

When you throw, respect your partner's ability to take a fall. Letting go protects both the thrown and the thrower. Beginners are often so shocked to see that a throw actually works, so startled at the sight of *uke* falling that they hold on harder with the intention of helping *uke* safely down to the mat. This is kindly meant, but can be dangerous. *Uke* must be free to roll or, for a brand-new beginner, to walk out of a throw.

The flip side is the danger to *nage*. Bending *over* to help *uke* can mean being kicked in the face by flying feet. If you wish to drop down to the mat,

- Bend at the knees and ankles.
- Drop *down* from the One-Point/Center.
- Imagine that you are doing these techniques on ice.
- Always keep / maintain awareness of One-Point/Center.

How to Be Uke

- Give the correct energy and follow through (page 181).
- Match the speed and energy of your attack to *nage*'s ability to protect you and your own ability to take a fall (page 181).
- Do not counter (page 182).
- Learn the technique well enough to "throw yourself" (page 183).

Do you see throwing as winning and falling as losing?

Uke is the most important person on the mat, *nage*'s teacher, the one who attacks and rolls so that *nage* can learn Aikido.

Give the Correct Energy and Follow-Through

We practice specific techniques to practice dealing with specific types of energy and motion. If *uke* does not supply the energy or motion for which the technique was designed, the technique may be forced, but it will not flow. It is like trying to sailboard or windsurf in a dead calm. Both partners need to understand the energy the technique is intended to deal with. If you are unsure of the correct energy, ask *Sensei* for help.

Tenkan techniques, for example, are intended for an attacker who is moving, pushing, shoving, punching forward. *Nage* turns (*tenkan*) and leads *uke* into a circle, at a speed that keeps the hand almost — but not quite — within grasp. *Uke* is kept reaching forward for the hand that is just a split second, just a hair, beyond his control[1].

You may attack slowly, but continue the motion — don't stop short. The raw material for many throws is the momentum, inertia, and change in balance of the follow-through. These increase with increasing speed and decrease or vanish with decreasing speed.

Walking slowly through a technique which relies on speed and momentum will not "work" in the sense of Uke Falls Down; it will "work" in the sense of establishing the individual steps of the technique. Once these are learned, increasing speed teaches rhythm and flow but there must be power and commitment behind the attack in order for a technique to work.

Aikidoist Jan Beyen compares this to the wind needed for successful sailboarding. Sailboarding doesn't work either — below windspeeds of around 15 knots.

Match Speed and Energy of Attack to Nage's Ability

Respect your partner's ability, never holding harder or attacking faster than *nage* can handle. The first few times through a new technique, move as easily and gently as you would through a new dance step. When your partner begins to feel the pattern and flow of the movements, you may give more of a challenge but always give the appropriate attack, especially when working with beginners — for their sake and yours. Too fierce an attack may be more than *nage* can handle and can result in injury. Part of

---

1. For what it should feel like, see the "Rag Doll Tenkan" on page 69.

nage's technique and practice is to protect *uke*. If the attack is beyond *nage*'s ability to do so and the results are beyond your skill to take *ukemi*, you may be injured.

> Q: I'm willing to make it an on-target strike, but I'm not willing to make it a "real" strike, one that I can't stop easily prior to contact. So am I screwing up their training or protecting them?
>
> A: You are describing what a considerate, caring student would do: determine what the level of training your opponent can handle and then "challenge" them a bit so they can grow. This has two results: You don't unnecessarily hurt a practice partner and you don't suffer the natural consequences of attacking with more force than you can handle when the appropriate technique is applied and you are sent flying
>
> I have seen more people hurt because they worked beyond their *ukemi* than because they were harshly attacked with more force than they could handle. I've seen pulled muscles, scrapes and one serious broken bone. All were a result of *ukemi* that didn't do what it was supposed to do, but I've never yet seen anyone get punched out.
>
> —George Simcox, Ki Society

Do Not Counter

As *uke* you are there to help and challenge your partner, not to engage in a contest.

Any Aikido technique can be countered. While it is very tempting to do so, that isn't the point of beginning practice. The point of practice is *practice*. Specific attacks involving specific energy are dealt with via specific techniques. Attacks are staged in class in order to practice a specific response, a particular placement of hands and feet, a specific point of rotation, even a particular mindset. An attack inappropriate to the material to be practiced will not work.

For example, *tenkan* techniques, designed to dissipate and redirect fast incoming energy by continuing the motion *forward*, do not work if *uke* pulls *back*. *Nage* may succeed in dragging *uke* around in a circle, but that is a pointless exercise which may lead you to the false conclusion that Aikido isn't "real" or that *nage* is fooling himself. In reality, the source of the problem is *uke* who may then add insult to injury by staging an elaborate imitation fall.

Countering is typical of the *uke* who does not understand his real role as helper and teacher or who does not understand or does not want to admit that changes in energy and direction are actually different attacks. If the exercise is to practice *tenkan*, and you counter with a hold appropriate for some other technique, it will be difficult, painful, or confusing for *nage* and your own learning will be impaired.

Or, you may learn more than you expected. A counter sets you up for an alternate technique. While you are thinking of the motion you are cleverly blocking rather than the new energy you are presenting, the counter to your counter tends to have more devastating consequences. As you go flying through the air you will be experiencing "Real Aikido."

The slyly accomplished Aikidoist will actually provide an opportunity then wait for *uke* to counter in order to take advantage of that specific energy. For example, in *Kokyu-Nage Basic nage* leads *uke* down then waits for him to counter by attempting to come up. *Nage* does not force *uke* up. He *waits* for him to come up, then *helps* him to come up, adding just a little extra energy to *uke*'s energy so that the final up is more than *uke* was expecting — or can deal with[1].

On the other hand, don't collapse just because *nage* appears to have completed the technique so now it must be time to fall down. While this can give *nage* a false sense of security, it can also give a *false insecurity* if your partner feels that you are merely collapsing on cue.

Never see your partner as competition; don't resist falling with the notion that if your partner succeeds in throwing you, you have somehow "lost." If you are *afraid* to fall, learn to fall, a critically valuable self-defense technique in and of itself. We also practice falling in order to help others learn. If you are *unwilling* to fall, examine your motives — you may find such hidden devils as fear, false pride, dignity, and the delusion of winning versus losing.

"Win" by being an effective teacher.

Learn the Technique Well Enough to Throw Yourself

The test of good *ukemi* is not whether you can counter ("Haha! You can't throw me!") but whether you understand the technique well enough to provide the correct energy and to guide an inexperienced *nage* through the technique and the throw. The ability to do so is not "tanking" and does not make the technique "phony" — it is a teaching technique, and once again, *uke* is the teacher.

On the other hand, beginners are often told not to fall unless they are actually thrown. This is because they don't know enough yet to be able to guide the throw and to avoid the habit of "tanking" even in response to bad technique. It is also because beginners often take terrible falls on their own. They may launch themselves into a mass of other students, or land in a way that risks injury. But there's another side to the issue.

> Senior students tend to go ahead and roll as soon as a junior student gets the technique even a little bit right, with the definition of "right" becoming more stringent as *nage* becomes more skilled. For complete beginners, it's real progress deserving of positive feedback if they move their feet and hips at all, even if they're still mostly using arm strength.
>
> Meanwhile, beginners don't yet have the awareness to protect *uke* and often don't realize that "Making *Uke* Fall" is not necessarily the same as "Good Aikido." I'm therefore likely to be much more protective of my joints and much more aware of my "landing zone" when I'm working with beginners. I might roll when I otherwise wouldn't in order to avoid getting damaged.
>
> —Katherine Derbyshire, Aikido Schools of Ueshiba

The flip side of teaching the throw from *ukemi* is learning the throw from *ukemi*.

Beginners are often distressed that many advanced students seem unwilling to work with them. This is often true, and often for all the wrong reasons, but very often it is because the newer student (who has not yet learned how to protect his partner) wants to concentrate on throwing the senior student who in turn needs time to work on other skills. Traditionally, beginners learned by taking years of *ukemi* for advanced students before doing the throws themselves[1].

---

1. For the same strategy applied to verbal techniques, see "Typecasting" on page 248.

Henry Kono insists that the basis of Aikido is *ukemi*. "When I went to Japan," he said, "they asked me: 'How long will you be here?'"

"Four years," I said.

"Then you take *ukemi* for three."

Kono was shocked and dismayed. Like everyone else, he expected to learn throwing techniques. We don't want to hear about years of *ukemi* as preparation for Aikido. In part, it fails to fit our cultural paradigm of the martial arts where all too often, *nage* is seen as winner and *uke* as loser. We go to class to study how to "win." We don't go to study "losing." Yet learning *ukemi* means learning to:

- Give the correct attack,
- Protect oneself while guarding against openings,
- Follow *nage*'s response in order to fall safely,
- Lose the fear of falling which otherwise results in the wrong attack or half-hearted attacks for fear of consequences,
- Convert the receiving and following skills of *ukemi* into the receiving and following skills critical in *nage* waza.

If you concentrate on *ukemi* skills and volunteer to *uke* for advanced students you will learn and you will never lack practice partners.

> Finding good players is easy. Getting them to play as a team is another story.
> —Casey Stengel

Ukemi is about engagement. It is about intent, attack, and continuation of the attack. It is about looking for the opening to take back control after you have been unbalanced, about keeping up the attack while keeping yourself safe. It is about sticking in there as long as possible to try to find a hole, so if *nage* makes some mistake you haven't bailed out and are no longer around. It is about separating from the other person when it becomes futile to continue, so that you can live to come back and attack again. It is constant awareness of all that is around you.

Many people just take falls. It's fun, and some people think it looks cool, but many times it's not *ukemi*. And often after the big jump the person either lies there or gets up without awareness, so that the person who just threw *uke* could in fact step on or attack from behind. This Awareness and connection with surroundings is what I find missing in most practice.

I took *ukemi* for a *shihan* at an *embu* recently. Afterwards, a guy told me "You never took your eyes off him!" Of course not. I never take my eyes off the person I am engaged with. If I did, I would have a large opening and he could kill me. Sometimes it is necessary to take some spectacular breakfall *ukemi*. For those rare instances, we must practice such falls but when practicing, not get sucked into the "I wanna take cool looking falls" trap.

Uke and *nage* both attack each other's Center, both must keep themselves safe, both must find a way to take the other's balance. Always engaged, always connected.

> —Lisa Tomoleoni, Aikido Shindo Dojo, Tokyo, Japan

---

1. See KIA, page 242, for the rest of the story and how to study *ukemi* in other ways.

CHAPTER 6   Locks and Throws

The secret behind the throws? Physical principles based on gravity, balance, and movement from Center. Good body mechanics based on the above plus issues of anatomy and physiology. Internal principles based on focus, relaxation, and calm. And Koichi Tohei's basic principles for the practice of Ki-Aikido.

1. **Extend Ki.** Extending awareness, attention, focus, intent, and goal.
2. **Know your opponent's mind (intent).**
   What exactly is it that *uke* wants to do? We are controlled by what we want . . .
3. **Respect your opponent's *ki* (energy/inertia/intent).**
   Per the physics of Aikido, practice being aware of and sensitive to speed, force, and direction in order to blend with it. Focus on these rather than on the attacker.
   Is the attack circular? Is it coming straight at you? Is it down? Up? Fast? Slow?
4. **Put yourself in your opponent's place.** Move into the position where uke would be stable, but can't because you and your Center are there. In tenkan it is the middle of the circle. In throws, it is the position where uke is supported, where supported only by you, or not supported at all.[1]
5. **Perform with confidence.** We are controlled by what we fear. Having confidence in your techniques requires that you have done them, practiced them, experienced them often enough that they are no longer a hopeful leap of faith into the void, but a confident use of known and trusted tools of mind and body.

Aikido techniques range from simple to complex, with infinite variation and nuance, but the basic techniques (*waza*) are divided into *katame-waza* ("immobilization techniques") and *nage-waza* ("throwing techniques").

Katame-waza are commonly known as "wristlocks" or "armlocks." Wrist, elbow, and shoulder joints are manipulated to control the attacker's balance and body.

Nage-waza are the actual "throws." The two categories overlap, but many *nage-waza* are based solely on redirection of weight, speed, and momentum.

> *Nage* slipping away
> Almost got 'em this time, Ha!
> Mat greets me loudly.
>
> —Kevin Beck

---

1. Always look for the invisible third leg that would keep *uke* from falling if only it were there and he could lean on it — but it isn't and he can't.

Ma-ai, Tenkan and Irimi

Ma-ai, tenkan and *irimi* are the most basic tools of Aikido. The differences between them can be thought of in terms of "danger zones." Most hostile humans are most dangerous in front, in the direction of the eyes. In general,

- *Irimi* is "entering" and pre-empting or turning *uke*'s danger zone away.
- *Tenkan is* "turning" *yourself* around and away from *uke*'s danger zone.
- *Ma-ai* is simply not being there, or being out of reach and out of the danger zone.

Ma-ai

I cannot begin to tell you the number of dumb looks I've seen by simply leaning back and letting a guy's fist fly past my face. Of all the reactions the dude was expecting, me getting out of the way wasn't one of them.

—Marc MacYoung, *Watch My Back*

The turn-of-the-century classic, *Secrets of the Sword,* by Baron César de Bazancourt, is a sort of Socratic dialogue on the most basic essentials of the sword and self-defense. Over the course of 11 evenings, the Baron proposes to strip away the techniques, the daunting foreign terminology (French), and reduce years of study to the most basic, root essential of swordsmanship. The essential that the Baron presents is *ma-ai.*

Literally *ma-ai* is "harmonious-distance," the natural or proper space maintained between bodies. *Ma-ai* is your first line of defense, the most important technique in your toolbox. It is space and time, rhythm, and flow.

- In traffic, the safe following distance between cars.
- In society, the distance that indicates neither inappropriate intimacy nor cold distance.
- In conversation, rhythm and timing and degree of familiarity.
- In graphics and layout, the "white space."

The *Ma-ai* of Space

Proper space is the distance required for safety from collision, reaction time in case of attack,[1] the position which requires a complete step and body commitment on the part of an attacker. If the attacker can connect with a strike without a step, you are much too close.

In Aikido, *ma-ai* is commonly thought of as the distance between two standing partners when they touch the fingertips of their outstretched arms, but this distance is not absolute; it is constantly modified by the situation.

---

1. Observe the use of *ma-ai* in computer games such as *Tetris*. As a rain of geometric blocks fall from the sky, the player must form a complete row. The program works to reduce *ma-ai* which in turn reduces available maneuvering space. With few incomplete rows on the screen, there is plenty of space to anticipate and maneuver. With a full screen of incomplete rows, the player's speed and reaction time must increase exponentially, while maneuverability decreases.

For armed partners, the distance is greater as sword or staff increase effective reach by several feet. Proper distance between partners using swords is with just the tips of the swords crossed. Closer means that a single step could result in a killing blow.

Ma-ai is different even for two partners of different size and reach. A short partner who cannot reach a long-armed partner may still be standing too close.

For *taigi* (paired exercises of choreographed attack and defense as practiced in the Ki Society) the proper starting distance between partners seated in *seiza* for the initial or final bow, is about 12 feet, or the distance of two *tatami* mats.

Ma-ai can also be thought of as the distance that allows you to see and take in a potential attacker's entire body, from head to foot. This is not only for time to react to an incoming punch or kick. It is to observe body language.

The human brain is exquisitely attuned to body language and the intent that underlies it. Don't believe it? If you are a commuter, consider that you may be negotiating the highway equivalent of a trip through an asteroid field on a daily basis, half awake and even before you've had your coffee. How do you know who is going to dart out of the next lane? Fail to stop? Wander across four lanes of traffic? How do you *know*?

You *know* because a tiny tilt of head, a drop of a shoulder is enough to tell you.

The same tiny motions are critical in martial arts and self defense. The more of them you can see, the better. Hence emphasis on full body view (rather than a set distance), to receive information — and to send it. Gavin de Becker (1997) explains a common violation of *ma-ai* in both information gathering and the message conveyed.

> Many do not use the full resources of their vision; they are reluctant to look squarely at strangers who concern them. Believing she is being followed, a woman might take just a tentative look, hoping to see if someone is visible in her peripheral vision. It is better to turn completely, take in everything, and look squarely at someone who concerns you.
>
> This not only gives you information, but it communicates to him that you are not a tentative frightened victim-in-waiting. You are an animal of nature, fully endowed with hearing, sight, intellect, and dangerous defenses. You are not easy prey, so don't act like you are.

Personal Space

People who have difficulty with the idea of self-defense are often those who have difficulty with or have been carefully trained out of the idea of their own right to personal space. They may roar into action when someone else is endangered but have extreme difficulty responding when they themselves are the target of hostile behavior. The following exercise tests and demonstrates personal boundaries.

At a table, in casual circumstances (and very carefully):

1. Push a glass of water, mug of beer, towards the table edge and "*nage's*" lap.
2. Observe the point at which *nage* takes action to prevent a spill.
   How long and how far does *nage* continue to ponder or rationalize intentions. For example, *"What in his background would make him act in this manner?"*
   "Why would she be doing this? She's really A Very Nice Person."
   Nage must simply deal with the situation before it lands in a lap. The point at which the unwitting subject *does* deal is a good rough guide to the limit of personal space, useful for a beginning point of awareness and assumptions.

Light-Bubble

1. Imagine you are standing in a bubble of light, with the consistency of thick honey or Neoprene, which extends at least to the palms of your extended hands, above your head and just below your feet, in front, to the sides and in back.
2. Drop arms to sides and with a partner approaching and backing away, practice maintaining the same distance throughout class time and throughout the day.

Variation

- On The Street, minimum size of your bubble of awareness should be four seconds in front of you, increasing and elongating forward with increasing speed. If you can't see four seconds of travel ahead, say in an area of curves and hills, you are going too fast. At 60 miles per hour your bubble of awareness should be as far ahead as you can see.
- Practice counting and timing your speed, spacing, and awareness of others, planning ahead for problems rather than cutting in and out at the last minute. And see Appendix B.

Ma-ai Jo

With a partner, place a *jo* between you. At the beginning stages, place it just above the belt; with practice, place it below the belt.

1. Take turns backing up, moving forward, and stepping side to side, moving in a circle maintaining distance so that the *jo* does not fall to the ground.
(Additional practice is gained by not letting the *jo* attack your toes).
2. Move slowly at first increasing speed only with success at keeping the *jo* in its position.

The *Ma-ai* of Time

> Time is God's way of keeping everything from happening at once.
>
> —Anon.

Common remarks about various violent acts . . .

> "It came out of the blue!" "There was absolutely no warning!" "He musta just snapped!"

. . . are rarely true, whether the attack is by flood, serial killers, the IRS, or *dojo* partners.

Part of blending is matching awareness of its *beginning*. No attack ever began at point of impact. Yet we often act as though they have no beginning, no past, no path of travel. Observe this in the following exercise.

Timing Belt

Uke sits *seiza* with a *gi* belt doubled in his right hand,

1. *Nage* walks or jogs past *uke*'s left side.
2. *Uke* whips the belt from right to left, parallel to mat, trying to catch *nage*'s ankles; *nage* tries to hop over the moving belt. Students often wait until they see the belt *at their ankles*. By then it is too late. The attack begins when *uke* begins to move and possibly sooner. The *nage* who hops at that point avoids the belt. Others will run through this exercise repeatedly never understanding why they continue to get smacked.

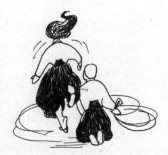

The defense against the overhead strike of *shomen-uchi* is *ikkyo-undo* in which *nage* swings arms up to meet and blend with the incoming strike. We often wait until the strike arrives, then try to rely on lightning reflexes and power despite little room to maneuver. Like the belt strike, *shomen-uchi* does not begin with the strike; it certainly does not begin at impact. It begins with the intent and never later than the upward motion. The beginning of effective defense is not at the impact, but at its birth and development; "Doing the exercise" of *ikkyo-undo* as *uke*'s arms rise allows blending before the downward motion can even begin.

Time Blending

1. *Uke* strike *shomen-uchi.*
2. *Nage* wait to respond until strike is on the way down.
3. Observe ease or difficulty of performing technique.

Variation

1. *Uke* swing arm repeatedly up overhead as if to strike *shomen-uchi.* Do not strike; just drop arm and repeat. *Nage* swing arms up (*ikkyo-undo*) matching *uke*'s speed and direction.
2. *Uke* strike with a complete *shomen-uchi.* *Nage* swing arms up (*ikkyo-undo*) matching *uke*'s speed, direction. Complete the motion with a technique.
3. Compare the ease of motion and control between the two approaches.

The *Ma-ai* of Balance and Flexibility

Balance, center, and body mechanics effect *ma-ai* in ways completely unrelated to actual distance. By controlling center it is possible to put *uke* at an angle where he cannot strike. *Uke* can see *nage*, close by, within easy reach, but any attempt at *atemi* will destroy his own balance. To demonstrate this principle:

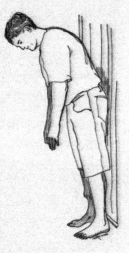

1. Stand with your back and heels against a wall.
2. Attempt to touch your toes. Observe what happens to balance.
   You *can* touch your toes (if that's something you can do normally) while falling forward, but do you really *want* to?
   Notice the parallel between this and lack of flexibility. A stiff uke with extremely tight hamstrings who can't flex hips and maintain balance when his hand is led downward essentially throws himself.

A few degrees of rotation makes a difference in vulnerability. For example, *tekubi-kosa-undo* can be applied in many ways to many grabs. Rotating the wrist while leading *uke*'s arm inward will cause the shoulder to drop. *Uke* may not realize it yet, but he's now off balance while his own arm and shoulder blocks his other arm and shields you. Likewise, rotating the wrist which rotates the arm and shoulder may cause the hip to shift too so that *uke* is no longer over Center and is off-balance.

As in *shiho-nage*, experiment with degrees of wrist rotation, and degrees of inward lead, also known as *irimi*. "Not being there" commonly appears as *tenkan*.

Tenkan

> Seeing me before him, the enemy attacks,
> But by that time I am already standing safely behind him.
>
> —Morihei Ueshiba

Tenkan is a means of rearranging yourself in space.[1] So is almost anything else, but *tenkan*, a simple turn, simultaneously removes you from immediate danger zone and makes you the center of a rotating circle.

In left *hanmi* (L foot and L hand forward)

1. *Nage* extends L hand, palm down.
2. *Uke* enfolds *nage*'s L wrist with the R hand.
   Grasp gently at first to provide a pivot point and a point of reference rather than an exercise in dealing with a "death grip."
3. *Nage* curls fingers back towards palm, then steps or slides forward with LF foot, bringing RF around to rear, pivoting hips 180 degrees to end approximately shoulder to shoulder with *uke* or slightly behind. Draw the LF back as necessary.
   LF is still forward and RF back (still in L *hanmi*); lead is forward.

Power Test Tenkan

In *tenkan* techniques beginners commonly back up instead of moving forward. A *nage* extending *ki* and moving forward is the center of the circle. *Uke*, rotating around the outside, is at a disadvantage.

Moving backward makes *uke* the center of the circle and puts *nage*, rotating around *uke*, at the disadvantage. The following exercise shows the difference.

With *uke* holding *nage*'s wrist and with eyes closed,

1. *Nage* performs an incorrect *tenkan*, by purposely backing up.
2. *Nage* performs a correct *tenkan*, motion and lead correctly forward.
3. *Uke* compare. Which one is more compelling?

Floating-Foot Tenkan

When doing a *tenkan*, *nage* commonly slides forward with the same-side (forward) foot, then turns. With a resistant *uke*, there may be collision. Instead of sliding directly forward, *nage* can,

1. Lift the front foot, then
2. Enter and turn 180 degrees (as for standard *tenkan*).
   The momentary balancing on one foot makes *nage*, like a balloon, sensitive to the slightest force or energy from *uke*. *Nage* naturally goes around and collision is avoided.

Starting and ending attacks, techniques, and rolls on one foot develops balance, timing, and a greater awareness of the energy involved[2].

---

1. For more *tenkan* exercises see KIA, Chapter 5, p. 140-149. See BA pp. 46-47, 30-31.
2. It also protects against the dreaded "Hakama Toe," toes tangled in the folds of the skirt worn by advanced students.

Dead Arm Tenkan

The flip side of a floating foot is a floating arm. Jim Baker *Sensei* (Aikikai) describes the relaxation of the arm in these terms: "Let the forward arm die."

Water Tenkan

It is often difficult for a student to realize when he is backing up, when he has left his circle, when the energy has changed from rotational to linear. Practicing small, tight turns in water encourages circular motion as linear motions are resisted by the water[1].

Tiny Tenkan

We often tend towards the large, swooping, *tenkan* during warm-up exercises. Practice small, quick, turns as well.

The late Don Lyons (Iwama style) used the image of attempting to "stab yourself in the stomach" with your own hand. Turn *tenkan* just before the hand can connect.

Snowboard Tenkan

There is nothing like being totally locked onto a single piece of board, tearing down a mountain to realize the importance of shifting vertical posture around a well-balanced center. I credit the lessons of my many *tenkans* for having survived the adventure.

—Michael Speece, Ki Society

---

1. For other advantages of "Poolkido" and practicing in water see page 14 and page 152.

Irimi

In Tom Clancy's thriller, *Hunt for Red October,* a Soviet submarine fires a torpedo to destroy the *Red October* before its officers can defect. To the shock of the crew, the captain's apparently suicidal response is to order full speed directly towards the oncoming torpedo — which impacts harmlessly against the hull. When the expected distance between source and target was abruptly closed, the torpedo had no time to arm itself. A nautical *irimi.*

In Aikido, certain *irimi* movements by *nage* appear to be nothing more than a direct frontal clash with *uke.* They are in fact, a redirecting of energy in a way that *uke* did not intend or expect by:

- Pre-empting an attack before *uke*'s full energy can be developed,
- Following motion in which *uke* is pulling in, rather than extending out, and
- Changing (redirecting) the motion or direction of the attack.

Pre-empting and redirecting energy and motion is especially clear in *shomen-uchi irimi.* In this technique,

1. *Uke* attacks with an overhead strike. *Nage* appears to simply block the incoming strike — no blending may be apparent at all.
2. *Uke* then appears to bounce violently off of his intended target, for no apparent reason, and is thrown.

It appears to be a full frontal clash of force against force. It is not. In part, *nage* pre-empts *uke*'s attack before the strike can develop its full potential[1] and the energy that is left is dealt with off-line and redirected.

Following the motion, energy or direction of attack will be familiar to those who have had to escape from a fish-hook or picked blackberries or other forms of roses armed with vicious thorns. If you pull directly away from the fierce, recurved thorns you will be ripped and torn. The best technique is *irimi,* entering and following the direction of the thorns just long enough to deflect, *redirect,* and disengage them.

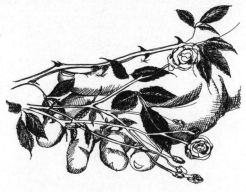

---

1. See "Shomen-Uchi Ikkyo Irimi" on page 217.
   Irimi is nicely described in TOT p. 18 and 60. See also BA pp. 30, 51.

Clotheslining and Tripping

If you ever rode your bicycle through backyards filled with laundry and caught a clothesline across throat or chest while the bottom half of your body kept on moving, you know what clotheslining is. Kokyu-nage Basic and its variations are "clotheslining" techniques.

In "tripping" techniques, the body hurtles forward while the legs remain behind. Examples are *zempo-nage*, *ikkyo-irimi* and any of their variations.

—George Simcox, Ki Society

Tenkan and *irimi* address the *horizontal* plane of movement. *Clotheslining* and *tripping* address the *vertical* plane of movement. While these terms or concepts do not appear to have official names in any style they are useful for categorizing throws and pre-empting common problems.

To new eyes, it appears obvious that the best way to get *uke* down to the mat is to push *uke* down, but this isn't the case. Understanding the underlying rationale helps to get the beginner past this point.

"Clotheslining" techniques involve leading *up*, allowing *space* and *time* for *uke*'s hips and legs to move forward of his torso. The best way to get *uke* down is not to push down, but to *lead uke* down then *lead up*. In Kokyu-Nage Basic, the final motion is *up*; as *uke* can't stay there, the "clothesline" that he trips on is thin air. In *tenchi-nage*, shown here, the clothesline is more readily visible: it is *nage*'s arm which *uke* has just run into.

In either technique, *nage*'s hand may follow *uke* to the mat, but it is a *follow* not a *force*. Attempting to force *uke down* neutralizes and defeats the spacial mechanics of *up* that these techniques are based on.

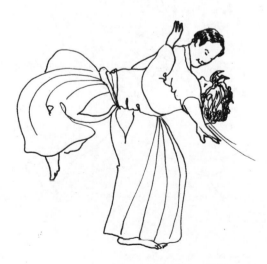

Another common mistake is trying to throw *uke* too soon, not allowing sufficient *time* for *uke*'s hips to pass his shoulders. This defeats the time mechanics of the throw, by actually helping uke regain balance and control.

"Tripping techniques" require leading *down*, moving *uke*'s upper body forward with legs and hips behind.

"Insufficient down" (often due to trying to throw *out*) defeats the mechanics of this particular technique. The advice to "drop *uke*'s hand down *through* the mat" as in *irimi* and *zempo-nage* reflects this issue[1].

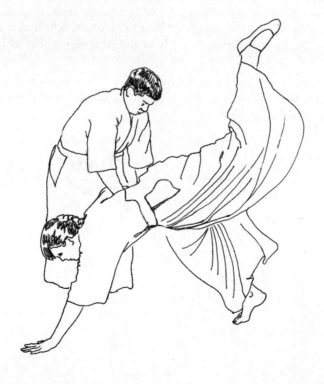

1. Because Aikidoists do not wear shoes on the mat, many readers have assumed that the one shoe in this picture was drawn in error. It was not. For the rest of the story, see page 126.

Katame-Waza

> Our sensei says that it's all very nice to cause pain, but not very useful if your attacker says "OWW!" and then bashes you because you hurt him which he could do because you were busy causing pain instead of controlling their center.
>
> —Dex Sinister, Aikikai

Katame-Waza ("Immobilizations") are commonly referred to as wrist-locks. Basics are:

- *Ikkyo* ("first-teaching"),
- *Nikyo* ("second-teaching"),
- *Sankyo* ("third-teaching"), and
- *Yonkyo* ("fourth-teaching").

Wristlocks are rarely an end in themselves; they are the first or intermediate step to a throw ("projection") such as *zempo-nage*, or a final pin (a modified wristlock). Wrist-locks can be exquisitely painful, especially to new students with tight inflexible wrists. But pain is not the ultimate goal. All locks aim to control the shoulder, by way of fingers, hand, wrist, and elbow joints. The lock may produce immobilization and control, sometimes via an implied threat of pain or discomfort — but the ultimate goal is control of *uke*'s center. Once that control is obtained, *nage* proceeds with a throw or a pin. In practice, the lock is applied until *uke* moves as intended or taps out.

The critical issue in a lock is *locking*, commonly referred to as "taking out the slack." This is where so many attempts fail.

How do you move a body attached to a wiggly flexible arm?

The same way you move a shoe at the end of a wiggly flexible chain.

If you simply push and shove, the links will collapse.

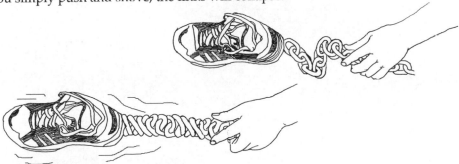

Lock the links and you can move the shoe (or other body) anywhere you want it to go.

Study the anatomy of wristlocks; study wristlocks in series to clarify the relationships between them. *Ikkyo* becomes *nikyo* becomes *sankyo* becomes *yonkyo* becomes *ikkyo* and so on. Combine with *shiho-nage* and *kote-gaeishi* to observe the patterns of entry, setup and application.

Practice wristlocks in *seiza* to isolate muscles, bones, and balance; this puts focus on the mechanics of the wristlock and away from the notion that "success" means Put Uke On The Mat. *Uke* is already there. For beginners, differentiating the name or the starting motions of one technique from another is tough enough without added inputs of technique and foot position, not to mention wasting time falling and getting up again. The *seiza* drill approach can be a big relief for beginning students and even the not-so-beginning students. Some students spend years in confusion because they were afraid to ask at first, later afraid to admit that they were still hazy on mechanics and application that they "should know by now."

A common problem is poor understanding of physiology. Martial arts books agree that a thorough understanding of underlying anatomy is critical to effectiveness but many stop there, offering no solid information. The best mechanical information is in Shioda's books[1]. The best anatomical information is by physiologist and Aikidoist Greg Olson who actually looked at, dissected, and studied the anatomy of shoulders, arms, and wrists. What's causing the pain? Manipulation of the ulnar and other nerves, but primarily the nerve-rich *periosteum* that "surrounds the bone" and is extremely sensitive to compression[2].

1. *Dynamic Aikido* (DA) and *Total Aikido* (TOT).
2. Greg Olson's articles on Aikido wristlocks are listed in the bibliography. For article reprints and related materials, contact Dr. Olson at golson@montana.edu.

The Cycle of Katame-Waza (Wrist Locks)

The four basic *katame-waza*[1] form a cycle of techniques. The choice of technique is based, as always, on the energy that *uke* offers. Every technique can be countered, but the motion necessary to do so sets *uke* up for the next lock in the series.

Practice the complete series slowly, as an exercise in hand placement, transition, and ultimately, effectiveness. Note that the cycle can flow in either direction.

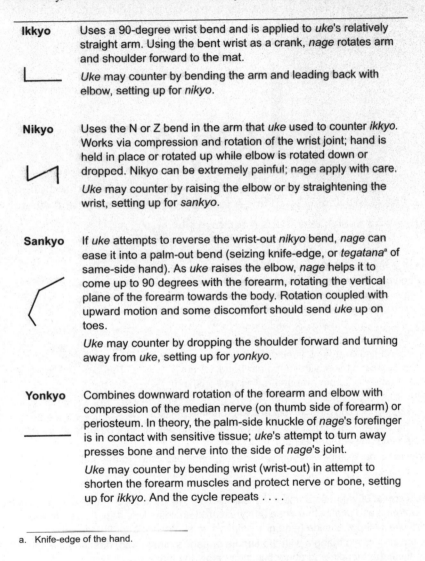

Ikkyo	Uses a 90-degree wrist bend and is applied to *uke*'s relatively straight arm. Using the bent wrist as a crank, *nage* rotates arm and shoulder forward to the mat.
	Uke may counter by bending the arm and leading back with elbow, setting up for *nikyo*.
Nikyo	Uses the N or Z bend in the arm that *uke* used to counter *ikkyo*. Works via compression and rotation of the wrist joint; hand is held in place or rotated up while elbow is rotated down or dropped. Nikyo can be extremely painful; *nage* apply with care.
	Uke may counter by raising the elbow or by straightening the wrist, setting up for *sankyo*.
Sankyo	If *uke* attempts to reverse the wrist-out *nikyo* bend, *nage* can ease it into a palm-out bend (seizing knife-edge, or *tegatana*[a] of same-side hand). As *uke* raises the elbow, *nage* helps it to come up to 90 degrees with the forearm, rotating the vertical plane of the forearm towards the body. Rotation coupled with upward motion and some discomfort should send *uke* up on toes.
	Uke may counter by dropping the shoulder forward and turning away from *uke*, setting up for *yonkyo*.
Yonkyo	Combines downward rotation of the forearm and elbow with compression of the median nerve (on thumb side of forearm) or periosteum. In theory, the palm-side knuckle of *nage*'s forefinger is in contact with sensitive tissue; *uke*'s attempt to turn away presses bone and nerve into the side of *nage*'s joint.
	Uke may counter by bending wrist (wrist-out) in attempt to shorten the forearm muscles and protect nerve or bone, setting up for *ikkyo*. And the cycle repeats . . . .

---

a. Knife-edge of the hand.

---

1. *Gokyo* is "Fifth Technique" but there is no reasonable counter that will return you to *ikkyo*. Some styles include a *ryokyo*. An instructor who begs to remain nameless claims that it is merely an arm bar and its elevation to "Sixth Technique" status is like the amplifier that goes up to 11 in Rob Reiner's rock spoof, *This is Spinal Tap*. "What does 11 get you?" "Well it's one louder, isn't it?"

Ikkyo

ADS: Immobilization #1 ("First Teaching") p. 166; TOT: Ikkajo, pp. 82-83; BA pp. 58-63.

> I rather like ikkyo. As *uke*, if I get tired I can just stay down and take a nap.
>
> —George Simcox, Ki Society

Ikkyo is the first of the wrist locks. It is usually applied to a straight arm and elbow in combination with a 90-degree bend of the wrist. To differentiate from other techniques, you may wish to remember it as:

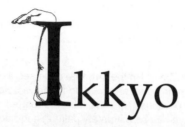

Ikkyo

Ikkyo is a relatively painless but effective technique which controls the shoulder (hence disrupting *uke*'s balance) by rolling it forward via fingers, wrist, and elbow.

If *uke* is holding your left hand with his right, to apply *ikkyo*:

Technique

1. As *uke* reaches for your left shoulder with his right hand, brush down on *uke*'s attacking hand with your right hand so that your fingers wrap over the knife edge of *uke*'s hand. Your thumb is aligned with *uke*'s thumb and index finger.
2. Step to the rear with LF. Draw back the forward foot.
3. Rotating *uke*'s wrist, thumb down and to a 90-degree bend, lead *uke*'s arm up and over his L shoulder in a circular path. Reinforce this circular motion with your other hand, coming up under *uke's* elbow or upper arm and *rolling* (not pushing) the arm over while . . .

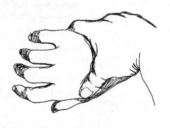

4. Stepping / skipping / sliding straight forward with outside (R) leg.
5. Rotate your hips so they are square and forward, dropping *uke* straight down to your arm's length, his shoulder lower than his hand.
6. Moving forward as necessary with your outside leg, bring *uke* down to the mat.

Pin

1. Extend *uke*'s arm at 90 degrees or more to his trunk. *Nage* faces in the same direction as *uke* with knee in armpit and *uke*'s other knee firmly secured against uke's arm. *Nage*'s inside hand covers *uke*'s elbow, outside hand grasps *uke*'s wrist. Wrist is bent 90 degrees.
2. With *uke*'s fingers, form a triangle with the fingers of *nage*'s other hand, directing them to a point at the tip of the triangle and about 6 inches below the mat.
   Release pressure immediately when *uke* slaps (taps out).

Variation:

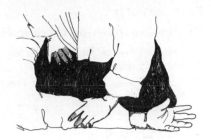

- With inside knee in *uke*'s armpit, *uke*'s arm secured against your knees, experiment with holding down the elbow only.
- In the "Gi Hold-down" *nage* places a knee in the armpit of *uke*'s *gi* to assist in pinning shoulder to the mat. This may be presented as a "Power of *Ki* Hold-down" but that is a spelling error.

The 90-degree wrist bend is an important part of the technique especially in response to a grab, and most especially if the attacker is much bigger and stronger[1]. See why with the OK Test.

The OK Test

For details and variations, see KIA, page 122.

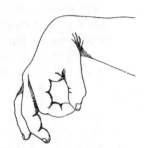

1. *Nage* touch thumb and forefinger in a circle. Try to hold the two fingers together while *uke* attempts to pull them apart.
2. *Nage* bend the wrist at 90 degrees.
    Uke compare force necessary to pull the fingers apart.
    Nage compare effort required to keep them together.
    Finger strength is poor when the wrist is sharply bent.
    This anatomical point applies directly to *ikkyo*[2] as follows.

The Ikkyo Elbow Pivot

1. *Uke* grab *nage*'s wrist.
2. *Nage*, with Unbendable Arm and leaving hand in place, pivot elbow down, hand up, catching *uke*'s wrist in the V of thumb and forefinger.
3. Notice *uke*'s wrist bend. Grasp *uke*'s hand with your other hand and compare the degree of strength or effort required to remove the hand; by *uke* to keep it there.
4. Compare effort required to bend *uke*'s wrist at the hand *without* dropping the elbow; compare ease or difficulty of removing *uke*'s hand.

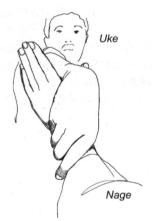

Uke

Nage

---

1. If attacker's hands are much bigger and stronger, small hands can grasp fingers.
2. It also applies to daily life. Opening a jar? Attempting to do so with wrist bent and fingers extended is an extremely weak position and can strain the hand. Straighten wrist, a far stronger position.

Back and Forth

Practice *ikkyo* (*irimi*) as a back and forth exercise to practice position and lead.

1. Partner 1 start by attacking with RH to Partner 2's left shoulder.
2. Partner 2 moves into *ikkyo irimi*, bending Partner 1 down to the mat, but before the throw,
3. Partner 1 rises, turning Partner 2 and applying ikkyo, bending Partner 2 down to the mat, but before the throw . . . .
4. And the cycle repeats.

Errors and Counters

Experiment with all of these, slowly. Compare to results obtained with good form.

In technique:

- Stepping forward with inside leg; *uke* may be able to grab it.
- Failure to drop *uke* far enough down. Think of first dropping him directly down *through* the mat and only then coming up to the proper position.
- Dropping *uke* down but with shoulder higher than hand. *Uke* can easily rise and turn the tables on *nage* (an action known as "conversion").
- Not maintaining your Center / One-Point; allowing *uke* to regain Center.

In pin:

- Do not lean forward over *uke*'s arm. A flexible and slithery*uke* — or a testing instructor — may unbalance and throw *nage* forward.
- Do not allow *uke* to regain control of elbow.

Although *nikyo, sankyo, yonkyo,* and *gokyo* are techniques in their own right, they are often thought of as the "second," "third," or "fourth" resort if *ikkyo* fails. *Uke*'s counter provides *nage* with the energy to flow into the next.

For example, if *uke* realizes that *nage* is moving into the basic *ikkyo irimi* described here, he might counter by tensing and blocking the forward movement of his arm. *Nage*'s counter to *uke*'s counter is to flow immediately into *ikkyo tenkan*[1] which uses the new force and energy being offered by *uke*.

---

1. This technique is one of several popularly known as "Airplane." See page 219.

Nikyo

ADS: Immobilization #2 ("Second-Teaching"), pp. 174-177; TOT: Nikajo, pp. 96-97.

Nikyo is the "Second Technique." *Uke* can counter by moving into *nage* and bending the elbow. Since the wrist is already bent in, this counter produces the N-shaped arm position ideal for *Nikyo*. To differentiate this lock from the others, remember:

Nikyo

Nikyo is a painful combination of rotation and pressure on wrist bones and nerves. It can be done in several ways, but key is relative motion of hand rotating up and forearm rotating down with compression of pain sensitive tissue. Two versions of *nikyo* are shown here. For the configuration and an idea of what it should feel like for *uke*, see "Nikyo-Undo" on page 106. Apply the lock gently, and release *immediately* upon hearing *uke*'s slap.

Nikyo 1

This is the first version of *nikyo* usually taught to beginners. Hand-on-chest position aids the beginner in keeping the attacking hand absolutely still, or perhaps "steel." As Chuck Gordon explains it, "the one hand is *steel*, the other is a *feather*." Many of us spend years allowing *uke*'s hand to rotate down with the elbow and wondering why the lock doesn't work. Because it isn't locked, that's why. For effective *nikyo*, watch for this tendency and eliminate it.

1. Place *uke*'s RH hand in the hollow of your L shoulder, *uke*'s fingers turned towards your armpit and hand (*tegatana*) vertical. *Uke*'s elbow should be bent into the "N" position.
2. Maintaining the bent-wrist *nikyo* position, move your other arm over *uke*'s arm until your fingers can pass over *uke*'s. This puts your elbow into position for moving downward onto *uke*'s arm.
3. Facing *uke* directly and imagining that the index finger of the holding hand is a sword, with a soft bow, slice *uke* from head to toe, down centerline of the body.

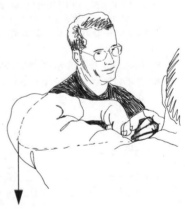

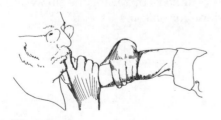

Variations

Consider the geologist's view of relative motion.

In designating movement along fault blocks of an earthquake, it doesn't matter if the left block went up and the right block stayed still, or if the right block went down and the left block stayed still. The relationships at the fault line (note arrows) are the same and are marked with the same symbols.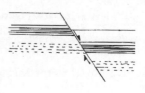

In *nikyo*, the hand may remain still while forearm rotates *down*, or hand may rotate *up* while the forearm remains still.

Either way, the results are the same if relative relationships are present.

Nikyo 2

Nage applies *nikyo* to *uke*'s same-side grab (LH grabbed by *uke*'s RH).

As *nage*,

1. Rest your RH atop *uke*'s hand to keep it in place.
2. Rotate your left wrist around to top of *uke*'s wrist, emphasizing the N or Z configuration in *uke*'s arm (wrist and elbow bent).
3. Cut down with palm of hand.
   Imagine that the middle finger of your holding hand is a sword, slicing *uke* from head to toe, straight down the centerline of the body.
   You must *really* cut rather than simply squooshing *uke*'s wrist (as happens when *nage* focuses on "causing pain"),

   • Mentally raise sword high, then
   • Slice down, to the horizon and down, cutting the sky in two.

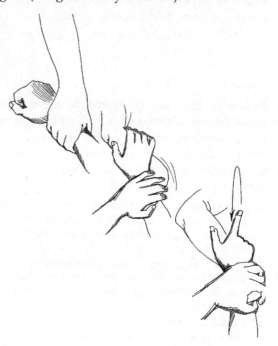

Didn't make it that far? *Uke* may counter your *nikyo* by raising the elbow and rolling the shoulder forward — the perfect position for *sankyo*.

Sankyo

ADS: Immobilization #3 (""Third-Teaching"), pp. 187-191; TOT: Sankajo, pp. 108-109.

Sankyo is the "third" wrist lock. To differentiate it from others, remember:

Sankyo and oykna**Z**

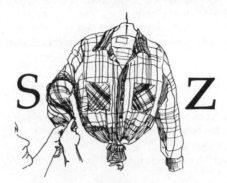

Sankyo locks the joints of wrist, elbow, and shoulder. For maximum effectiveness all must be stretched to their limit. Several motions are involved in taking up slack, all of which add another small part to the whole

As *uke* seizes your hand (same-side or cross).

1. Touch lightly to keep the hand in place.
2. Enter, passing under his arm and rotating it.

   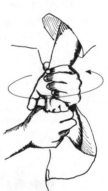

   If you are applying *sankyo* on the left side (from your point of view) you will be moving around and ducking under *uke*'s right arm in a counterclockwise direction. If you are applying *sankyo* on your right side (his left arm) you will be ducking under *uke*'s arm and turning so that you face in the same direction as *uke*. This rotates *uke*'s arm towards his body. For *uke*, it is the same motion of turning the hands inward as in "Ushiro-Tori Undo" on page 96[1]. See also "Swankyo" on page 71.

   Nage's upper hand controls *uke*'s wrist, thumb, and four fingers above the wrist, palm of the hand on *uke*'s knuckles. Keep slack out of *uke*'s wrist, elbow, and shoulder by applying torque with hands and hips. Point your own index finger at *uke*'s armpit.

   Nage's lower hand (outer hand) lightly holds *uke*'s fingers, keeping them slightly hyper-extended (bent back) below the forearm. Your hand applies torque on *uke*'s hand; the axis of rotation is *uke*'s middle finger.
3. Bring *uke* up on his toes.

---

1. For a practice partner, see "Closet Uke" in "Weapons, Tools, and Toys" on page 227. In a plaid shirt, the S or Z configuration can be clearly seen. But how is a Z of "Zankyo" different from the N of *nikyo*? *Nikyo*'s N is more horizontal, *sankyo*'s Z more vertical. You will see the twist in muscles and skin, as when you wring out a towel. S and Z designate direction of twist in vines in botany, and of fibers in textile arts. It can work here too.

Any throw from *sankyo* should be done from this tip-toe position. Once *uke* is on his toes (and probably slapping) . . .

4. Cut straight down.

Traditionally, this is a sword cut. In more modern terms, imagine tapping home plate with your baseball bat. For either situation, the motion is to rotate the tip of the sword or the bat down, not the handle.

The tiny interval between the beginning of the cut and the actual throw gives *uke* the momentary illusion of relief and he will come down to earth. Continue this motion by flowing into the actual throw. Taking *uke* up on his toes, then allowing him to come down, then starting the throw (three separate moves) is not nearly as effective as using *uke's* natural downward movement in one continuous downward flowing motion.

Variations

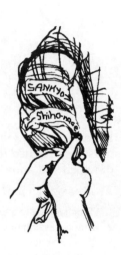

- Because beginners often confuse the approaches to *sankyo* and *shiho-nage* (page 207) practice going back and forth between these two. Observe that *shiho-nage* rotates the arm *outward* away from the body (supination); *sankyo inward* towards the body (pronation).
- Practicing with a shirt? A masking tape label can show direction of movement.
- *Sankyo* requires rotation and locking of all three joints so count them in order as 1-2-3 as you apply them: Wrist, elbow (forearm), and shoulder.
- Practice moving smoothly from *up* to *down* into throw.
- Establish *nage's* correct ending point; *nage* point at *uke's* armpit with extended index finger.

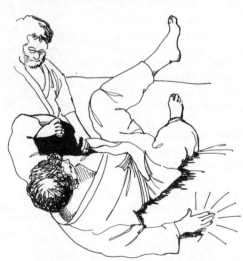

If you do not have all the slack out, or if the fingers can flex, *uke* can counter by turning in the direction of his free shoulder, seize your wrist, converting it to a *kote-gaeishi,* and converting you to a flying *uke. Uke* may also counter *sankyo* by pushing away and straightening the arm, but this is the position for *yonkyo.*

Yonkyo

ADS: Immobilization #4 ("Fourth-Teaching"), pp. 198-199; TOT: Yonkajo, pp. 118-119.

Yonkyo controls *uke*'s Center through the elbow, but also involves compression of the periosteum and nerves (usually the radial nerve) whose location and accessibility may vary with individual and musculature. It tends to be practiced less commonly than other wristlocks, because when successful it is so exquisitely painful for *uke*. Do it well and *uke* may be unable to use his hands for several minutes and may be sore for days. Hence the kind-hearted *nage* is reluctant to impose on friends; persons of fiercer nature may reflect that *nage* always becomes *uke*.

⅄onkyo

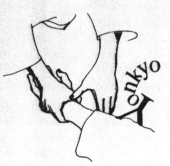

To differentiate *yonkyo* from other wristlocks, observe the **Y** position of thumb and forefinger.

The knuckle or joint used in *yonkyo* is the base of the index finger on the palm side. If you drive a car with a manual shift, you can practice the feeling of pressing with this joint by moving the gearshift with this point instead of pulling with the fingers.

Part of the difficulty of *yonkyo* is transition of hand position from the *sankyo* to *yonkyo*. Practice transitions first with no finish.

From *sankyo*, when *uke* counters by straightening the elbow/arm,

1. Leave lower hand on *uke*'s hand, sliding upper hand up to catch *uke's* forearm in V of thumb and index finger.
2. Rather than trying to compress nerves or cause pain, focus on rotating *uke*'s elbow down to the mat. The feeling is like tapping a baseball bat on home plate.
3. Do not try to force with arms; rotate from hips. The motion presses the base joint of *nage*'s index finger into *uke*'s arm.

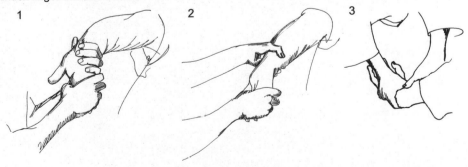

Sankyo-yonkyo transition: 1) *Sankyo*, 2) *Uke* counters by straightening arm, 3) *Nage* slides V of thumb and forefinger of upper hand up forearm.

Yonkyo is effective when *uke* has a straight arm with fingers extending straight out.

If you allow slack, *uke* may counter by bending the wrist. This shortens and thickens the flexor muscles of the forearm, protecting the radial nerve. But the resulting straight arm with bent wrist is the ideal position for *nage* to counter the counter by returning to *ikkyo*.

And the cycle repeats . . . .

"No, that's not quite right, let me show you, OK? Now you do it . . . No, you're still just squashing the wrist, do it like this, OK? Come on, get up, it doesn't hurt that bad, try again. No, cut through the elbow like this . . tell you what, why don't you practice with Big Earl (the one with wrists thicker than a kindergartner and nerves, if he has any, buried so deep you'd probably strike oil before you found them)?" After about six years they start getting it right.

—Tim Griffiths, Iwama

Variation

Arm-bar waza neatly combines practice of all wristlocks with after class beer.

1. *Uke*, seated on a revolving bar stool, hold *nage*'s wrist while turning slowly.
2. Observe the relationships between pronation and supination.
   Where is *ikkyo* and *sankyo*? Where does *shiho-nage* live?
3. Notice that if *uke* continues to turn, the lock appears automatically.
   Ideally, this is how Aikido really works. *Nage* does not force a lock on a resistant *uke*. The opportunity is there and *uke* walks into it.

Shiho-Nage

ADS. Immobilization #6 ("Four Direction Throw"), pp. 206-208; TOT: p. 71; BA p. 48-49, 54-57.

Shiho-nage is one of the most fundamental techniques in the Aikido repertoire. It doesn't require the precise attention to anatomy seen in the other wristlocks but the lead tends to evaporate at the "top" of the technique.

Alan Drysdale offers this exercise[1] to practice lead in a way that does *not* require *uke* to choose between a broken elbow or jumping over his own arm."

The Barbarella Lead

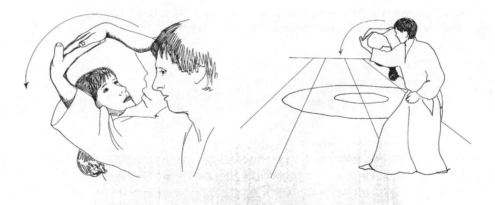

1. Stand in *ai-hanmi* (both *uke* and *nage* with their RF feet and RH forward). *Nage* offers RH palm up; *uke* lays hand palm down on *nage*'s hand.
   Uke's job is to maintain light palm-to-palm pressure and not let the hands separate. *Nage* will move through *shiho-nage*, pressing lightly against *uke*'s hand also, and moving so that the pressure is maintained.
   To start the movement,
2. *Nage* turns hand over, easing *uke*'s hand down and out into position for *shiho-nage*.
3. *Nage* steps in, maintaining pressure, leading hand up and over. This is where most people lose the contact, and resort to grabbing *uke*'s fingers.
4. Nage leads *uke*'s hand out behind shoulder.. . . then down back and towards the mat.

---

1. Alan notes that he "stole it from Chuck Clark." For why it's named after "Barbarella," rent the movie. You might also think of it as Alan's *Rocky Horror Picture Show Shiho-Nage*. "The Palm-to-Palm thing reminded me of RiffRaff and Columbia getting ready to do "The Time Warp." — Eric Tilles

Kote-Gaeshi

ADS: Immobilization #7 ("Wrist-Bend"), pp. 216-218; TOT: pp. 144-145.

> I remember getting certified for Two-person CPR and water rescue. In one lesson, we were learning how to deal with a drowning victim trying to pull you down.
> I kote-gaeshi-ed him. I passed.
>
> —David C. Pan

> Grizzly crunching sound
> Like tigers eating marrow
> Oh! was that your wrist?
>
> —Joel Zimba

Kote-gaeshi ("wrist-bend") is considered a wristlock although it doesn't fit well into the basic foursome of *Katame-Waza*. It also differs from these in that it is an actual throw, rather than an intermediary technique on the way to the throw.

It is similar in another unfortunate respect. Because of dynamic forces leading up to the technique, a student can muddle through it for years without ever quite understanding what makes it work or why it went wrong. This is especially true if emphasis is on Making Uke Fall Down rather than on learning effective technique.

Practice the mechanics from *seiza*, eliminating the throw, while learning what works, what doesn't, and why.

Kote-Gaeshi 1

1. Holding *uke*'s right wrist with your left hand....
2. Take up the slack.
3. Roll/rotate wrist and fingers, especially the index finger, toward the forearm.
4. Lead *uke*'s hand towards your center and down leaving room for him to fall.

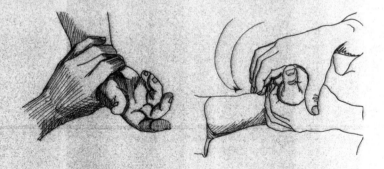

Variations

This version of *kote-gaeshi* is a natural for an uppercut punch or any other situation where the wrist is already bent. By removing slack, and controlling *uke*'s index finger, *kote-gaeshi* becomes a one-finger throw. This is because of two muscles controlling the index finger (the extensor digitorum and extensor indicis) and associated tendons.

The longer extensor digitorum begins above the elbow. It ends at the tip of the index finger. Hence it crosses *four* joints: the elbow, the wrist, the knuckle of the hand, and the two joints of the index finger.

Kote-Gaeshi 1 isn't just a matter of curling "the fingers" but of specifically curling the index finger. The outer three fingers share flexor tendons (which are necessarily relatively loose and floppy). The index finger has its very own dedicated tendon. Not only is this tighter then the others, but the more joints it must flex over, the tighter it becomes.

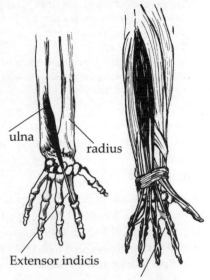

ulna

radius

Extensor indicis

Extensor digitorum

To feel the difference,

1. Bend your wrist to 90 degrees or as sharply as you can. Notice the natural position of fingers: index finger more extended, last three digits more relaxed. Try touching your palm with each finger in turn. Which is easiest? More difficult?
2. Push the large knuckle of the index finger towards your forearm in the direction of your palm; see how far it goes without discomfort.
3. Repeat with the middle, ring and little fingers and compare; you will be able to bend them much farther with no discomfort.
4. Repeat the above curling one or two finger joints versus curling all three.
5. Repeat the above with wrist held straight (no bend).

To see the difference (what is actually happening inside),

1. Lay two pieces of tape on your arm in positions of the two tendons.
2. Repeat the exercises above.
3. Notice what happens when you bend your wrist; when you bend the knuckles. What happens when you add a twist?

When beginners see *kote-gaeshi* most interpret it as "wrench elbow out to the side in to haul *uke* off his feet." It seems logical that this would be most effective. That approach is dangerous to *uke* (it can snap the elbow, the old version of this technique), much harder work for *nage* and a far less efficient motion.

To compare "wrenching" versus "curling,"

With partners in *seiza, uke* with arm extended,

1. *Nage* slowly apply *kote-gaeshi* by curling up *uke*'s hand with attention to the index finger while bringing *uke*'s hand towards own Center or One-Point.
2. *Uke* observe and report the point at which he begins to feel discomfort and the point at which he begins to fall.
3. For the *uke* who refuses to acknowledge discomfort, *nage* may simply observe the point at which the shoulder begins to drop and *uke* begins to lose balance.
4. Repeat by slowly twisting *uke*'s elbow out to the side (the "common sense" *kote-gaeishi*). Observe the point at which the shoulder begins to drop and *uke* begins to lose balance.

5. Repeat both of the above while "giving the slack back" to *uke*; that is, *nage*'s arms are extended, *uke*'s arms are close in to the body.

6. Compare relative motion and effort required to unbalance *uke* in all cases. Compare with *Kote-Gaeshi* 2 and 3.

   To actually do the throw from *seiza* (making it a *suwari-waza* technique*) nage must move, pivoting on the knee opposite the kote-gaeshi to allow room to keep uke's arm extended and space for uke to fall.*

Generally you will find that properly done, proper application of *Kote-Gaeshi* involves only a few inches of lateral motion and little effort.

Finding the Wrist

Targeting the wrist and grabbing for it is far less reliable than targeting the entire arm. An arm, after all, is much larger and leads directly to the wrist. Start the motion like an open-handed block, then allow the hand to soften and cup *uke*'s arm, sliding towards *uke*'s wrist. Uke's hand will stop nage's motion in exactly the proper position, much like a knot at the end of a rope. In pairs,

1. *Uke* attack with a slow *mune-tsuki punch.*
2. *Nage* turn *tenkan* and experiment with:

   a) Grabbing directly for *uke*'s wrist versus ("catch the wrist").

   b) Sliding arm down *uke*'s arm from upper arm to wrist. To be really sporting,
3. Repeat *with eyes closed* at different speeds.

Giving Back Slack

Rolling arm, wrist and hand back towards *uke* "gives back slack." With slack in the arm, wrist, and fingers, the throw won't work. Or, it will offer the opportunity of a reversal; that is, it will enable *uke* to flow into another technique (such as Kokyu-Nage Basic) to throw the now extended and off-balance *nage*.

Think of *kote-gaeshi* like going fishing. Rolling the wrist, hand, and fingers is like rolling up the reel on a fishing rod.

- You are weaker and *uke* stronger when you are reaching out to *uke*'s Center.
- *Uke* is weaker and you are stronger when you draw *uke* in to *your* Center.
- Do you go to the fish? Or do you bring the fish to you?
- Try both approaches. See which works better and why.

Hips and Legs

Landing the fish is made still more effective by adding hips and legs.

1. Imagine that *uke*'s hand is linked to your same-side forward foot.
2. As you curl wrist and fingers, bring them to your Center while sweeping your same-side foot and hip back; with them flow your arms and hands as if attached to the foot. You can practice this motion alone. With a partner, be sure to allow space for *uke* to fall safely and to protect your own toes.

   The "hand linked to foot" motion is the vertical version of the motion (horizontal) used to make a toy walk. (See "Standing, Stepping and Stance" on page 44.)

Kote-Gaeshi 2

TOT: pp. 144-145.

This version of *kote-gaeshi*[1] is similar to Kote-Gaeshi 1, except that it is actually a wrist turnout. Instead of rolling up the index finger,

1. *Nage* curls *uke*'s little finger outward and towards the foot that is swooping back, leading *uke*'s straight but locked arm forward and down towards what is now the back foot.
2. Note again that arm is *extended*, not wrenched to the side.

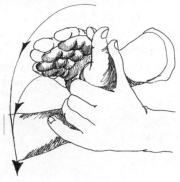

Kote-Gaeshi 3

This version is based on *tekubi-kosa undo*, the wrist-crossing exercise (see page 88).

As *uke* holds *nage*'s left hand with right hand,

1. *Nage* curl fingers, rotate and cross wrists,
2. Reach under *nage*'s hand to grasp *teyatana* of *nage*'s hand.
3. With other hand, make a "hand-sandwich," *uke*'s hand enclosed in yours.
4. Like cutting down with a sword, bring *uke*'s hand to your Center while stepping back, hand coordinated with foot as described in "Hips and Legs" above.

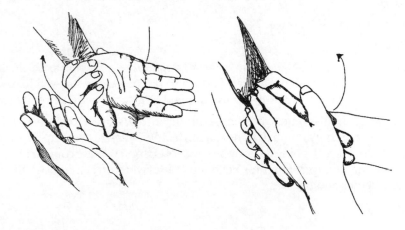

---

1. Also known as the *August Kote-Gaeshi* because the finger-curl of *Kote-Gaeshi 1* can be very slippery when hands are wet with sweat. A more secure grip is provided by *Kote-Gaeshi 2* and *3*.

Aikido Throws (Nage-Waza)

One does not do Aikido *to* someone, one does Aikido *with* someone. [You can't do] Aikido to people as if it were a definable technique. Technique has form, form has function, the content of the function is Aikido. Not the Form or its Function but the "content" defines the art. Don't react but interact, don't do things *to* someone but *with* someone.

—Dennis Hooker, Aikido Schools of Ueshiba

The following basic throws are presented primarily as an overview to relate to the Hitori-Waza exercises presented in Chapter 4 and the training exercises presented here. Directions are generalized descriptions of Ki Society style (because that is what I am most familiar with) and in no way intended to serve as the definitive description of any technique. This set of techniques makes up the 5th *kyu* (first adult level) test at the Virginia Ki Society.

You, your instructor, or your individual style may emphasize other points, processes, or procedures. Adapt as necessary.

Kokyu-Nage

ADS: Projection #1 ("Breath Throw"), pp. 224-226.

Kokyu-nage comprises a family of "breath-throws," or "timing-throws." There are many different applications of this concept, but the underlying principle is that the attacker is thrown by manipulation of timing and balance rather than by a wrist lock or immobilization. Similarly, *kokyu-nage* techniques are never followed by pins.

In *kokyu-nage* the attacker holds *nage*. *Nage* does not hold the attacker. In fact, *nage* does so little to the attacker that if the attacker were to let go — cease his attack — he could simply walk away without consequence. This issue must be clearly understood by the student. Otherwise beginners tend to devolve into a "This would never work because I could just . . . "

Just what? Let go? Walk away?

Yes. Exactly.

In the Ki Society, Kokyu-Nage Basic (*katate kosa-tori kokyu-nage irimi tobikomi*) is the first technique at the beginning of every test during the course of your Aikido career. This "20-year technique" is a "breath-throw" applied to a "grab to the opposite wrist."

Kokyu-nage techniques tend to be "clotheslining" throws, based on a lead *up*. Take care not to not rush the *up* motion. *Uke*, not nage, decides when to come up. Trying to force *uke* up when *uke* is still going *down* opposes *uke*'s energy; you are countering your own throw. Forcing *uke* up before hips have moved forward of Center actually helps *uke* to regain Center and balance.

Katate-Kosa-Tori Kokyu-Nage Irimi Tobikomi[1] (Kokyu-Nage Basic)

ADS: Projection #2 ("Cross-hand attack, dealt with by entering and jumping in") p. 230.

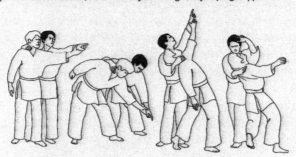

Uke:	L *hanmi*, grabs *nage*'s LH with his LH, reaching forward throughout course of technique.
Nage:	L *hanmi*, presents LH, little-finger-side down.
Mechanics:	*Nage* redirects incoming energy around then *up* (a place where *uke* can't stay long). Torso goes up, legs continue forward ("clotheslining," page 193).
Hitori waza:	*Ude-mawashi-undo, ude-furi undo.*
A. K. A.	"The Hello Hug and A Tour of the Dojo." (*See our nice walls, nice mat? Nice ceiling? Oops!*)

1. As *uke* grabs *nage*'s L wrist, *nage* leaves the seized hand in place and moves straight in (*irimi*) until resistance is felt in *uke*'s arm.
2. With RF step behind *uke*; RH thumb and index finger cradle base of *uke*'s head, a soft, effective but barely noticeable hug, not a jerk or torque to the chin or neck.
3. Leading and circling to the L (extending forward, never backing up) seized arm drops straight down, rises up, then follows *uke* downward with weight underside.
4. When *uke* attempts to stand up, *nage* "helps" by leading arm to a point on the ceiling while simultaneously dropping R arm with weight underside on *uke*'s R shoulder. *Uke*'s upper body follows the "up" while his legs continue forward, moving out from under him.
5. As *uke* falls, invert R hand, following *uke* down to the mat with the little finger.

Variations

- **Placement**. *Nage* repeats stepping into position, leaving hand in place.
  - *Uke* note whether *nage*, in the course of turning, pulls back.
  - Work to eliminate any tugging and make the move as smooth as possible.
- **Attack and Lead.** *Uke* feel difference in lead between:
  - Extending forward (correct) or pulling sideways or back (incorrect).
  - *Uke* let *nage* know if the lead is not forward. A string or cord (rather than a wrist grab) makes direction of force clearly visible. A forward lead is easier if you are looking in the direction that you are going.

---

1. Jim Baker Sensei (Aikikai) describes this as "The French Waiter Irimi-Nage." "Greetings Madame! Let me lead you to your table. What? No tip? You fall down!"

- **Up and Down**. "Down" to a 6-footer may be "up" to a 5-footer. Tall *nage* with short *uke* must check to see that lead has actually dropped enough to disrupt *uke*'s center.

  If you and your partner are a "Mutt and Jeff":

  -Standing shoulder to shoulder, where are your hands? Where are your hips?

  -How far down does the taller person have to reach to be "down" to the shorter one?

  -How far down does the shorter one have to bring *uke* to have an effective "up"?

  -What happens if the tall *nage* drops to his knees? To *suwari-waza?*

Kuzushi ("unbalancing ") is disruption of weight and Center into a fall. But different bodies have different Centers and balance break points. Even bodies of the same height may respond differently due to body shape, weight distribution, and gender.

- In men, the break point is at the top of the hip bone (at the waist), often above the belt.
- In women, the break point is at the level of the hip socket or lower.

What Can Go Wrong

This "first technique" is one of the most dangerous when done improperly.

Kokyu-nage techniques rely on balance and timing which beginners (and some more advanced students) fail to see. They *think* they see *nage* flinging *uke* around by head and neck. Often when *uke* fails to fall, tall, strong students tend to grab shorter ones by the neck and just fling *harder*.

If *nage* continues to turn while completing the throw, centrifugal forces cause *uke* to fly out of *nage's* circle, often spiraling wildly across the mat. *Nage* may then attempt to correct the perceived problem by holding ever more tightly to *uke*'s head and neck "for control[1]."

The rationale is that "where head goes, body will follow" but improperly done (and especially if done for the wrong reasons) the result can be serious injury to *uke*'s neck and symptoms ranging from back, arm, and hand pain to herniated disks[2]. Personally I feel that beginners should stick to shoulder and not touch neck and head at all.

There are better solutions for control than headlocks. The best solution is to simply change the physics. If *nage* steps out of the circle (as for "Tenkan Ude-Oroshi" on page 221) *uke* can be laid down on a line and under perfect control.

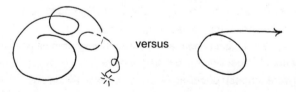

versus

---

1. See footnote on rotational physics on page 77 for what happens to spinning bodies. This is an odd notion that *uke* is falling "prematurely" and must be controlled until it is *nage*'s time for *uke* to fall.
2. See symptoms of scalene injuries on page 156.

Shiho-Nage

ADS: Immobilization #6 ("Four Direction Throw"), pp. 206-208; TOT: p. 71.

Pivoting of the hips, complete redirection of attacking energy, and the unusual fact that it can be applied to almost any attack, from energetic to static, make *shiho-nage*[1] one of the most fundamental Aikido techniques.

Yokomen-Uchi Shiho-Nage Irimi

ADS: ("Diagonal-strike to head with entering four-direction throw") pp. 214-215; TOT: pp. 76-77.

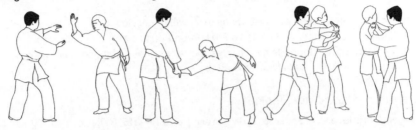

Uke:	L *hanmi*, stepping into R *hanmi* striking *yokomen* with RH.
Nage:	L *hanmi*, pivoting back into R *hanmi* to avoid strike.
Mechanics:	*Nage* continues incoming motion and by changing direction, guides strike to *uke's* rear where *nage* is stable but *uke* is not.
Hitori waza:	*Ikkyo-undo, tenkan.*
A.K.A.	*"London "Bridge" as mnemonic for ducking under the arm during the turn."*

1. *Nage* step back, arms rising into *ikkyo undo*, guiding striking arm down.
2. Touching *uke's* wrist with your RH and switching to R *hanmi*; rotate *uke's* wrist by turning your LH hand palm up. Step toward *uke* with RF crossing his body, turning it. (Remember, in *irimi*, *nage* turns *uke*. In *tenkan*, *nage* turns himself).
3. Lead *uke's* arm up and around, turning under your arm so that *uke's* hand and forearm are curled over *uke's* own shoulder, palm down.
4. *Nage* rotates hips to the R while dropping Center; end looking into *uke's* ear.
5. Drop *uke's* arm over *uke's* same-side shoulder, down *uke's* back and straight down to mat.

Variations

In practicing the above *shiho-nage* technique, you are continuing the lead. But first note where the lead should go.

---

1. The name is usually interpreted as "four-direction throw," but in Japanese culture, *shiho* suggests "around the world in all directions" just as we refer to the "four corners of the earth" but mean "around the whole circle or globe of the earth." From *shiho* came *shippo*, a symbol composed of interlocking circles and representing expansiveness.

Yokomen Only

1. *Uke* strike *yokomen* several times.
2. *Nage* observe the path of *uke*'s arm and hand.
   This is the path that *nage* should follow.

Feeler Shiho-Nage

It is common (and dangerous) to force *uke*'s arm out to the side during the turn or the throw but this occurs when *nage* is unsure where *uke* actually is. Practice with eyes closed. Keeping in constant contact with *uke,* roll around *uke*'s arm and shoulder, feeling *nage*'s position constantly.

1. Repeat the Barbarella Lead exercise (page 207) with eyes closed.
2. Feel the lead, and feel the *contact* as you roll around *nage*'s arm and shoulder.
   This exercise removes dependence on eyes, activates sense of touch. You will know, because you *must* know, *exactly* where *uke* is.

Yokomen-Uchi Shiho-Nage Tenkan

ADS: ("Diagonal-strike to head, four-direction throw with turn"), pp. 214—215; TOT: p. 75; BA p. 80. .

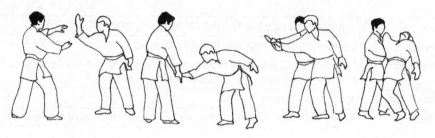

Uke:	L *hanmi*, stepping into R *hanmi* and striking *yokomen* with RH.
Nage:	L *hanmi*, pivoting back into R *hanmi*.
Mechanics:	*Nage* turns *tenkan* around striking arm, and guides it to rear where *nage* is stable but *uke* is not.
Hitori waza:	*Ikkyo-undo, tenkan-undo.*
A.K.A.	*"London Bridge."*

1. Begin as in *yokomen-uchi shiho-nage irimi* above, but turn *tenkan* around *uke*'s hand.
2. Lead *uke*'s arm up and around, turning under it so that hand and forearm are curled over his shoulder, palm down.
3. Step through, leading hand over *uke*'s shoulder and down back to mat.

Shiho-nage irimi is a natural for the *yokomen* motion as it simply continues and wraps *uke*'s arm up in its own motion. The *tenkan* version appears to clash with this motion but actually extends and deflects the *yokomen* strike into *tenkan* rather than suddenly reversing direction. Experiment with *extending* the strike into a *tenkan,* as compared to stopping the motion then reversing and doing a *tenkan* as separate motions.

Ikkyo

ADS: Immobilization #1 ("First Teaching") pp. 166-167; TOT: Ikkajo, pp. 82-83.

Ikkyo is a fundamental Aikido technique, the first of the cycle of wrist-locks.

Shomen-Uchi Ikkyo Irimi

ADS: ("Front-strike to head, first wrist-lock technique done by entering") pp. 171-172; TOT: shomen-uchi ikkajo osae ichi, pp. 84-85.

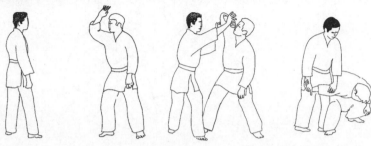

Uke:	L *hanmi*, stepping forward into R *hanmi* to strike *nage*'s head.
Nage:	R *hanmi*.
Mechanics:	Reversal of *uke*'s incoming strike.
Hitori waza:	*Ikkyo-undo*

1. Swing arms up into *ikkyo undo*, not blocking but extending in the direction of *uke*'s fingertips. Make contact with *uke*'s arm before forearm has passed the vertical, deflecting it in direction of *uke*'s fingertips. The more horizontal the arm, the more power behind the blow.
2. Circle *uke*'s arm up in front of his face and body then forward and down; your LH around uke's upper arm stabilizes and rolls his shoulder forward.
   Uke should pivot off center around a new point of rotation — the shoulder.
3. Stepping or skipping forward with RF (outside foot), lead *uke* down to the mat.

Variations

This technique and its results appear magical because we tend to assume that attacks are linear. That is not the case here. This is clarified by striking with a *jo*. Notice that:

- The lines of force are circular.
- The most powerful (and dangerous) point is tip of hand or *jo*, not the upper arm.
- At time of *nage's* contact with *uke's* arm, the *jo* is not yet a danger.

Perhaps the best way to understand *ikkyo-irimi* is to first do it wrong.

1. Partners assume a static position.
2. *Nage* push directly in against *uke*'s power.
   Observe that this approach accomplishes nothing. Where is the way out?
3. Notice the direction of *uke*'s fingers; lead in *that* direction instead.
   Observe results.

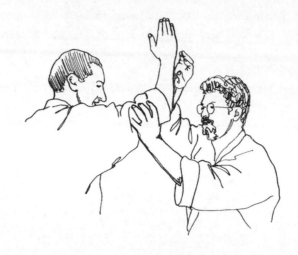

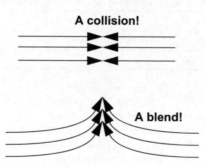

A collision!

A blend!

Shomen-Uchi Ikkyo Tenkan

ADS: ("Front strike to head, first wrist-lock technique done with turning") pp. 166-167. Commonly known as "Airplane."; TOT: shomen-uchi ikkajo osae ni, pp. 86-87.

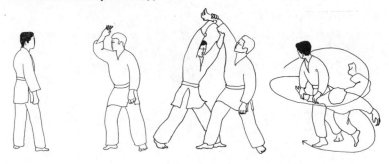

Uke:	L *hanmi* stepping forward into R *hanmi* to strike *nage*'s head.
Nage:	R *hanmi*.
Mechanics:	A counter to *uke*'s attempt to counter *ikkyo-irimi*. Redirects resisting forward energy into a *tenkan* spin.
Hitori waza:	*Ikkyo-undo, tenkan-undo.*
A. K. A.	*"Airplane"*

1. Begin as in with *ikkyo-irimi,* but as *uke*'s arm reaches highest point of the circle, step forward with LF to stand just behind *uke*'s shoulder.
2. Swing RF back and around (*tenkan*) rotating the hips; simultaneously . . .
3. Drop *uke*'s arm 90 degrees down to mat. (Try for a 180-degree turn).

Variations

This technique can be done on its own, but it is often used as a counter to a counter to *ikkyo-irimi. Uke* knows what's about to happen and blocks by pushing forward to resist *nage*'s attempt to send his arm over his shoulder in *nage*'s forward direction. Practice the following:

- *Uke* strike *shomen-uchi* then hold arm firmly pushing forward.

  Practice the feel of directing that energy forward and around into a tenkan.
- Experiment with *nage*'s ending position. What happens if you end your *tenkan:*

  -Standing in front of *uke*?

  -Even with *uke*?

  -Slightly behind *uke*?

Kote-Gaeshi

ADS: Immobilization #7 ("Wrist-Bend") pp. 216-218; TOT: p. 57.

Mune-Tsuki Kote-Gaeshi Tenkan

ADS: ("Mid-level punch with wrist-bend and turn") p. 223; TOT: Shomen-tsuki kote-gaeshi ("Front-punch with wrist-bend") pp. 146-147.

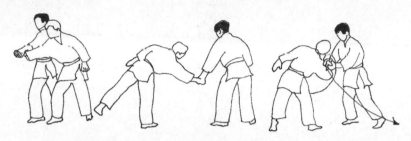

Uke:	From L *hanmi*, *uke* steps forward into R *hanmi*, and punches to *nage*'s midsection with RH.
Nage:	L *hanmi*.
Mechanics:	*Nage* leads incoming energy around in a circle, redirecting it into a wristlock forward of *uke*'s center ("Tripping," page 193).
Hitori waza:	*Kote-gaeshi-undo, ude-furi-undo, tenkan-undo.*

1. As *uke* punches, *nage* sweeps hand down *uke*'s arm to wrist and turns *tenkan,* hand at hip.
2. *Nage* absorbs energy of punch, leading in circle until *uke* is felt to be unstable and directed strongly forward.
3. Applying *kote-gaeshi*, *nage* reverses direction, such that *uke* walks into the wristlock at the same time that *nage* sweeps back the same-side leg, unbalancing *uke* while simultaneously opening up a place for *uke* to fall.

Variation

It is common to grab for the hand, a small target that is easily missed. Instead,

- Practice sweeping your hand down *uke*'s arm while grasping lightly. Think of making a "U" with thumb and forefinger. The bottleneck of the wrist will stop your hand in exactly the right position.
- Now try the above with your eyes closed.

Ude-Oroshi

ADS: Projection #2 ("Arm-Drop") p. 244.

One of the family of "clotheslining" throws, *ude-oroshi* ("arm-drop") uses the same motions seen in the *sayu-undo* exercise. No beginner ever believes that this technique could "really" work (especially "On the Street"). It requires effective dynamic *tenkan* and precise timing but is devastatingly effective. Students commonly try to push *uke* over with an arm but the arm should merely lead. Aikidoist Dan Henry likens the arm to the bowsprit on a ship: "It leads, it extends, but it's the vessel itself (the Center) that does the real work."

Katate-Tori Kokyu-Nage Tenkan Ude-Oroshi

ADS: ("Same-side grab, breath-throw, with turn and arm-drop"), also known as "Emperor's Clothes," pp. 244-245)

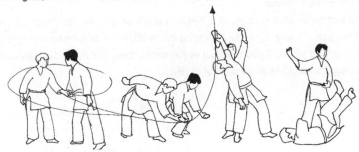

Uke:	L *hanmi*, seizing nage's R wrist, energy forward.
Nage:	R *hanmi*, RH palm down.
Mechanics:	Incoming energy is deflected and redirected in a circle which leads to "Clotheslining."
Hitori waza:	*Tenkan-undo, sayu-undo*
A. K. A.	*"Emperor's Clothes"*

1. *Uke* grabs *nage*'s R wrist with his LH.
2. Pivoting on RF, *nage* turns palm up turning *tenkan* around the seized hand ending shoulder to shoulder with *uke*.
3. With fingertips extended forward forming a V with Center (as if carrying a stack of laundry or a basketball), *nage* leads *uke* around Center until *uke* is in dynamic motion.
4. Stepping out of circle, *nage* bends knees, dropping One-Point and leading *uke* down and forward of his Center. The motion is very similar to that of bowling.
5. As *uke*, descending towards the mat, begins to attempt to rise to regain his balance, *nage* swings both arms upward as for *ude-mawashi*.
6. End in *sayu-undo*, weight and One-Point dropping down onto RF.

Variation

- *Nage*'s body must be in full contact with *uke*'s body so that weight of *nage*'s body and arm are dropped onto *uke*'s unbalanced upper torso when the knee is bent in *sayu-undo*. Lacking this contact, *nage* ends up trying to force *uke* down with a one-arm push while standing on the wrong end of the lever arm. Experiment with trying to do the technique at a distance. Compare with close contact.

Philip Akin (Yoshinkan) comments: "I can use strength and push down with my arm or I can let my knee go soft and bend." Notice that in *sayu-undo*, arms are not *forced* down, they *drop* down with a drop of Center and a bend of the knee. Do the exercise! (page 94).

- Arms do not act alone. They rise in coordination with upward thrust of legs, rise of One-Point. They descend with downward drop of One-Point and body weight. If *tenkan* and downward lead are done well, the upward lead will leave *uke's* upper body off-balance to the rear while legs continue hurtling forward. Experiment with isolating arms, exaggerating upward lead, eliminating upward lead, combining with upward thrust of legs.

- Notice that *tenkan* proceeds in a horizontal circle to develop momentum. Once *uke* is moving, *nage* steps out, transforming the horizontal circle into a vertical circle. *Uke* is laid down in a sliding fall perpendicular to *nage*. Compare with "Katate-Kosa-Tori Kokyu-Nage Irimi Tobikomi (Kokyu-Nage Basic)" on page 213 per continuing to spiral versus stepping out of the circle to throw.

-Do the technique on the seam of a mat or a chalk or tape line to check positioning.

-What happens to *uke* if you do the entire throw while continuing to turn *tenkan*?

-What happens to *uke* if you step out of the circle, then throw, as described above?

-Which approach offers more control of *uke*?

Zempo-Nage

ADS: Projection #22 ("Forward-Throw"), p. 308.

This is a large family of "forward throws." In the Ki Society, they are done not by hurling *uke* forward like pitching a baseball into the outfield, but by moving your own center forward then simply dropping the leading arm (*ude-mawashi-undo*) 90 degrees down to the mat. *Zempo-nage* are common as final techniques in *Taigi* (Ki Society) so that *nage* can help return *uke* to his proper position for the final bow.

Ryote-Mochi Kokyu-Nage Zempo-Nage Tenkan

ADS: ("Both-hands grab, breath-throw, throwing forward-throw with a turn") pp. 308-309.

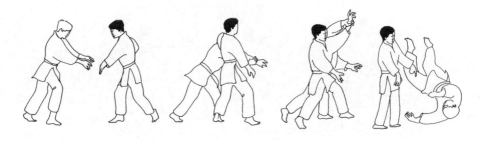

Uke:	R *hanmi*, seizing both of *nage*'s wrists, energy forward.
Nage:	L *hanmi*.
Mechanics:	A "tripping" throw. *Uke*'s Center is lead up, forward, and then down ahead of his supporting feet
Hitori waza:	*Tekubi-kosa undo, tenkan-undo, udemawashi-undo, funekogi-undo.*

1. Nage turn with full *tenkan* to *uke*'s R side.
2. Moving Center/One-Point forward, raise *uke*'s hands, then drop leading hand 90 degrees straight down to mat.
   Students think they see uke being thrown forward, but this is deceptive. *Uke* slides off the arm carried by his own forward momentum just as rapidly moving water thundering over a 90-degree cliff does not fall straight down, but flows forward and down.

Ushiro-Nage

ADS: Projection #16 ("Rear-Throw") p. 295.

Ushiro is used to refer to any throws done in response to attacks from "behind."

The wrist grab from behind was intended to disarm or neutralize an attacker armed with swords or knives. Techniques usually begin by bringing the attacker forward, then flow into any number of other possibilities from *ikkyo*, to *kote-gaeshi*, to *kokyu-nage* to *zempo*.

Ushiro-Tori Tekubi-Tori Ura-Gaeshi

ADS: ("Rear-attack to wrists, with a turning to the rear") p. 295.

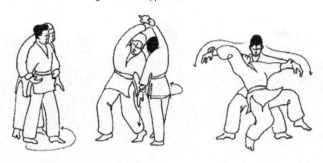

Uke:	Behind *nage*, holding both wrists, pulling down.
Nage:	*Shizentai.*
Mechanics:	Rotation of *uke* around *nage*'s "earth" hand.
Hitori waza:	*Tekubi-kosa-undo, ushiro tekubi-kosa-undo.*
A. K. A.	*"Inside Out."*

1. *Nage* extend LH straight down, forming center of *uke*'s rotation.
2. Leading from fingertips, bring RH to Center then up centerline of body, fingers pointing up.
3. As hand leads over *uke*'s head, pivot on LF to your L side.
4. Step to *uke*'s rear (*ura*), turning him "inside out."
5. Extend both arms out and drop One-Point 90 degrees to mat.

Tenchi-Nage

ADS: Projection #9 ("Heaven-and-Earth Throw") p. 274.

A basic exercise in weight upperside, weight underside, and unbalancing.

Katate-Tori Ryote-Mochi Kokyu-Nage Tenchi-Nage

ADS: ("Both-hands grab, heaven-and-earth breath-throw") pp. 274-275; TOT: pp. 164-165; BA p. 70, p. 92.

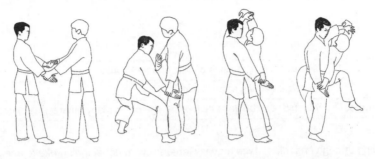

Uke:	L *hanmi*, seizing both of *nage*'s hands, energy neutral or back and down.
Nage:	R *hanmi*.
Mechanics:	"Clotheslining" by moving *uke*'s torso backward of feet.
Hitori waza:	*Udemawashi-undo*
A. K. A.	*"Heaven and Earth"*

1. *Nage* drops L elbow, Center/One-Point,
2. With LH *atemi* motion to *uke*'s One-Point (to draw *uke*'s attention), *nage* leads LH up, RH down and forward.
3. *Nage* slides past *uke's* forward *LF* with RF continuing LH upward in an "S" pattern as if throwing *ki* (or a cream pie) up and over *uke*'s shoulder.
4. Step through and up with LF then drop Center/One-Point down to the earth.

Variation

- There is often confusion about which is the throwing hand. It is actually the "earth" hand. The "heaven" hand leads *uke* "upperside" making *uke* easier to move (see "Swankyo" on page 71) while the "earth hand" moves *uke*'s torso forward of his stable center.

  This is also known as the "pizza and dollar bill" throw. Most beginners try to knock *uke* over with the "heaven" hand. To return focus to the "earth" hand, imagine — or place — a dollar bill on the mat for *nage* to pick up. Live pizza is optional.

- Students often attempt to force their way through *uke*. To prevent this, and return focus to unbalancing and dynamics, *nage* offer just two fingers to *uke*.

  Fingers aren't as strong as wrists: trying to muscle through a technique risks a sprained finger. Start with index fingers. With practice, go to pinky fingers.

Zagi Kokyu-Dosa

Not a wrestling match, but an exercise in relaxation, expansion, balance and control.

ADS: ("Seated Breath-movement") pp. 109-111; TOT: Kokyu-ho, pp. 168-173; KIA p. 50-54.

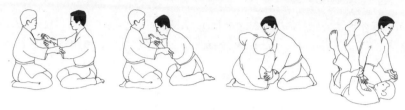

Uke:	In *seiza*, seizing outside of both of *nage*'s wrists.
Nage:	In *seiza*, offering arms to *uke*.
Mechanics:	Variable. Can be done as *tenchi-nage* or via many other forms of unbalancing.

1. Extending through fingertips, *nage* moves Centerforward unbalancing *uke* to one side. Do not throw straight back in *seiza;* it is awkward and painful for *uke*.
2. As *uke* falls, follow motion with whole body, ending in *seiza* with your R knee in his R armpit.
3. Hold-down: In *seiza* on toes with back erect, gently press *uke*'s L wrist and R shoulder with knife-edges of your hands (if on *uke's* right side; reverse for L side).

Variations

- Try this exercise with *nage* and *uke* clasping hands around a basketball.
- To see the steering-wheel motion, try the exercise with a hula-hoop.
- Experiment with consciously sending every push or thrust of energy down to your Center or to the center of the earth.
- What happens if you imagine that you are bigger, larger, and sitting deeper under the mat than *uke*? Imagine only your eyes peering over the top of the mat.

Taigi #5

Ki Society's Taigi 5 combines five of the above techniques (or their variations). Uke attacks first with right hand, then left hand for each technique.

1. *Shomen-uchi kokyu-nage*
2. *Yokomen-uchi shiho-nage irimi*
3. *Mune-tsuki kote-gaeshi tenkan* (with turnover and hold-down)
4. *Kata-tori-ikkyo irimi*
5. *Kokyu-Dosa*

CHAPTER 7

Weapons, Tools, and Toys

The techniques you learn in Aikido are not weapons. They are tools which can be used to save a life. If you use them as weapons, you will get cut by them. You will hurt somebody or get hurt. If you use them with virtuous intention, you will go right through the opposition.

I stole this theory from 150 Japanese sword teachers.

—Terry Dobson, *It's a Lot Like Dancing*

Weapons

Aikido offers training in the traditional Japanese weapons — sword (*katana* or *bokken*) and staff (*jo*, similar to the Old English quarter-staff of Robin Hood and Little John)[1]. Sword and staff are a tad archaic as "weapons" but as tools they teach the concepts of extension, alignment, rotation, leverage and *ma-ai* more effectively than empty hand techniques alone. They are also the original source of many Aikido techniques in which the empty hand emulates the rise and fall of a sword. They also emulate Real Life better than the empty hand. There is nothing quite like a whack across exposed knuckles to teach proper position or make its reasons more luminously clear.

Kata are choreographed exercises designed for individual practice of flow, balance, and timing, and often contrast the control of rapid motion with the calm relaxation of the beginning and the end. When practicing individually, visualize an opponent. Practice with a real opponent will raise your forms from a purely theoretical art to an artfully applied science.

Note that the count is not a count as we usually think of it. Numbers serve as guidelines to what more than to when. Follow the natural rhythm of the *kata* and do not try to force it into rigid time constraints.

---

1. Aikido includes knife techniques, but they aren't as heavily emphasized. Peter W. Boylan notes: "Traditionally, the knife wasn't even considered a serious weapon in Japan. Recall that until the 1870s, Japan was a country where part of the population was required by their social position to walk around with two long, sharp pieces of steel in their belts. Anything shorter than about 1.5 ft. (40 cm) would have gotten a big grin, and then the person holding it would have been bisected."

   In modern Japan, the knife is the Number 1 murder weapon; for Number 2 and why defenses against swords aren't so archaic after all, see "Bokken (Wooden Sword)" on page 228.

Ideally, *kata* begin and end at the same point. Practice this by dropping a marker at your starting point; see how close you can come to finishing at the same point — with your eyes closed.

In learning a *kata,* divide practice into stages.

1. Begin in a group of four or more experienced people so that no matter which way you turn there will be someone to follow.
2. Practice on your own, without relying on someone else's motions. Split steps into sections, but preferably *backwards* (such as 15-20, 10-15, 5-10, 1-5) or any natural combination of motions). Recombine the small sections into larger segments and practice these.
3. After you have the sequence under control, practice with your eyes closed. This removes the visual clues (i.e. "when facing the door, I poke. . . ") on which you may unconsciously rely.
4. Practice in opposition with a partner.
   Now your motions are opposite; time and space must be perfectly coordinated.

Bokken (Wooden Sword)

Practicing against sword attacks is actually useful, even if not for defending against swords. One of the most common weapons around is the baseball bat (in Japan, it is the second most common murder weapon behind kitchen knives). The basic strike with a bat is usually a wild helicopter *men* cut.

—Peter W. Boylan

Principles for Sword Training

1. Hold the sword softly with LH at base of the hilt; put your RH at the top of the hilt to steady it. Power comes from the base hand.
2. Keep the tip calm and steady.
3. Use the weight of the sword and gravity to cut. Do not force the blade down — unbalanced forces will tilt the blade and tension in your arm will slow it.
4. Raise sword overhead whether you intend to strike *shomen* or *yokomen.*
5. Maintain attention and focus.
6. Cut first with the mind, then with the sword.

Yokomen Strikes and Tenkan

1. Starting in L *hanmi* (N) step R, strike L/R *yokomen.*[1]
   You will end up in R *hanmi* facing S.
2. In R *hanmi* (S) step L, striking L\R *yokomen.*
   You will end in L *hanmi* facing N.
3. Repeat the above practicing in pairs.
   The result is a series of alternating clockwise and counterclockwise turns. Practice on a mat seam, a chalk line or a piece of tape to control direction.

---

1. A *yokomen* starting on the R side and striking to the L. A L/R *yokomen* starts on L and strikes down to the R. Letters are for directions. N=North, S=South, E=East, W=West.

Yokomen Strikes and Blocks

In pairs,

1. Strike *yokomen* and block across the mat.
2. *Nage* alternates R and L *yokomen* while *uke* blocks.
3. Switch then return in the opposite direction.
   It is helpful to work down a mat seam or other marker such as tape or a chalk line.

Sword goes over the head for a *yokomen* strike, not from the side as in baseball.

Live Blade

No matter how often I was told to "put my mind at the tip" and "extend *ki*," the *bokken* was just a hunk of wood until the day I had to chop down a tree with a machete. The blade cut into the wood with ease when I simply let it go; with difficulty the more I tried to force it. Suddenly those lessons became luminously clear.

With a machete (from Army surplus or outdoor store) and a log[1]:

1. Strike target with the middle of the blade.
2. Strike target with the tip of the blade.
3. Repeat while forcing blade down or allowing it to drop.
4. Compare effort and effectiveness.

Happo Undo for Sword

Happo Undo ("Eight-Way Exercise") is done on the eight points of the compass. For basic exercise, see page 102).

The first set of four positions (A) may be thought of as facing the four square walls and is characterized by sword thrusts or pokes. During thrusts, the "blade" faces away from the forward foot.

The next set of four (B) on the diagonal, are strikes done in immediate succession.

From *seiza*, sword at left side, blade out, *nage* bows, draws sword, rises into R *hanmi*.

(A) On the Square,

1. From R *hanmi* ready position, strike *shomen*; step forward with LF and poke (blade faces R.) Note: the full step is done this time only).
2. *Zengo* to R *hanmi* while raising sword; strike *shomen*; slide forward with RF and poke (blade faces L).
3. Step into L *hanmi* while raising sword; slide LF forward and poke (blade faces R).
4. *Zengo* to R *hanmi* while raising sword; slide RF forward and poke (blade faces L). *Zengo* to L *hanmi* while raising sword.

---

1. Notice that must cut wood at an angle; chopping straight into the wood leaves nowhere for the chips to go. You can also make a target of a tire (see page 234) to replace the log. Provide vertical support for cutting lengths of bamboo with a *tameshigiri dai* (see *page 233*).

(B) On the diagonal,

5. In L *hanmi*, strike *shomen*. *Zengo* to R *hanmi* while raising sword.
6. In R *hanmi*, strike *shomen*. *Zengo* to L hanmi while raising sword.
7. In L hanmi, strike *shomen*. *Zengo* to R *hanmi* while raising sword.
8. In R *hanmi*, strike *shomen*. With sword in RH only, fully extended and parallel to mat,
   - Turn 360 degrees to starting position ending in L *hanmi* sweeping sword back with RF.
   - Step back into L *hanmi*, ready position, and
   - Return to *seiza*.

Variation:

Do the entire exercise with *uke* testing every step, from

- Attempting to block the forward bow.
- Holding the blade throughout the cuts and swings of the exercise.

Jo (Wooden Staff)

1. Hold the *jo* lightly, move the *jo* freely.
2. Control *jo* with the rear hand.
3. The line traced by the *jo* is never broken.

The previous exercises listed for *bokken* can also be done with the *jo*. Start by swooping the *jo* through the path of a figure 8, changing from hand to hand. This helps develop balance, sure-handedness, and familiarity with the center of the *jo* and its relationship to your center before adding humans or other movements to it. Focus on principles rather than on the characteristics of a particular weapon. The materials below vary from steel bars, to wood, to PVC piping.

- **Heavy Jo**. Weight requires efficiency of motion, but again, use good sense. This exercise was eventually halted due to a rash of muscles sprains and tears. Not so heavy! *Many years ago we practiced jo kata with the steel bar from a set of weights. It weighed 10 Kg by itself. We used to repeat the kata and pass the metal one up the line one place till it got to the end, and then pass it back down again. There was always a scramble to be at either end of the line, because then you only had to have the heavy jo once or twice. We once made a lead jo by filling one-inch copper pipe with molten shot, but someone "accidentally" lost it. — Jonathan Diesch*

- **The Fluid Dynamic Jo**. Fill a length of 1-1/2 PVC with water and sand, cap it, and seal it. The weight and fluid motion of the interior require large circles, nicely curved *tenkan* and *irimi*. Sharp or bumpy movements? It will jump out of your hands like a live thing.

- **The 1/8" Dowel Jo**. For an interesting switch on the weighted workout of the heavier designs above, try working with a delicate 1/8" dowel.

- **The Silk Scarf Jo**. To watch circles and flow, attach a silk ribbon or scarf to the each end of the *jo*. Flowing, circular motions are clear, as are short-cut or choppy motions.

Teaching Tools and Toys

This homely game of life we play, covers, under what seem foolish details, principles that
astonish. The child amidst his baubles, is learning the action of light, motion, gravity,
muscular force.

—Ralph Waldo Emerson

Effective teaching commonly draws analogies between the topic and already-familiar
objects and situations. The following items are useful for demonstrating basic concepts of Aikido. Items in sight and in hand makes them still more real.

- **Balancing Baby / Tightrope Walker**. A classic science toy for demonstration of weight
  underside. See what happens if you flip the model over and attempt to balance it on its
  head with weight clearly upperside. See also "Daruma" on page 232.

- **Balloons**. A balloon senses what you cannot. Try turning *tenkan*
  around a balloon cupped (not held) in your hand. The feeling is like
  holding the ball in a lacrosse stick or scooping fish in a net. Also useful
  for breathing practice.

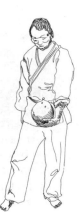

- **Balls**. Useful for illustrating the "roundness of motion" Large exercise
  balls such as the "Physioball" are also useful for teaching rolling.
  Rather than merely instructing the apprehensive new student to make
  himself "round like a ball," let him actually feel it.

  To demonstrate roundness of motion in *kokyu-dosa nage* holds the
  ball while *uke* grasp wrists. Smaller balls can be used to demonstrate
  circularity of *sankyo*, *nikyo*, *shiho-nage* and other exercises. See also:
  http://onlinesports.com for balls and equipment.

  Balls or bean bags can also be used for dodge ball to teach another
  useful Aikido lesson: it doesn't matter how hard an opponent hits if you
  aren't there.

- **Bean Bags.** Use for "catch" (see *tekubi-tori*-with-beanbag exercise on page 88) an act
  even less self-conscious and more psychologically compelling than "fix glasses" or
  "scratch head." Try to throw the bag into the air, roll, and catch. A great exercise for timing
  and focus.

- **Bio-Feedback Sensors**. Available from various sources at widely varying prices.
  Edmund Scientific has a wide range. An illuminating illustration of the differences
  between tension and relaxation and their impact on stability, balance, and technique.

- **Bonsai**. In Aikido, a classic exercise is expansion/contraction.*Bonsai* is a different form of
  the same exercise. Through root pruning, adult trees centuries old, complete in every
  way, are mere inches tall. Tradition has it that this art was taught by Buddhist monks to
  demonstrate change in point of view. A similar concept in the West is the gazing ball, not
  just a shiny ball on a post in the yard, but a different point of view: a reflection of the garden itself blooming in miniature in the depths of a mirrored glass. See also Escher's classic etching of a fish in a pond. Expand, contract, choose your focus.

- **Breakfall Pole**. Tony Fitts uses a ceiling support pole in the *dojo* for *ukemi* practice. Padded and covered with carpet, it allows individual practice of "clothesline" breakfalls or sliding falls as from *tenchi-nage* and *tenkan ude-oroshi*. This is a similar idea to the
  traditional Japanese *makiwara* (from *maku* "to wrap" and *wara* "hay"), a padded target for

various types of practice. Make your own from layers of cloth or leather or other padding tacked to a wall or wrapped around a board. See Punching Bags on page 233.

- **Boxing Clown / Daruma**. For demonstration of Center and Weight Underside. The weighted bottoms of the classic children's toys, boxing clown or balancing baby, return them to upright position after being knocked over.

  The Japanese *Daruma* doll is the same idea; a rounded figure made of paper maché with a weighted bottom. When knocked over, it rolls around then returns to upright, representing triumph over adversity.

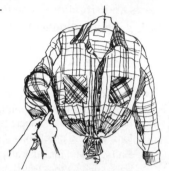

- **Closet Uke**. Stuff a shirt with rags or crumpled newspapers; add a head of paper bag, pillow, or balloon if desired. Hang on a cord or a hanger to swivel from a door frame and you have your own live-in *uke* to practice positioning and procedure. If you aren't yet at the point of being able to visualize and dance through the techniques on your own, this provides valuable feedback. Keep him around for garden or Halloween.

  You might also consider adding directions with masking tape. Can't remember the difference between *sankyo* and *shiho-nage*? Why not tape directions on the sleeve? *Sankyo*, turn arm in; *shiho-nage*, turn arm out.

- **Cord / String**. For jump rope, either a great warm-up and aerobic exercise, or for practicing leads and direction. For example, the lead on a *tenkan* should be forward. When cord is stretched out to the side, the problem becomes clearly visible. Also useful for the "Timing Belt" exercise (page 188) although a *gi* belt can also be used.

- **Gyroscope / Top**. A vivid demonstration of the stability of motion.

- **Hula Hoop**. Great for illustrating circles of motion such as the "steering wheel" motion of *en-undo* throws and others.

- **Masking Tape/Chalk**. Use to mark starting and ending points, lines of travel or other guidelines on the mat where a permanent mark is not desired. It's often useful to work along the seam of a mat to establish direction and position, to demonstrate whether you're moving forward or backing up. A large canvas mat may have seams in only one direction; smaller joined mat sections may catch toes in their multiple seams.

  Tape and chalk work very nicely to provide guidelines. See Shioda's *Total Aikido (TOT);* positions and movements are greatly clarified by photographing figures and partners from different angles and overhead against a quadrant of masking tape.

  By extension, consider the Sword Dances found in many cultures. In Scotland (and elsewhere), the dancer performs intricate steps over two swords crossed on the ground. The romantic tale is that a victorious Scottish Chieftain threw down his enemy's sword, topped it with his claymore, and danced around them in victory. But where did he learn that dance, eh? It seems to me that an excellent approach to teaching position, direction, and the center of a circle in a pre-masking tape society might be simply to throw down crossed swords. (The danger to bare toes might also develop an awareness similar to that developed by joined vinyl mats.)

- **Mirrors**. Mirrors are always valuable for observing body position on your own or in contrast to an instructor. If long expanses of mirrors are impossible, two mirrors on adjacent walls in a corner allows side and front views. Use as tool, not a crutch, that is, translate what you see in the mirror into what you can *feel* in your body on your own.

- **Paper Towels**. A twisted paper towel is useful for practicing leads. Lacking the strength of a washcloth or a cord, even when twisted, it helps to inspire cooperation between nage and *uke*. If *nage* yanks forward it will break. If *uke* pulls back it will break.

- **Plastic Bats**. Extremely useful for teaching *ikkyo*. The plastic bats produce an impressive THWACK! but no harm is done aside from a slight sting, enough to encourage the student to do the exercise even better. This is the same idea as traditional Japanese bound bamboo slats but cheaper and splinter-free.

- **Punching Bags**. A heavy bag or the traditional Japanese *makiwara* (a padded target for punching and striking) are both useful for teaching students how to actually punch with power and focus. Although Aikido doesn't usually use punches in its defensive techniques, other martial arts do. Before *nage* can effectively practice a defense against a punch *uke* must be able to produce one. See also **Tires**.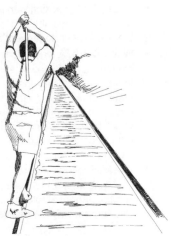

- **PVC Tubing**. A length of PVC tubing filled with water and sand, capped and sealed, gives a whole new feel for the flow and movement of *jo kata*. If you shortcut motions, the *jo* will practically leap out of your hands. For visual input, a silk scarf or ribbon at each end will highlight movements that are circular and those that are not.

Larger diameters of sturdy PVC pipe are useful as carriers to protect weapons and swords in iffy situations such as airline luggage.

It can also make a utilitarian *tameshigiri dai* for sword practice. Stand a length of PVC in the center of a large bucket. Check with a level to make it perfectly vertical. Fill the bucket with angular gravel such as bluestone, or pour in concrete to secure the pipe and weight the bucket. A length of bamboo or other material standing in the tube provides a vertical target for sword practice.

- **Railroad Tracks**. A permanent balance beam for practicing strikes, *kata*, and other exercises with *bokken* or *jo*, with balance and awareness.[1]

Fred Younger, who laments the scarcity of Iwama-style training partners in northern Iowa, reports: "I do all 7 sword *suburi*, paying particular attention to 5-7 as I feel they are the most challenging. I have also gotten a lot out of doing a *shomen* cut, pivoting 180 degrees, *shomen* cut, pivoting again, I start in *migi hanmi*, usually 8 pivots and cuts, then repeat in *hidari hanmi*. Keep in mind that when working in this situation you aren't working to perfect your forms. You are working on maintaining your Center on difficult footing. I also like to do *jo kata* and *suburi* on steep hillsides (close to 45 degrees) from different starting positions; uphill, downhill, and parallel to the hill. It adds a different facet to your training. "

---

1. Compare this to Aiki-Pitching training methods with balance beam on page 62. Saotome *Sensei* has a similar structure, a balance beam, for training built in his *dojo*.

- **Rubber Knives**. Mechanically it matters little what the training tool looks like. Psychologically and emotionally it matters a great deal. It is one thing to practice knife techniques with a block of wood, quite another to face sharp steel.

  Tony Fitts has students bring in all the real knives they can find, the scarier the better, just for the emotional shock value. "When you're faced with a real knife, you're going to be shocked. Do it here. Get over it. Get on with practice." Rubber knives from theatrical supply shops are serve as an intermediate step between the visually unreal and the visually very real.

- **Skates, Skis, and Bicycles**. Great for "cross-training" basic physical concepts / sensations. Try turning or riding in a circle while testing (with care) the effects of eye direction, attention, extension and focus.

- **Swings**. Small children on rope, tire, or bag swings can always use a push.

  Fred Younger suggests striking the rope or chain with a *jo*. Great practice for focus and extension and great fun for the kids.

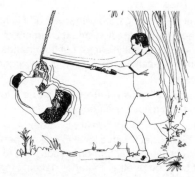

- **Tires**. For thwacking with *jo* and *bokken*. A frame-mounted or hanging tire (weighted to dampen swings) will serve nicely. Wrap tire with a cloth to prevent black marks on weapons.

- **Wash Cloth**. A wash cloth tucked in the *gi* has myriad uses. Most obvious is patting away sweat when hot and drippy but it is also a teaching tool. Many instructors use it to illustrate the relaxed, 90-degree drop down (rather than a forward hurl)) that makes *zemponage*. An *uke* with small hands may be unable to hold on to large wrists but both partners can hold the ends of a cloth. In *tenkan* techniques done this way, the washcloth also gives immediate visual feedback if *nage* is backing up rather than moving forward.

- **Water**. Support for persons who cannot practice easily on land. Possible uses range from providing support for people with bad knees or heavy weight to checking balance and position. For example, if you do an exercise off-balance in water you will drift. Water is also a great way to practice rolls and breakfalls without the consequences of landfalls.

CHAPTER 8

Off the Mat, in Real Life

I didn't have anyone to practice with.
My first partner in Aikido wasn't even human. It was a tree.
—Terry Dobson, *It's a Lot Like Dancing*

There's more to Aikido than mat time. Practically speaking, there will never be enough time on the mat to practice all that needs to be done. Rolls, balance, breathing, the physics and internal attitudes of Aikido should be a continuous and meaningful part of daily life. Consider the practice of harmonizing and blending applied to social skills and verbal self-dense. Sometimes we think we need special equipment, special environments to make the practice worthwhile. Actually not. Why wait for mat time if you can practice *funekogi-undo* with a lawn mower? Or *tenkan* in the kitchen or hall? Not enough room?

> Kenji Tomiki was imprisoned for three years[1] after WWII. He spent most of that time in solitary confinement in a cell 3 meters square. There he developed the *unsoku* and *tegatana* exercises. It boggles the mind to think of the number of times he performed these but they are perfect for the average hotel room. You develop *tai sabaki*, fluidity, and a good sweat (beware of rug burns on your feet). Repetitive *tenkan* and *irimi* exercises would serve just as well. Since all of the above exercises are considered basic, traveling is a good opportunity to work on something that many don't emphasize during regular training (i.e., "Let's get to the *waza*!")
>
> —Peter Rehse, Shodokan Aikido

Practicing Alone

Travelling? Working? Shopping? or at home? Consider the following.

- **Breathing**. Some say breathing is the most important part of Aikido practice, that anything less than several hours of practice a day is inadequate, indicating a less-than-serious student. Whatever your opinion of appropriate time, it probably won't happen on the mat. Outside self-practice required[2].

- **Stretching**. You don't need extreme flexibility to do Aikido but the more limber you are, the easier it is to blend and flow. The stiffer you are, the easier you are to throw and to

---

1. He had taught Aikido to senior army officers, but was apparently imprisoned due to his position as Professor at the Manchuria Kenkoku University lecturing in Bugaku ("martial studies"). "Possibly," says Rehse, "the Russians distinguished this from English literature."

2. See KDL, pp. 61-69. KIA Chapter 6, "Breathing and Meditation" for the biology of breathing and breathing exercises. See also Lessac (1996) and Zi (1986).

damage. Yet stretching cold muscles can be counterproductive and dangerous. Better done *after exercise*, following a brisk walk, run, or combined with hot-tub sitting.

- **Rolling**. You can practice all kinds of rolls on your own on grass, soft carpet, or even hard floor. I began on industrial carpet over a concrete floor. Not the best for flying forward rolls, but excellent for back rolls and learning how to round and tuck. The "thump-thump" that indicates poor rounding may be absorbed by a more forgiving mat or mattress. Do not roll on a bed. Put the mattress on the floor. See Chapter 5 for rolling exercises.

- **Sword Cuts and Strikes**. Consider 100 sword cuts or a series of staff exercises as a regular daily exercise. But sure, however, that you're doing them properly. Practice doesn't just make perfect, it makes *permanent*.

- **Dancing the Techniques**. Practice techniques by imagining an attacker and stepping through the motions. If you need a more visual support, a stuffed shirt on a hanger will help you practice the names and positions of various attacks, the difference in approach between *shiho-nage* and *sankyo* between *irimi* and *tenkan*. You can also "dance" the attacker's part. Why would you want to do that? Because *uke* is the teacher. Especially when dealing with a beginning nage, the test of good *ukemi* is not ability to block a technique. The test is: Do you understand a technique well enough to guide an unfamiliar nage through the technique and the throw — without the visual and physical support of a partner? Find out by visualizing or dancing the attack, seeing and blending with the incoming energy, performing the technique and the hold-down.

- **Mind Dancing**. Can't sleep? Go through a list of techniques mentally, from the attack through finish. Work up to an entire test list without losing concentration.

- **Surfing the Subway**. Subway or bus is a great opportunity to practice balance and blending. Observe the difference between stiff legs and tense shoulders versus bent knees and relaxed shoulders. Notice how you can transform the forward inertia of hard braking into an "up" or a "down." For safety, do these exercises with a stable support at hand and in situations where you will not alarm other passengers.

- **Funekogi Mower**. The "rowing exercise" can be applied to rowing machines at the gym or by setting heavy equipment (including boats) in motion. Walking lawn mowers are an excellent tool for showing the difference between pushing with arms and moving with One-Point. Equally applicable to opening heavy doors, heavy file drawers, and more.

- **Dogs and Cats**. Try turning *tenkan* with your dog, keeping the hand, the stick, the ball, just ahead. The dog will love it and you get good practice in judging distances and ma-ai. I first came to really understand *tenkan* the day a free-running German Shepherd attacked my puppy on his leash. Puppy with shorter wheel base, less mass, and a leash to hold him in, could stay ahead of the larger dog. I found myself standing in the center turning slowly as a furious cyclone of activity swirled around me. When grown, this would-be sled-dog taught me other lessons. Controlling him with upper body was exhausting; with leash at my hips, easy. Feel the difference. And note that the first touch of the leash on your thigh is signal to practice *tenkan* to avoid a tangle.

- **Horses**. "Any experienced horseman/woman uses *aiki*," says Cady Goldfield. Although a measure of "equine psychology" is part of the mix, a large part of horsemanship is to "become one" with the horse. Your body becomes exquisitely sensitive to the horse's every move, every intended move and every behavior. Likewise, the horse feels and senses his rider's body, weight shifts and signals, however subtle."

- **Groceries**. Groceries and the resulting bags of trash can be heavy awkward loads. Paper bags, which must be held in the arms, have given way to plastic sacks that hang from the hands, their weight completely "underside" in perfect alignment with gravity; arms need serve no purpose other than to form a connection between body and load.

Observe the weight and bulk of groceries that you can carry hanging compared to what you can hold up in paper bags. Compare the effort required to do so.

- **Garbage**. Lifting heavy bags into a tall bin may be beyond the capabilities of a small person of moderate strength — if statically lifted directly up against gravity. If a moving load is directed up rather than lifted up, the situation changes. Notice that almost any movement (even that of dropping) to get the bag moving and then redirecting that motion, makes the bag easier to lift up. With care (strong bag, non-messy load, and easy target to avoid disaster) experiment with turning tenkan to get the bag moving, direct it upwards and into the can. Feel the difference between muscling a heavy load and a one-handed flick of the wrist. Compare a full tenkan to a partial turn. This is the power behind karate's spinning kicks and of Aikido tenkan techniques.

- **Jaywalking**. Some view it as the ultimate exercise of awareness, blending, and flowing. The point is not only to cross the street safely, but to do so without disturbing the consciousness or flow of oncoming drivers or police.

- **Chess and Go**. "Chess is war." The Japanese game of *Go* and the worldwide game of chess both teach strategy and were popular with the military of their respective cultures. An interesting detail of the *Highlander* TV series was emphasis on *strategy*[1] (rather than the usual super-hero frontal assaults) and a chess-board visible in nearly every episode.

- **Focus and the Tupperware™ Randori**. Pick a point and focus. Drive a nail with one blow. Pick a single voice out of a choir. Follow a presentation from beginning to end without diverging to daydreams. You can train in many subtle ways. Focus, awareness of space and position, balance and direction. When an attack is not an attack, when it is, and what its component parts may be. I once stored too many plastic containers atop the refrigerator. Every so often there was a *shomen-uchi* avalanche of Tupperware. Eventually I was surprised to realize that after several years of Aikido I no longer saw these incidents as chaotic avalanches of countless unmanageable things; I saw it as a bowl, a cover, individual items of definite speed and direction.

- **Juggling**. There is no art that is, from the very beginning, so extremely reliant on correct interpretation of distance, speed, and position[2] as the art of juggling. You can see many video examples at YouTube.com. Imagine that the incoming balls, bowls, and clubs are hands, feet, or sword strikes.

- **Weigh Your Head.** How much does your head weigh? Add an equivalent weight to your head (if not a five-pound medieval helm, perhaps a motorcycle helmet or a sandbag). Notice how your neck feels when head is held in any position other than balanced atop neck and Center. A motorcycle helmet may weigh only 3-4 pounds, yet notice how off-balance and disoriented you may feel if you try to do a technique without good posture. Consider then, the importance of good posture on balance and energy efficiency.

- **Taping the Test**. Consider videotaping tests of senior students and your own tests. Follow through all the test requirements, dancing the techniques, concentrating on timing and flow. Make an audio tape of the test (the dress-rehearsal) on one side, explanations of the test techniques and what you are looking for on the flip side (training side).

If you are helping a fellow student prepare for the test, go through the entire test, from start to finish, from presentation to return to place in line. For beginners, the terror of the first test is often less a matter of the actual techniques than stage fright and uncertainty about the *procedure* — where to stand, when to bow, and what to do when finished. More new students have dropped out of classes due to terror of the unknown, then from boredom or disinterest. Help them any way you can.

---

1. From the Greek word for a military general.
2. See Lessons from *The Art of Juggling* by aikidoists Gelb and Buzan (1996).

- **Meditations and Changing Point of View**. What is the value of a different point of view? Observe the difference between professional and home movies. How many cameras? How many seconds, on the average, do you think the standard scene lasts in a professional move? Watch a movie and see. The standard number of cameras in professional work is three (and there may be more). In modern movies, individual shots last only about 3 to 5 seconds before switching cameras and point of view[1]. Shots in commercials last about one second. The viewer is constantly given new information or insight that would be impossible with just one camera from a single viewpoint. In techniques and exercises, be a camera.

  Try placing point of view overhead or to the side then "watching" yourself as if moving through water complete with bubble trail. We all like to videotape tests, but how about filming from overhead?

  In daily life, pick a topic and argue it from both sides.

- **D-Days**. What are the 20 things you want to do before you die? Plan now.

---

1. Individual scenes in older movies, closer to the live-stage tradition, tended to last much longer.

Verbal Self-Defense

Voice and speech are our first lines of defense and our chief weapons of offense
—-Arthur Lessac, Voice Coach

Dr. Bashir:	I can't believe you're not pressing charges.
Garak:	Constable Odo and Captain Sisko expressed a similar concern, but really doctor, there was no harm done.
Dr. Bashir:	They broke seven of your transverse ribs and fractured your clavicle!
Garak:	Ah, but I got off several cutting remarks which no doubt did serious damage to their egos. Thanks to your ministrations, I am almost completely healed. But the damage I did to them will last a lifetime. What I can't understand is their inexplicable hostility towards me . . . .

— On Garak's pummeling by a band of enraged Klingons
Star Trek Deep Space 9, "The Way of the Warrior"

We often think of language as we think of a fan — a frivolous sort of accessory for wafting hot air about. Pretty, decorative, pleasant, but largely insignificant.

The *samurai* fan (*tessen*[1]) however, was something more. It was an efficient and deadly weapon in its own right, replacing more overtly offensive weapons in situations where swords and knives were strictly forbidden. Beautiful and elegant, under its cover of painted silk and shining black lacquer were ribs and spines of sword steel. The outer ribs were heavy enough to fend off strikes from a sword. The thin inner ribs, hidden under the thin silk covering, ended in sharp points that could stab and slash when opened. Closed, it served as a bludgeon or billy to jab at vital points.

Language is a similar tool in many ways. It can be the most vicious of attack weapons. It can also be an enormously effective defense. Like the deceptively delicate *tessen* in trained hands, verbal self-defense skills are appropriate in situations where swords, knives, and other physical solutions are wildly inappropriate or simply do not work.

The truth is that verbal and emotional attacks are far more common than mere physical attack, usually precede physical attack when physical attacks actually occur, and are often far more difficult to deal with. The phrase "On the Street" as commonly heard and interpreted in martial arts classes is mostly nonsense. The real battlegrounds are in the shop, the office, the boardroom, the kitchen, the bedroom, the bar, the beltway. The weapons are words, and their underlying messages. Consider verbal skills as a critical part of martial arts training. You had better, because Bad Guys use them too, even On the Street.

Much of the desperate "shopping for a Black Belt" is certainly because the prized belt is seen as a status symbol but it may also be seen as the solution to problems that are verbal in origin. That is, "When I am a Black Belt people will respect me and won't bother me anymore."

---

1. For use of the *tessen*, see Mizukoshi (1997).

It doesn't work of course, because physical solutions don't address the non-physical origins of the problem. Furthermore they can (and often do) make the problem even worse. Verbal problems require verbal solutions, yet training in effective verbal skills is rare. Linguist Suzette Elgin notes:

> We're not taught about language as a *system* but as a vague sort of thing hanging out in the air somewhere. We have the feeling that only the highly trained expert, the trial lawyer, or those with "the gift of gab," "the silver tongue" can know anything about language. This is a shame because you are by definition an expert in your language, simply because you speak it. You just need a little more information, terms, principles, concepts that will let you put to use information that is not currently available at the level of conscious awareness.

Elgin considers verbal skills to be so critical to self-defense that their study qualifies as a martial art in its own right. Compare the linguistic concept of matching Sensory and Satir modes (page 243) with the Aikido concept of matching speed and direction, blending with the partner or attacker before actual execution of a technique.

Essay: The Martial Art of Verbal Self-Defense

You're in a bar with friends, enjoying a pleasant evening. Suddenly a man in a booth near you shoves his date roughly against the wall and pulls back his hand as if to smack her hard across the face. You move fast. Before he can even begin to follow through on the threat, you're standing over him. "That's enough!" you say, quietly but firmly. But it's not enough for this joker. First he whirls around and tells you to mind your own business, and then — when you shake your head and say, "Sorry, I can't do that" — he comes roaring up out of the booth and goes for you. This is a serious mistake on his part; in seconds you have him down and begging for mercy, and you aren't even sweating. You hold him there while his date gets up to go call and cab and head safely for home. When she tries to thank you, you smile and shake your head. "No thanks required," you tell her.

This is what martial arts are for, right? This is walking the warrior walk, following the *bushido* path, doing the *tao/do*. With quiet confidence in your skills, you can go anywhere and know that when violence comes your way you'll be able to deal with it efficiently, effectively, and honorably. You're ready for anything. Right? Maybe. Let's consider a different scenario.

You're in a business meeting, working through a new sales plan your boss has put together. And the boss keeps picking on one of your colleagues — making sarcastic remarks, interrupting her, ridiculing everything she says, doing his best to make her look foolish and stupid in front of everybody at the table. The woman looks at you, hurt and fear in her eyes, and her message is clear — she's asking for your help. Now what? Well, you could of course move fast and have your boss down and begging for mercy in seconds. You could hold him there on the floor, saying (quietly but firmly), "All right — apologize!" and not let him up until he did as you told him. And then when the woman he'd targeted tried to thank you, you could smile and shake your head. "No thanks required," you would tell her.

Ridiculous? Absolutely! You might feel that what I've just described is exactly what you'd like to do in such a situation. But you know it's out of the question. And that's the problem, of course. Unless you're someone who spends all your time in physically permissive environments such as bars and mean streets, most of the situations of conflict you run into in modern life are going to be like the second scenario. They're going to be situations in which the use of physical force — no matter how skilled, no matter how controlled and restrained, no matter how classical and respected a set of moves it may include — won't be appropriate. They're going to be situations in which using your martial arts skills is more likely to get you fired or arrested, or both, than to win you honor and respect. Situations in which what's needed is not physical skills but *verbal* ones. What does that mean for you as a martial artist?

All too often, in my experience, it means that in the majority of conflict situations in your life you will either do nothing at all or you will do something that makes matters worse and none of your hard-earned martial arts skill will be of any use to you.

Physical violence, the most visible and obvious chunk of this problem, almost always begins with verbal violence — with arguments, and hostile language. It's more efficient and enormously cheaper to deal with violence while it is still verbal.

Among the classical martial arts there are some which are intended specifically as systems of combat; their goal is to subdue enemies by the use of physical force. Other martial arts, however, are supposed to be different. Their core principle is that real victory means never needing to use physical force, because you are (as Joe Hyams puts it in *Zen in the Martial Arts*) "so strong inside that you don't have any need to demonstrate your power."

In these systems, the best outcome for encounters of potential conflict is an *honorable* resolution without using any of the physical techniques of that particular martial art. Notice, please, that I stress "honorable." Avoiding the use of physical force by running away, or by lying, or by toadying, is not honorable, and none of those actions is an acceptable choice except in the rarest of life-or-death situations. We have many excellent schools and teachers of these arts in the Western world today. But I see two problems in the way that their students are being prepared for life.

- Most of the students don't appear to be learning that core principle. So far as anyone can tell by observing their behavior, their primary goal is to win in combat, whether real or staged, just as if their chosen discipline were one of the killing arts.
- Even when the principle is remembered and learned the students are not being taught what to do instead of using physical moves[1]. Just saying: "Don't use physical force until you've tried talking and that has failed," is accurate, but is not enough. No one would tell a student: "Just keep using some kind of effective physical force until the opponent is subdued" and consider that enough. Making it up as you go along is not a martial art.

Terry Dobson and Victor Miller[2] wrote that "What we need is a new definition of conflict, a new way of looking at it, a new way of experiencing it, and a new way of responding to it." They were absolutely right — except in one small detail. It's not so much that we need new ways; not yet. That is not the most economical solution to the problem. What we need is to relearn some very old ways of looking at, experiencing, and responding to conflict, ways that are new to us now only because we have forgotten about them. We need to relearn the principles and strategies and tactics that make up the neglected martial art of verbal self-defense.

The Gentle Art of Verbal Self-Defense is a precise system like any other martial art. Its foundations are in those very old ways combined with the adjustments that are necessary to make them work in today's world. Its goals are to teach just two things:

---

1. Consider Sun-Tzu's famous statement that "the highest skill is not winning one hundred victories in battle but subduing the enemy without fighting." Until very recently, most combatants died from their festering wounds rather than from direct trauma. Verbal violence can kill in the same way. — CMS
2. See Introduction in Dobson (1987).

- How to establish and maintain a language environment in which verbal violence almost never happens. That is, to have such personal presence — such *sai* — that people around you would not even think of trying verbal violence there.
- How, in those rare situations when verbal violence cannot be avoided, to deal with it efficiently, effectively, and honorably — with no loss of face on either side of the conflict.

Yes — with no loss of face on either side. That may strike you as a strange idea. Dobson and Miller put it very well: "You've bought into an imaginary, arbitrary system where everything's a contest and there are no ties — just sudden-death play-offs and a long walk to the showers."

The idea that every difference of opinion, no matter how trivial, has to end with a clear Winner and a clear Loser, is imaginary, arbitrary, and really is "something new." Although it may seem as natural to you as the air you breathe and as inevitable, this is in fact an idea that we have invented for ourselves, only recently and it has brought us nothing but trouble and misery. It's time to admit that it's an idea whose time has come — and gone — and that it has been a failure. We've been there, we've done that, and it was a mistake; time to move on.

Verbal self-defense has an advantage that no physical martial art is blessed with: its core tactics and techniques and strategies, even its principles, are already known by the students. They are included in the grammar of the students' language, already stored in the students' long-term memories. They don't have to be learned the way kicks and holds and throws must be learned. All students must learn is new ways of indexing and organizing those elements — plus the strategy of making conscious decisions in verbal conflict just as they would in physical conflict. The basic principles of verbal self-defense are identical to the basic principles used in physical self-defense and in Aikido.

- Know that you are under attack.
- Know what kind of attack you're facing.
- Know how to make your defense fit the attack.
- Know how to follow through.
- Know that anything you feed will grow.

But wouldn't you know if you were under attack? Not necessarily. The attacker may not fit your image of an attacker: a small child, a frail elderly relative[1], or someone who is ill. The attacker is often someone that you are in a close relationship with. As on the mat, you must judge intensity, strength, the degree of violence that you are actually facing in order to adapt your defense to use just enough force, no more and no less, in response to the attack. Don't go after butterflies with a machine gun.

The Language and Grammar of Verbal Attack

Just as there is an English grammar for questions and commands, there's a grammar for verbal attacks. In English they are not so much in the words as in the music. If you hear language with the abnormal stresses indicated below, you are under attack. But an attack isn't the shouting, curses, or epithets people usually think of. Yelling of garbage is just part of a bigger physical abuse pattern. Verbal Abusers are more subtle. The English verbal attack has a two-part pattern.

---

1. The ultimate example of attack by a frail elderly relative is surely *Tatie Danielle*. See page 264.

1. **Bait**. The part that gets your attention, the part you're expected to fall for (equivalent to a feint or *atemi* in Aikido), and
2. **Presupposition**. Something that a native speaker knows is part of the meaning of a sequence of words, even if it isn't there on the surface. For example.
Even JOHN could pass THAT class.

As a native speaker of English, you already know that two other sentences are included here. You know that John is no great shakes and that the class isn't worth much either. You don't have to say that "Even John whom everybody knows can hardly reason his way out of a paper bag . . . " The pattern alone says there's something wrong with both John and the class[1]. A common example of baiting is: "If you REALLY loved me . . ." For example:

If you REALLY loved me, you wouldn't waste MONey the way you do.

- **Bait**: "Wasting money."
- **Presupposition**: "You don't love me."
- **Response**: Ignore the bait.

    Respond to the presupposition rather than to the bait as the attacker intends and expects you to do.

When you take the bait, you feed the pattern. Here's what happens.

Speaker 1:	Whaddya MEAN, waste MONey? I'm very CAREFUL with our money!
Speaker 2:	OH YEAH? Well how come it's only THURSday and we're BROKE?
Speaker 1:	It's not MY fault you can't make a decent living!

There's going to be a fight, a row, and it's not going to be pretty.

To deal with a physical attack, the Aikidoist matches speed and direction and chooses an appropriate technique. How is it possible to match a verbal attack?

By matching the attacker's Sensory Mode and choosing an appropriate Satir Mode.

Sensory Modes

People who prefer sight, hearing, taste/smell, or touch use language reflecting that mode.

People can and do shift between modes when relaxed. Under stress, they will not only lock into a preferred mode, they will even have difficulty expressing themselves or understanding language coming at them in another sensory mode. For example,

Speaker 1:	This looks bad.
Speaker 2:	I don't feel that this is a problem.

---

1. If you doubt the significance of tone in English, find a copy of the classic audio skit "John and Marsha" by humorist Stan Freberg. "John," says the female voice. "Marsha," says the male.

    These two words *only* are repeated throughout the recording. On the written page this "dialogue" conveys absolutely nothing. To the listener, messages conveyed by timing, tone, pitch, and emphasis are so very clear that the skit was banned from the airwaves. —CMS

Speaker 1 has used SIGHT Mode. Speaker 2 has mismatched with TOUCH Mode. Mismatch destroys rapport. On the other hand . . .

| Speaker 1: | This looks bad. |
| Speaker 2: | I don't see that this is a problem. |

Speaker 2 has matched with SIGHT Mode. Matching builds rapport by blending with incoming language. Remember that anything you feed will grow. If you don't know what to do, don't use any sensory mode language at all, but if you can, match.

Satir Modes

The second tool classifies language into Satir Modes[1] which include body language to match.

- **Blaming**. "Why don't you EVER . . . ?" Why do you ALWAYS . . . ?" perhaps including fist-shaking, jabbing, threatening body stance.
- **Placating**. " I don't care, you know me, whatever you want, " with cringing and squirming.
- **Computing**. Third-person and vague generalizations avoiding words like I, Me, Mine, You, Yours. "There is undoubtedly good reason for this delay. No reasonable person could . . ." or "Many people find that . . . ." Minimal body language, very Mr. Spock.
- **Distracting**. Cycles through all of the other Modes and their respective body languages. It is verbal panic.
- **Leveling**. Simple truth expressed as faithfully as possible for the speaker. Lacks the word emphasis of other Modes.

People can cycle through Satir modes or lock into one under stress just as they do for Sensory modes. Do you match Satir Modes as you match Sensory Modes? Not necessarily. Once you've recognized the Satir Mode coming at you, decide:

"Do I want this to grow?"

If you *do* want it to grow, *match* that mode.

If you *do not* want it to grow, *do not match* that mode.

Here's what happens if you do match.

- Blaming at a blamer will always lead to a scene, a fight.
- Two placators PLACATING at each other will starve to death before deciding on a restaurant.
- Two computers COMPUTING introduce dignified delay. (Typical of committee meetings which is why so little gets done.)
- Two distractors DISTRACTING build a feedback loop of panic feeding panic.
- Two levelers LEVELING have simple truth going in both directions. It will grow.

What does it mean to say that something involving only language — no kicks, no jumps, no punches, nothing of that kind — is a *martial art*? Please look at the following dialogue, which takes place at a hospital "checkout counter." Try to hear the language in your head as you

---

1. These classify language only, not personality type.

read (applying emphasis to sections in capital letters). The speakers are the angry wife of a hospitalized patient, and a hospital clerk.

Wife:	How can you POSSibly ask me for money when my husband is lying in there in AGony??! DON'T you have any human feelings at ALL??
Clerk:	Now wait just a minute! I don't make the rules around here, and I don't set the fees! I'm ONly doing my JOB!
Wife:	Oh, sure! SURE you are! And you're getting a big KICK out of it TOO! My husband and I aren't human beings to you, we're just NUMBERS! Just a couple of staTIStics, THAT's all we are! And YOU . . . !
Clerk:	LISten! I don't have to take that kind of talk from you! Who do you think you ARE, ANYway?!?

The hospital staffer in this dialogue is under attack, but would be in big trouble if he responded by leaping over the counter and immobilizing the furious attacker with a choice move or two. However, responding the way he has — by what we call "giving as good as he gets" — isn't working either. It's undignified, it wastes valuable time, it throws fuel on the fire and makes things worse, and it's likely to end with the wife suing the clerk, the hospital, or both. There has to be a better way — and there is.

The type of language behavior used by both of these people is Blaming. We know what happens when a Blaming attack gets a Blaming response, as in the dialogue here: a Blaming Loop is set up. It feeds on itself, and it guarantees combat. Let's do something else instead, as in this revision.

Wife:	How can you POSSibly ask me for money when my husband is lying in there in AGony??! DON'T you have any human feelings at ALL??
Clerk:	People have a very hard time thinking about money when someone they love is in pain.
Wife:	(Sighs.) Yes. They do. And that's what's wrong with me right now. I'm sorry I took your head off like that.
Clerk:	That's all right. No problem.

The wife has opened this language interaction with Blaming, as in the original dialogue. But rather than blaming back, the clerk has chosen to use a response of a very different kind: Computing. The result is also very different. The next two utterances, instead of being yet more Blaming, are Leveling — the plain unadorned truth, going both directions. They show us two people who are now talking to one another, successfully, rather than fighting.

This example is familiar to almost everyone and a perfect demonstration of one of the most common patterns of verbal self-defense. It looks like this:

Speaker 1:	Opens with a blaming utterance.
Speaker 2:	Responds with a Computing utterance.
Speaker 1:	Switches to a Leveling utterance.
Speaker 2:	Responds with a Leveling utterance.

Everyone uses these tools as part of the grammar of English. But there are three ways to use them.

1. **Just wing it.** Do whatever feels right to you at the time and depend on blind luck. That's not safe, and it's not smart.
2. **Pick one tool.** Use it all the time, no matter what the situation. Of course any martial artist knows where that is sure to get you.
3. **Make systematic and strategic choices.** Choose modes based on your knowledge of the situation, your skills, and your experience. This is the way it is supposed to be done.

When you have mastered both a physical martial art and the martial art of verbal self-defense, you are no longer at a loss in the multitude of conflict situations in which physical moves are inappropriate or forbidden. Now, it's true: with quiet confidence in your skills, you can go anywhere and know that when violence of any kind comes your way you'll be able to deal with it efficiently, effectively, and honorably. You truly are ready for anything.

—Suzette Haden Elgin, Ph.D

When I was first dating Jim I had to gather my courage in both hands to tell him that I was angry at him. I don't remember the issue, but I remember working myself up to mentioning it for the better part of a week. Naturally when I finally got it out, it came out with much more force and anger than was actually needed. I said fiercely to Jim:
"I really HATE IT when you do [X]!" (whatever it was).
And Jim said thoughtfully, "Yes, Hal doesn't like it when I do that either."
He didn't offer submission. He didn't meet anger with anger. He didn't block. He didn't apologize. He came from 90 degrees and redirected the anger. I remember the sensation of floating, as if in a void — unable to attack any further.

—Wendy Gunther

Garak to Tain:	You seem to have left your retirement far behind unless you're simply on a pleasure cruise with your pointed-eared friends.
Tain to Odo:	Cunning isn't he? He makes a racial slur within earshot of two Romulans putting me in the position of either defending them, thus giving away my allegiance to them, or letting the comment pass, in which case he has managed to plant a seed of discord between us.

— Enabran Tain comments on Elim Garak's interrogation skills,
Star Trek Deep Space 9, "The Die is Cast"

The Interview Language of Physical Attack

As Billy walked away down the aisle, I asked the girl [a young teenager traveling alone] if I could talk to her for a moment, and she hesitantly said yes. It speaks to the power of predatory strategies that she was glad to talk to Billy but a bit wary of the passenger (me) who asked permission to speak with her. "He is going to offer you a ride from the airport," I told her, "and he's not a good guy."

—Gavin de Becker, *The Gift of Fear*

Is violence random? Did an attack just "come out of the blue"?

Probably not.

Why? Because first you may be *interviewed*.

Bad Guys use the same verbal skills as a means of interviewing, building rapport with, and setting up a victim. Patterns presented by Dr. Elgin above are used in verbal attacks perpetrated *in place of* (although they may escalate to) physical violence.

The patterns below are preparation for planned physical violence. The predator who is fishing, preparing to reel in a potential victim, may use the same Sensory and Satir Modes so useful for blending and establishing rapport, to please and to charm. Unlike the verbal patterns of every-day social encounters, these are played as a prelude to physical violence, mugging, murder. Counselors who work with criminals must be constantly aware of their attempts to control the conversation — and by extension, the counselor — through verbal manipulation and attack. Remember Dr. Elgin's Number One rule of verbal self-defense: Know that you are under attack.

A hidden goal of physical attack often relies heavily on language[1]. Common verbal patterns of a "pre-attack interview" are as follows.

- **Forced Teaming**. Blending and intentional development of rapport for ill purposes. "We're in the same boat," "*we* need to," "*we* are," "*we* will" . . . when it is premature and inappropriate, and sometimes even where it might not seem to be. In the film *House of Games*, a psychologist is led by a skilled professional con man to believe that in studying con games together, the two are a "we." They are not.

  In Aikido, "teaming" appears in blending with the partner, matching speed, direction and the apparent goal[2].

- **Charm and Niceness**. Think of *charm* as a verb rather than a noun, then consider what the verb "to charm" really means. As de Becker notes: "He was *so nice*" is a comment I

---

1. Based on Gavin de Becker's *The Gift of Fear*. The title refers to the intuitive sense of fear or foreboding that something is wrong or about to happen. This response is often trained out of us as "good manners" or dismissed because "feelings" are not "logical." Actually they can be a phenomenally accurate reading of intent via body language, verbal patterns and more.

2. On approaching a graphics house as a first-time walk-in customer, I asked whether payment was due up front or after 30 days or so. Instead of replying directly, the owner looked at me searchingly and asked when the project was due. "In three weeks," I replied. He brightened and immediately extended credit on a thousand-dollar job to a complete stranger. Why?

   "Because," he said, "people who give you lead time are working from a schedule, behave calmly and are rarely out to stiff you. The ones who come in with 'emergency' jobs, short turn-around times, and who work to pull you into a sense of urgency that keeps you up all night working on their projects are the ones who disappear, never to be seen again."

often hear from people describing the man who, moments or months after his niceness, attacked them." Charm is a behavior choice, a social *strategy*. It is not personality, it is not an indicator of intent. It is not the same as *goodness*.

In Aikido it is perfectly possible to throw *uke* with a gentle smile, great maliciousness of heart and intent to do terrible harm. It is possible in many other situations as well.

"She was charming and it took me many years to learn that her charm was not goodness. I paid dearly for not catching on sooner." — T. B.

- **Too Many Details**. Telling the truth? The teller won't feel doubted. Lying? The teller knows it. Even if it sounds believable to you, it doesn't sound believable to the liar because he knows better — so he continues to throw in additional details, explanations, and self-justifications, many designed to appeal to emotion. There may be more than a touch of Satir's Distractor Mode thrown in to keep the interviewee off-balance, less able to focus on the situation at hand.

In Aikido it might be *atemi* and *ki-a*i, plus the three other things that always go on in almost any Aikido technique. Combined, these produce sensory overload and confusion.

- **Typecasting**. Typecasting involves a derogatory remark or faint insult to which you are expected to respond so as to prove it untrue. "You're probably too young, too old, too stuck up, anal, bitchy, inhibited, too [x] to do [y]." That is, you are to "prove" that you aren't [x] by doing exactly what the perpetrator hopes you will do which is [y].

Equivalent to the Aikido strategy of providing a move to counter, for example, dropping down, then waiting for *uke* to counter by coming up. *Nage* adds just enough energy that the final up is more than *uke* was expecting — or can deal with.

- **Loan Sharking**. Inappropriate psychic debt. The classic example from the dating world is the fellow who offers dinner; when his date does not deliver on his intended but previously unstated goal, she is reminded that he "paid for dinner." It attempts to exploit via the target's sense of obligation, no matter how wildly inappropriate that may be.

- **Unsolicited Promises**. One of the most reliable signals of questionable motives. It ties in with "Too Many Details" (above). The predator knows he's not reliable; he may be trying desperately to convince you that he is.

As Elgin directs, "respond to the presupposition" which is: "You Don't Trust Me." Do not, however, respond to it as something that must be proven wrong (as in "Typecasting") in order for you to be approved as "nice" by a potential attacker with an agenda. Instead, consider that this person has noticed that you do not trust him. Why is that? You may have good reason not to trust. When someone says "I promise," consider the presupposed distrust to which you are supposed to respond and then consider that your distrust may be exactly the correct response.

- **Discounting "No."** Refusal to hear and to accept NO is a blatant violation of *ma-ai*, an attempt to gain control or unwillingness to give it up. In the victim selection interview, it is an active attempt to find the person whose boundaries and autonomy can be violated, the easier the better, safer and more efficient for the perpetrator.

In Aikido, violation of *ma-ai* is time for technique. It may be simply moving out of that space (in a direction that does not qualify as "effective herding" from the attacker's point of view). It may be re-establishing *ma-ai*. It may be forceful physical action.

But either way . . . the interview is over.

Life Etiquette

The etiquette taught in Aikido [is] mutual respect, consideration for others.
—Kisshomaru Ueshiba

No matter how many mean things you say or do to someone,
they still aren't going to like you for it.
—J. E.

The future is neither ahead nor behind, on one side or another. Nor is it dark or light. It is contained within ourselves; it is drawn from ourselves; its evil and its good are perpetually within us. The future that we seek from oracles, whether it be war or peace, starvation or plenty, disaster or happiness, is not forward to be come upon. Rather its gestation is now, and from the confrontation of that terrible immediacy we turn away . . . as though the future were fixed, unmalleable to the human will, and to be come upon only as a 17th century voyager might descry, through his spyglass, smoke rising from a distant isle.
—Loren Eiseley, *The Night Country*

Is violence random and unpredictable?

No. It is actually quite predictable. The problems and their consequences often come back to etiquette, the standards of proper behavior for a society and life and what you personally choose to nurture and grow.

Working with thousands of married couples over many years, Dr. John Gottman found that he could predict — with 90 percent accuracy — which couples would stay together and which would divorce based on just 15 minutes of verbal interaction. Gottman focused on verbal cues, what he calls the Four Horsemen: defensiveness, stonewalling, criticism, and most especially, *contempt*. Gottman and his associates found that for a relationship to survive, the ratio of positive to negative emotion in a given encounter must be at least five to one. Negative verbal behavior alone can have a powerful impact the immune system. Using the same 15-minutes of shame, the researchers could even predict who would suffer colds and flu — and distrust, despair, and divorce.

Rudeness in the office causes anxiety, depression, and illness. It hurts the bottom line with greater absenteeism, decreased work, effort, and commitment to the company.

Rudeness on the road has led to tragic crashes and deaths, most of which were easily avoidable and just as easily triggered. Studies have shown that persons waiting at a left-turn signal light linger just a wee bit longer if there are cars behind them; that people who know someone is waiting for their parking space take a distinctly longer time to pull out than those who have no one to keep waiting. Although they are small breaches of etiquette, small subtle attacks, the recipients recognize them for what they are, if not consciously, at least at the gut level.

A common plea following violent verbal or physical confrontation is: "But I just couldn't let him get away with it!" If an escalating situation leaves you or others dead, injured, or facing legal fees and lost time for no reason other than raging ego and hurt pride, he has gotten away with it. More accurately, everyone loses. The discipline of good manners and good sense is part of the toolbox for self-defense, defense of others, safety and well-being of all. In real life as in the dojo, *ma-ai* and etiquette, good manners and responsibility, are your first line of defense and a powerful tool.

This weekend I drove into a crowded parking lot and pulled into a space. When I got out this guy in a car was livid. I had taken his space and didn't I see that he was waiting for it. I walked over to his car and my first reaction was to tell him to get lost. It then came to me in a flash like Saul of Tarsus on the road to Damascus that maybe I was in the wrong and not him.

"I'm sorry," I said. "I didn't see you waiting. I'll move my car and find another space."

"What did you say?" he asked.

"I'll move my car," I said again, "and I'm very sorry."

"Oh," he said, "Look, never mind."

"No I insist! It was my fault. I'll move my car."

"No man, it's okay!" And he drove away looking perplexed, but mellow.

—Philip Akin *Sensei*, 5th *dan*, Aikido Yoshinkai Canada

The Way of a Warrior, The Art of Politics, is to stop trouble before it starts.
The Way of a Warrior is to establish harmony.

—Morihei Ueshiba

Gardens

I learned more about economics from one South Dakota dust storm than I did in all my years in college.

—Hubert Humphrey

In one of his Renai Saga books, David Gemmell's character "Druss the Legend" says that he would rather be a warrior than a farmer because he felt he lacked the courage to be a farmer.

—Neil McKellar

"Farming is *budo*," said *O-Sensei*, and for the enormous amount of emphasis he put on farming and gardening, there is surprisingly little commentary on his reasons or his thoughts in that area.

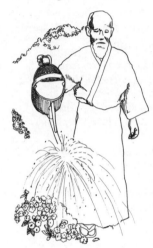

Armies and farmers have always been linked. The first formal armies were in Sumer, their role was the design, upkeep and maintenance of the life-giving system of canals. Subsequently, most wars have been fought over who gets to keep the food the farmers grow. In Greco-Roman mythology, Ares/Mars, the god of war, was originally a god of agriculture. The practical need to protect the crops and life is also the root of the Japanese samurai and martial arts from other lands.

Gardening and farming are also acts of creation. For northerners, February is the worst of months when we let our minds stop at the dark and cold. It is the gardener who sees the buds, observes that the sun has been coming back for well over a month now, that we are leaving the dark and turning again towards the light. Knowing that, February becomes the most fervent time for dreaming and planning. When everyone else is still huddled inside, the gardener is out in the cold and damp planting the seeds of what will be the colors and shapes and smells of the coming spring. it is creation and dedication — and often brutally hard work.

The "farming" *O-Sensei* was talking about and the "farming" that is done now (even on a small scale) are very different. I know nothing about 19th century Japanese farming techniques, but I know quite a bit about 19th century American farming techniques. I learned them from my great uncle and my grandfather and they are hideously, viciously, exhaustingly labor intensive. That huge labor element may be one of the things *O-Sensei* was referring to inasmuch as when you are doing things that are laborious and repetitive you learn to use your body in the most efficient way possible. When my grandfather replaced fence posts, driving them into the ground with a sledgehammer, he'd swing the hammer in an arc and pull it into his center at the very end of the swing, just before he hit the post. It is exactly the same motion we use when we swing a *bokken*, then draw it in towards our center at the end of the swing. When my great uncle finished milking he'd carry four milk cans from the cow barn to the pump house to immerse them in well water to keep them cold. They must have weight around one hundred or more pounds apiece. He simply learned how to use his body efficiently.

—Ken Speed

I'm no farmer, nor historian of Japanese culture, but I think it's reasonable to assume that *O-Sensei* had an agenda of unifying the class hierarchy somewhat. It's my understanding that the warrior class and the farm folk did not historically mix well. I'm speculating, of course, but my take on it is that it would have had a good deal to do with his vision of a world family.

We know from his writings and personal anecdotes that his *budo* became increasingly oriented toward nurturing and cultivation, attempting to revolutionize the old view of *budo* as a means of destruction. While farmers must also plow, uproot, weed out, clear the land, the ultimate aim is to engender life.

Although not a gardener myself, as a musician and composer I find thinking of "growing" songs more productive than trying to "write" or "construct" them. Much of what would not work is thrown on the "compost heap" and later on something may grow out of it. So agriculture can be a very useful metaphor for many endeavors.

—Ross Robertson

A common remark on weapons work: "Ha! He looks like he's using a hoe!" suggests that neither knows how to use a hoe. Proper use of a hoe and other farm tools is similar to proper use of the sword. Bob burns of San Diego Aikikai comments:

In 1989 I suffered an injury that kept me from working. Being raised on a farm as a boy I got back into the soil where being an organic farmer allows one to be *uke* for Mother Earth. I began a small garden working in it four hours a day. I noticed when I went to training that my body, after being in the garden, was more supple and flexible. When I did not garden, my body was more stiff. I am sixty years old and must pay close attention to what my body tells me.

It also felt that the *tenchi* (heaven-and-earth) dynamic of gardening was directly related to my training. I utilize the Jeavons French double digging technique (Jon Jeavons is my garden *Sensei*) and I began to make the tip of the fork, shovel, or hoe alive. I sent my body energy through it, feeling the earth from the tip. Bending my front leg, keeping my spine straight while digging, I found I could double-dig all morning non-stop, with a rhythm, breathing as we do when we train. It was then that I realized that framing and Aikido are the same thing. The life force was identical.

Ironically, my weapons work changed.

Chiba *Sensei* had told me that I could not do weapons. His reason was that it seemed that I wanted to kill my mate during practice. I went one year without touching *jo*, *bokken*, or *katana*. Thus my feeling for the hoe, shovel, and fork became tender, loving and sensitive. It also became more powerful and efficient. When I came back to weapons they felt light and beautiful. I was able to strike fast, but be soft at the same time. This sense went back to the garden tools.

The excitement and the bond between the garden and Aikido is so dynamic. My dream is to one day open a dojo where students farm as part of the training, to feel the life force that comes from the earth and that feeds us.

Voltaire's wickedly hilarious novelette *Candide* lampoons the idealistic philosopher Rousseau while galloping from class prejudice, war and murder, treachery and deceit, to sword fights and syphilis, the Catholic Church and its heretics, piracy and shipwreck, slavery, the Lisbon earthquake and cannibalism. Beneath the wild plot twists and fast action there is an underlying motif of gardens. Candide spends a brief time in a classical Utopian paradise, but for love of Miss Cunegund, cannot stay.

Many trials and adventures later, the tale ends in Voltaire's more modest vision of earthly paradise, another garden. All members of the little group help and contribute, not just in gardening but by sharing their own individual talents of baking, textiles, carpentry, and husbandry. Dr. Pangloss (despite a faith badly shaken) used to say now and then to Candide:

> There is a concatenation of all evens in this best of all possible worlds; for, in short, had you not been kicked out of a fine castle for the love of Miss Cunegund; had you not been put into the Inquisition; had you not traveled over America on foot; had you not run the Baron through the body; and had you not lost all your sheep, which you brought from the good country of El Dorado, you would not have been here to eat preserved citrons and pistachio nuts."
>
> "Excellently observed," answered Candide; "but let us cultivate our garden."

And so they do. It is a miniature model of the world — with a clear contrast drawn between those who bloody the earth and those who cultivate it. And meanwhile, is everything for the best? Are there no accidents? Do murder and hatred, gain and loss all happen for a reason and come to the best of all possible ends?

Perhaps. Perhaps not.

Nevertheless, says many a wise old man, let us cultivate our garden.

Another passionate gardener, the late, great Henry Mitchell, offered the garden as another parable for life. "How often in great gardens," wrote Mitchell,

> . . . do we see some inspired grouping of plants that only the highest art could have placed just so; that only the most informed and delicate taste could have arranged in just that combination of texture, color, bulk.
>
> And almost always it turns out it was not specifically planned that way at all. Usually the original planter had included a revolting assortment of this and that (all of which has died or been chopped down because of desperate overcrowding) and the thing we admire in the great garden is not some glorious composition come at leas to maturity. Instead it is merely the feeble survivor of all that had once been intended, but which never worked out at all.
>
> In this respect the garden is very like life itself. The coherence, the pattern, the glory even, is rarely planned and steadily approached, but is instead merely what at last is seen from the rubble of false starts, absurd ambitions and clumsy efforts.

The Timeframe of Violence

Whatever you feed will grow.

—Suzette Elgin

Medical conditions are lumped into two categories: *acute* and *chronic*[1].

An *acute* condition is one of sudden onset at a given point in time. A *chronic* condition is one that occurs over *time*. an aspirin may be good for an acute, sudden headache; for long-term migraine or cancer, a broken heart or a broken mind, other treatments are needed.

As there is a time frame of physical ills, there is also a time frame of violence.

Martial arts students in particular love to see themselves as noble warriors, waging heroic battles against Eeviiiil with thrilling action-hero derring-do. Yet every great strategist, from Sun-Tzu to Musashi to *O-Sensei* has insisted that the greatest art is stopping trouble before it starts, either by nipping problems in the bud, or by dealing with the long-term view of the situation. The violently explosive, adrenalin-charged, heroic remedies we often imagine are actually little more than fantasy. Brain candy. Even when applicable they are too often mere band-aid remedies, too little too late, applied to acute situations years after the chronic problem began its long, slow march through time. As in the "timing Belt" exercise (page 188) it is equivalent to ignoring the origin and waiting until the blow meets its target.

Suppose you are attacked On The Street but succeed in disarming and controlling your attacker. He is tried, convicted, and sent to prison for a very long time. Case closed? Think again. The assault is only the contact point. As in every other attack, there is a time-line. Consider the time-line in both directions.

Consider the future. Every year, we spend more resources on violence and its consequences. The U. S. has more people in prison (and more people per capita in prison) than any other Western industrialized nation. In 1997, we spent $28.9 billion on 1.2 million prisoners. That is approximately $24,000 a year per prisoner— more than a year of tuition and fees at most Universities. The tab for an elderly prisoner in poor health is still higher, some $65,000 a year. You will pay that in tax money to support the attacker and his fellow inmates, perhaps while struggling to cover your own rent, food, and tuition and expenses for your own life and children. Meanwhile, lives are disrupted or lost on both sides of the equation.

Consider the past. The attack, the crime, the hatred and anger and fear or exploitation behind it did not appear out of nowhere. On examining serial killers on death row, Dorothy Lewis and Jonathan Pincus found that all had a history of horrific abuse as children. Following the time line back shows that these and other children were not snatched from the street to be damaged by evil perverted strangers. They were abused by their own families, with the quiet consent of neighbors, friends, and others who allowed the cycle of abuse to continue[2] and set the stage for the future.

---

1. *Acute*, from Greek *ake*, a point; Latin *acutus*, something sharp. *Chronic*, from Greek *chronos*, time.
2. See *Guilty by Reason of Insanity* (Lewis, D. O., 1998)

The murderous Cain demanded of God: "Am I my brother's keeper"?

And the response through the ages, through the laws of worthy men and worthy gods has always been: "Well *yes*, actually, you *are*."

The same is true of that brother's children and all the other lives, souls, and futures that hang in the balance.

It is often said that defending a spouse or child from an abusive partner or parent is a no-win game as the defended will turn on the defender. Why? Because that person has come to confuse abuse with love. The cycle will continue through generations.

You must defend against attack, destruction, and murder, but you need not wait until the point of contact. Stopping trouble before it starts, turning the situation from the Dark towards the Light is the higher art. Helping and caring for the lost ones and for those who will be lost without help requires more dedication, more caring, more hard work than mere punches, kata and kicks.

Aikido is supposed to be great for this. However, despite much idealistic wishful thinking, Aikido doesn't automatically make you wise or kind or noble. It doesn't make you Yoda or Obi-Wan. It doesn't make you morally superior to Karate students, Judo players, golfers, or even the local gymnastics team.

Aikido is a tool. It teaches lessons to those who are paying attention and, like Garrison Keillor's Power Milk Biscuits, might give shy persons the courage to get up and do what must be done but cannot be done when afraid to speak out, afraid to move, afraid of being battered and broken, afraid of dying.

Innumerable martial artists who began their studies through fear of abuse or a need to "prove" their toughness or manliness have remarked that after acquiring their skills, they no longer needed to use them. Simply knowing that they were in the tool-box was enough.

Aikido gives you tools for war, for peace, for building and beautifying lives, or just for moving the grass. And besides all that it's great fun.

Come play!

It changed the future and it changed us.
It taught us that we have to create the future or others will do it for us.
It showed us that we have to care for one another because if we don't, who will?
And that true strength sometimes comes from the most unlikely places.
Mostly, though, I think it gave us hope, that there can always be new beginnings,
even for people like us.
—Susan Ivanova, "Sleeping in Light," *Babylon 5*

Resources

Magazines

Aikido Journal
  Online at www.aikidojournal.com.
Journal of Asian Martial Arts
  An academic and historical approach to martial arts history and practice. E-mail: info@goviamedia.com.
Journal of Japanese Sword Arts
  JJSA deals with all aspects of the Japanese Sword Arts. Online at: www.uoguelph.ca/~iaido/

Books, Websites, Organizations

Alexander, R (1999), "Jackson — zen and now": *The Washington Post*, Nov. 9, D-1.
  Shaquille O'Neal in the lotus position? A profile of basketball coach Phil Jackson, brought on to revitalize the ailing Los Angeles Lakers via yoga, zen, and meditation. A far-out approach? It worked for Michael Jordan and the Bulls. Coach Jackson's regular season winning percentage set an NBA record.

Anderson, Bob (1980), *Stretching*
  A comprehensive manual on stretching.

Associated Press (1997), "Angry moose brought to its knees by politician's oratory". Jan. 2
  On defeating an angry moose while armed only with a rabbit gun and a *ki-ai*.

Baker AJ and others (1993), Excitatory amino acids in cerebrospinal fluid following traumatic brain injury in humans: *Journal of Neurosurgery*, Vol. 79, pp. 369-372.
  Researchers measured concentrations of the excitatory amino acid glutamate in the cerebrospinal fluid of patients with traumatic brain injuries. See Zhang and others (2001).

Bazancourt, Baron César (1862/1998), *Secrets of the Sword*.
  A sharp point [is a reality that] makes short work of illusions.

  A Socratic dialogue concerning the sword. Topics range through fencing basics, the hard realities of armed combat, and life itself. Charming and sensible.

Born, Jan et al (1999), *Nature*: Jan.7.
  Per the ability of certain people to wake up at a designated time without setting an alarm clock, a clear example of mind-body coordination, a link between expectation, consciousness, and hormones.

Dalby, Lisa (1993), *Kimono : Fashioning Culture*.
  The history, aesthetics, and meaning of Japanese clothing, from its Chinese inspiration to present-day.

Davies, Claire and Davies, Amber (2004), *The Trigger Point Therapy Workbook*.
  A hands-on treatment manual for myofascial pain and dysfunction. For those who think in terms of *kiatsu* based on meridians, consider the high correlation between "lines" and trigger points, apparently because both are related to fascia (connective tissue). For medical background, see Simons (1993).

De Becker, Gavin (1997), *The Gift of Fear*.
  The human violence we abhor and fear the most, that which we call 'random' and 'senseless,' is neither . . . We want to believe that human violence is somehow beyond our understanding, because as long as it remains a mystery, we have no duty to avoid it, explore it, or anticipate it. We need feel no responsibility for failing to read signals if there are none to read. We can tell

ourselves that violence just happens without warning, and usually to others, but in service of these comfortable myths, victims suffer and criminals prosper.

Is violence random and unpredictable? No. A thorough discussion of the myths, profiles, and even protocols of violence. From verbal tools and forms used by Bad Guys to perceptions of time and risk . Also explores the making and makeup of "monsters" — why "they" are us and how we create them.

Dobson, Terry, and Miller, Victor (1987), *Aikido in Everyday Life—Giving in To Get Your Way.*

Translates aggression and defense into the visible realm through the geometry and symbolism of Aikido's triangle, circle, square.

Elgin, Suzette Haden (1980), *The Gentle Art of Verbal Self-Defense.*

On the mat we learn to recognize a physical attack for what it is and to respond appropriately. Here is Aikido applied to verbal and emotional attacks which are far more common than mere physical attack and far more difficult to deal with because training is so rare. The phrase "On The Street" (as commonly heard and interpreted in martial arts classes) is usually nonsense. The real battlegrounds are in the shop, the office, the kitchen, the bedroom, the bar, the beltway. The weapons are words and attitudes. Excerpts from books at: www.adrr.com/aa/excerpts.html. See also Sullivan, EF (1993).

___ (1997), *Try to Feel It My Way.*

Some students deal best with written and visual input; others need to hear. Others are "feelers" who can't "see" it and "don't get it" partly because they are operating in another mode entirely. These are touch dominants, people who must "get their hands on things" in order to "grasp" new material. Rephrasing visual images will help get the point across as will going through technique with eyes closed.

Fudebakudo. The world's greatest Aikido cartoons at www.fudebakudo.com.

Gaines, Patrice (1999), "Hitting the head pin — blindbowlers ready to make a mark": *The Washington Post,* Saturday, November 13, B-1.

An article on blind bowlers who must and do extend and target with the mind's eye.

Gelb, Michael J and Buzan, Tony (1996), *Lessons from the Art of Juggling.*

Gelb, juggler and learning consultant, and Buzan, author of *Use Both Sides of Your Brain* and *The Mind Map Book*, co-wrote this trail guide to learning to draw skills from both sides of the brain.

Glassner, Barry (1999), *The Culture of Fear.*

Why we fear all the wrong things: crime, drugs, minorities, teen moms, killer kids, mutant microbes, plane crashes, road rage, and so much more. See this and a current almanac for the real statistics behind the news. See also Ripley, Amanda (2008) for surviving the real disasters.

Gluck, Jay (1996), *Zen Combat.*

The late Jay Gluck was the author of "Masters of the Bare Hand Kill," the 1957 *True* magazine article that introduced Karate to America. The article become a chapter of the original (1962) edition of *Zen Combat.* He was asked to photograph Ueshiba for a similar article on Aikido, but when editors saw the resulting photos of American military police, Karate blackbelts, and sword-wielding *kendoka*, all "looking everywhere but at the little old target," they rejected the photos as "posed" or "rigged." "Modern Zen Fools" details an encounter between Morihei Ueshiba and the cartoonist/engineer Rube Goldberg.

Grayson, Betty and Stein, Morris (1981), "Attracting assault— victims' nonverbal cues": *Journal of Communication*: Vol. 31, n. 1, p. 68.

How do muggers select their victims on the street? It is fast (about 7 seconds). It may be unconscious, but it is heavily based on posture and body movement. Also reviewed in the August 1980 *Psychology Today*: "Body Language that Speaks to Muggers."

Herdman, S. J. (2000), *Vestibular Rehabilitation.*

On the Cawthorne-Cooksey exercises and more.

Homma, Gaku (1993), *Children and the Martial Arts — An Aikido Point of View.*

On the pros and cons of martial arts for children and for those who care about them on and off the mat.

___ (1990), *Aikido for Life.*

On beginning Aikido, from the point of view of the new student and instructor. Succinct and insightful.

IMPACT Personal Safety and PREPARE, Inc.

This program comprises several programs including that formerly known as Model Mugging. For programs in your area visit their web page at: http://www.PREPAREINC.com.

Internet Aikido

www.aikiweb.com is Jun Akiyama's Aikido Web, the most popular Aikido site on the web. To find a dojo, see http://www.aikisearch.com. See also: www.aikido-l.org for information on the Aikido-L mailing list.

Lessac, Arthur (1960), *The Use and Training of the Human Voice* .

___ (1978), *Body Wisdom*.

Lessac is one of the most famous voice coaches in the theatre and acting world. Many years ago, he taught voice by teaching Unbendable Arm. Many of his lessons on "floating" took place in a pool to actually experience the feeling followed by "recreate the feeling" on land and in air. He talked of "radiating energy" (we would talk of "Extending *Ki*") and of buoyant energy (we would talk of "Weight Underside") which he explains as "gravity down, but air up."

MacYoung, Marc (1993), *Ending Violence Quickly:How Bouncers, Bodyguards, and Other Security Professionals Handle Ugly Situations*.

Emphasis on recognizing the *verbal signals* of impending aggression. For verbal skills, see Elgin. For the futility of being logical with drunks, plus street smarts and how not to be a target, see this.

Mizukoshi, Hiro (1997), *Aiki Tessenjutsu*:

Using the *tessen* (iron fan) as a weapon. Aavailable from www.budogu.com.

Moseley, GL, Parsons, TJ, and Spence, Charles (2008), "Visual distortion of a limb modulates the pain and swelling evoked by movement": *Current Biology*, Vol. 18, n. 22 (Nov. 25), R1047-R1048.

Model Mugging. See Impact Personal Safety.

Myers, T W (2008), *Anatomy Trains*

A brilliant work on "myofascial meridians," the relationships and continuity between muscles and fascia.

Nagrin, Daniel (1988), *How to Dance Forever:* William Morrow and Co.

We practiced our dance numbers for eight hours a day for six weeks prior to principal photography. — Ginger Rogers

Is Aikido "a lot like dancing?" Not exactly. Dancing is harder. If you're having problems with fatigue or injury with a heavy practice schedule of say, 10-12 hours per week, consider the professional dancer who may now practice for 10-12 hours per day for weeks or months on end. Nagrin began his distinguished solo performance career in 1957 at age 40, which popular wisdom considers retirement age for dancers and other athletes. Practical and pithy advice from the trenches on what works, what doesn't, why and how to keep you dancing — on the stage or on the mat — forever.

NAMTPT, National Association of Trigger Point Myotherapists.

This is the professional certifying body for persons trained in treating trigger points and myofascial pain. Website: www.MyofascialTherapy.org. See also Simons (199

Olson, GD, Seitz, FC, and Guldbrandsen, FC (1996), "An inquiry into application of gokyo (Aikido's fifth teaching) on human anatomy": *Perceptual & Motor Skills*, Vol. 82, pp. 1299-1303.

An anatomical investigation to determine the source of pain in wrist locks. See also Seitz, F. C.

___ and Seitz, Frank C. (1994) "What's causing the pain? A re-examination of the Aikido nikyo technique": *Perceptual & Motor Skills*, Vol. 79, pp. 1585-1586.

Presents the conclusions of two separate investigations (one being Olson and Seitz' 1993 paper) of *nikyo* and the possible reasons for discrepancies in their results.

___ and Seitz, FC, and Guldbrandsen, FC (1994) "An anatomical analysis of Aikido's third teaching — An investigation of sankyo": *Perceptual & Motor Skills*, Vol. 78, pp.1347-1352.

___ and Seitz, FC (1993), "An anatomical analysis of Aikido's second teaching: an investigation of nikyo": *Perceptual & Motor Skills*, Vol. 77, pp. 123-131.

___ (1990), "An examination of Aikido's fourth teaching: an anatomical study of the tissues of the forearm": *Perceptual & Motor Skills*, Vol. 71, pp. 1059-1066.

Pryor, Karen (1999), *Don't Shoot the Dog*

Pryor, a marine mammal specialist and a former trainer at Sea World, shows how to be truly, effectively positive in life and teaching — and the benefits that come from that. Here are the secrets behind "talking to the animals": teaching a dolphin to jump, a chicken to dance, the secrets of "the horse whisperer." Here's why your students or children may not be "getting it" and how to remedy that, kindly and effectively. It works whether you're dealing with a tuna or a *taigi*. Pryor's approach is now known as "clicker" training. If nothing else, it's a stunning revelation of how standard teaching styles unwittingly encourage failure or unwanted behavior. Here's how to actually encourage and reward desired skills. It helps the subject learn and helps *you* to realize exactly what you are reinforcing—or not.

Raman SS, Osuagwu FC, Kadell B, Cryer H, Sayre J, Lu DS (2008), "Effect of CT on False Positive Diagnosis of Appendicitis and Perforation: *New England Journal of Medicine*, Vol. 358, n. 9 (February 28), pp. 972-973
On false diagnoses of appendicitis (and improving rates with pre-appendectomy imaging).

Ripley, Amanda (2008), *The Unthinkable: Who Survives When Disaster Strikes and Why*:
A superb review of real emergencies, real disasters. The real people who survived them and why. From 9/11 and explosions to air crashes and hurricanes.

Samenow, Stanton E (2004), *Inside the Criminal Mind*.
Samenow's program is renowned for having beaten the statistics on recidivism. Invaluable insight on criminal choices and behavior, its origin in children, and an opportunity for we, the supposedly "Good People," to take a long, hard look into the mirror at our own hearts and minds.

Saotome, Mitsugi (1993), *Aikido and the Harmony of Nature*.
History and anecdotes of Aikido founder Morihei Ueshiba by a former live-in students (*uchi-deshi*). Ranges from the ideals of honor and service in the *samurai* tradition, to the elements of "reality," waveforms, gravity, and spirituality woven into the descriptions of individual Aikido techniques.

___ (1989), *The Principles of Aikido*.
Aikido philosophy and techniques. Particularly remarkable for the chapters on "The Sword" and "Ukemi." If you are caught in the common beginners' delusion of *nage* as "winner" and *uke* as "loser," this will help you see *ukemi* as discipline and art in its own right.

Seitz, FC, Olson, GD, and Stenzel, TE (1991), "A martial arts exploration of elbow anatomy — Ikkyo (Aikido's first teaching)": *Perceptual & Motor Skills*, Vol. 73, pp. 1227-1234.
See also Olson, GD.

Shifflett, CM (2009), *Ki in Aikido : A Sampler of Ki Exercises*.
Exercises used in the Ki Society for stability, balance, and relaxation, and for the patterning of Aikido techniques. Step-by-step testing and exercises. The 2nd edition includes information on the history and application of biofeedback techniques that make the tests and the results visible onscreen.

Shioda, Gozo (1996) [Trans. David Rubens] *Total Aikido : The Master Course*.
Excellent enlargement of the Yoshinkan style *Dynamic Aikido*. The photos lack the close-up detail of the first book but this is because so much more material is presented. Many techniques are shot from overhead against a grid; text emphasizes important points and common mistakes. One problem: in some pictures, the point the picture is trying to make is about half a second later than the snapshot. Especially useful for the notes on how not to do it. A valuable resource for all styles.

___(1968) [Trans.: Geoffrey Hamilton], *Dynamic Aikido*.
Aikido Yoshinkan style, with clear, close-up photographs. Invaluable for notations of lines of force. Some consider this to be "Aikido Lite" compared to Shioda's subsequent *Total Aikido*. Both are valuable. *Dynamic Aikido* has larger pictures. *Total Aikido* has more illustrations but these were reduced to fit available space and the photographs do not include the lines of force and direction shown in *Dynamic Aikido* drawings. Consider including both in your Aikido library.

Simons, David G, Travell, Janet G, Simons, (1993 / 1999), *Travell & Simons' Myofascial Pain and Dysfunction: The Trigger Point Manual*
This is the Bible of myofascial pain (dysfunction arising from muscle and fascia, or connective tissue). Includes thorough medical documentation. Volume 1 addresses upper body; Volume 2, lower body. The treatment information is heavily based on trigger point injection. For manual self-treatment methods, see Davies (2004). See also NAMTPT (National Association of Trigger Point Myotherapists, named by Travell) to find a therapist in your area.

Stevens, John (1984), *Aikido — The Way of Harmony*.
Biographies of the Founder of Aikido, Morihei Ueshiba, and of Shirata Rinjiro, the author's instructor. Detailed analysis of Aikido philosophy and techniques with such basics as proper bowing, sitting, standing, breathing. Extensive photographs.

Sullivan, Edward F (1993), *Necessary and Reasonable Force*.

It is always disturbing to meet frightened beginners who think they need killing techniques. Consider the common notion that "On The Mat" a technique is done one way, but "On The Street" you can and should destroy an attacker. The people who are *really* there, police and emergency personnel, know this popular fantasy for what it is — fantasy. Here a veteran Chicago police officer discusses the legal meaning of "necessary and reasonable force" and issues of responsibility and liability. Techniques for de-escalating situations (with anecdotes of rookies who failed to do so) apparently due to watching too many cop shows). Take-away's and controls for the times when physical techniques are necessary. Notice the emphasis on *ma-ai,* stepping off-line, and affirming that 95 percent of the job is verbal.

Thompson, Geoff (1994), *Watch My Back: A Bouncer's Story*.

Physical violence of the bar-bully type is almost always preceded by distinct verbal and postural rituals.

Tohei, Koichi (1978), *Ki in Daily Life*.

I was pleased to have read this book just for the commentary on the Japanese phrase *suisei-mushi,* meaning "to be born drunk and to die while still dreaming." Koichi Tohei was student, *uchi-deshi, and* designated Chief instructor for Aikido founder Morihei Ueshiba. He is the founder of *Shin-shin Toitsu Aikido* (Aikido with Mind-Body Coordination).Here are standard Aikido exercises linked to daily living.

___ (1976), *Book of Ki : Coordinating Mind and Body in Daily Life*.

From training body, mind, and soul to raising a golf handicap. Includes an introduction to *kiatzu,* a method of healing with *ki*.

Twigger, Robert (1997), *Angry White Pyjamas*.

Sara thought martial arts were pretty silly. To a trendy young Japanese, aikido was about as sexy as morris dancing.

Twigger combines insight, inanity, history, hilarity and commentary on traditional and modern Japanese culture. Many Yoshinkan practitioners have been outraged by its apparently myopic point of view, while others have privately giggled over his descriptions. Whatever your conclusions, it's a highly entertaining read centering around a brutally demanding course "where any ascetic motivation soon comes up against blood-stained dogis and fractured collarbones." Surely the only Aikido book combining goldfish, Mike Tyson, mildew, and martial arts all in one.

Ueshiba, Kisshomaru (1987), *The Spirit of Aikido*.

The late Kisshomaru Ueshiba was the son of Morihei Ueshiba, Founder of Aikido. Presents a detailed review of the underlying philosophy of Aikido and its pre-WWII history.

U. S. Dept. of Transportation (1997), *An Investigation of the Safety Implications of Wireless Communications in Vehicles*: National Highway Traffic Safety Administration.

Cell-phones and their distractions to driving, and compared to equivalent impairment by high blood-alcohol levels. If you have trouble believing the benefits of focus, consider the consequences of distraction. Research concluded that talking on the phone while driving was equivalent to blood alcohol levels of at least the legal limit. Available online at: www.nhtsa.dot.gov/people/injury/research/wireless/

Walker, Jearl (1985), "Roundabout — The Physics of Rotation in the Everyday World" [Readings from "The Amateur Scientist" in *Scientific American*].

The physics (lever arms and centers of rotation) behind the techniques. Walker discusses the physics of *yokomen-uchi, ushiro-nage,* the Judo hip-throw, and why as a Small Person he gave up Karate for Aikido. How we do what we do on the purely mechanical level.

Westbrook, Adelle, and Ratti, Oscar (1970), *Aikido and the Dynamic Sphere*.

The classic Aikido textbook, written when Koichi Tohei was Chief Instructor at Honbu *dojo* in Tokyo. Invaluable for Ratti's famous line-drawings which emphasize the circular motions.

Zi, Nancy (1986), *The Art of Breathing*.

Exercises with visualizations for improved breathing by a professional singer and voice coach. In Aikido, as in yoga and other arts, breathing is a discipline in and of itself. Website: www.theartofbreathing.com.

Zhang H, Zhang X, Zhang T, Chen L (2001), Excitatory amino acids in cerebrospinal fluid of patients with acute head injuries: *Clinical Chemistry*, Vol. 47, n. 8, pp. 1458-62.

Excitatory amino acids glutamate and aspartate play a clear role in post-traumatic brain injury: they destroy brain cells . Researchers measured glutamate and aspartate in patients with acute head injury and in healthy control adults. Peak values appeared within 48 hours and were still elevated a week later. The more severe the injuries, the higher the concentrations of these toxic chemicals. The more severe the trauma, the worse is the neural destruction and patient outcome.

Movies and Videos

While most movies and videos presented here are fictional, the ideas behind them and the people who choose to convey these particular ideas are real or may become real. Observe purpose and intent.

Bad Day at Black Rock (Director: John Sturges, 1954)

Merely by appearing unannounced and unexpected, a mild-mannered stranger (Spencer Tracey) sends a small town with a dark secret into a frenzy of suspicion and fear. A story of choices: the shame and guilt of having made the wrong ones, the terror and opportunity of a second chance. Includes Karate versus the classic Western Bully when karate was still a rare and exotic oriental art. See Gluck (1996).

Deep Space 9 (Producers: Ira Steven Behr, Rick Berman, Michael Piller, 1993-1999)

The last and best of the Star Trek series addressed hard topics of politics, religion, racism, and war. Brilliant dialogue and language skills are showcased in "simple tailor" Garak, the duplicitous Kai Winn, and others. Observe the parallel relationships of Kira and Odo, of Kai Winn and Dukat, one based on mutual respect and appreciation, the other on resentment and mutual lust for power. Over the course of this seven year tale, some chose the darkness and more than one monster turned to the Light.

Exposed! Pro-Wrestling's Greatest Secrets (Don Wiener, 1998)

A fascinating review of the performance art known as "pro-wrestling." Between the hype, the shills, the cartoon costumes, and the scripted wins and losses, it's easy to say that "it's all fake." Well it isn't. It is real, industrial-strength *ukemi*. No one is supposed to get hurt, but should anything go wrong, the risk of accidental injury is very real. The physics are real. The *ukemi* is real. These men are real athletes and this is one really tough way to make a living. Compare with Bruce Bookman's *Ukemi* tapes.

Grand Canyon (Director: Lawrence Kasdan, 1992)

A strange and beautiful look at violence, real and imaginary, the interrelationships between lives and the things that actually matter. In the beginning moments of this film you will see a great Aikido Master working as a towtruck driver (Danny Glover). Watch what he does and how he does it then compare his actions with Terry Dobson's diagrams for attack and defense. (See Dobson, 1987.) Another haunting scene follows Steve Martin's portrayal of a movie maker exploiting the lucrative genre of make-believe violence; after a real mugging he sees the light — then chooses to walk back into the darkness.

Groundhog Day (Director: Harold Ramis, 1993)

A charming remake of the legend of the Flying Dutchman of folklore with a kinder, gentler, wiser ending. The profoundly unlovable and unloving Bill Murray is trapped within the same day, apparently doomed to live it over and over — forever. See *Highlander*.

Hidden Fortress (Director: Akira Kurosawa, 1958)

This 1958 Japanese film by Akira Kurosawa inspired George Lucas' 1977 movie *Star Wars*. Lucas saw it in film school and never forgot it. Toshiro Mifune is general Rokurota Makabe, who in *Star Wars* becomes Obi-wan Kenobi and Han Solo. Princess Yukihime becomes Princess Leia Organa, and the two hapless wandering foot soldiers who come to the aid of the fugitive princess become C3PO and R2D2. The Source of the Force. Many reviewers have referred to the "deadpan expressions." Actually those are "masklike expressions" which come (with much of the movie's symbolism) from *Noh* theater tradition.

Highlander (Producers: Panzer and Davis)

The more experienced you are in any martial art, whether taiji or Tae Kwon Do or Aikido, the more it becomes like a game of chess. This is a universal combat principle. And, when you get to the high levels of any art, you see that aggression is replaced with pure strategy.

— *Cady Goldfield*

"It isn't about fighting," says immortal Duncan McLeod, while training for a coming battle. "It's about strategy." He's often outclassed and outnumbered but what comes up again and again is strategy, awareness, and a chessboard that shows up somewhere in almost every episode.

The *Highlander* TV series was a long-running version of *Groundhog Day:* What would you do if you could live forever? How long before money, manipulation, and preying on others become very very boring? The science-fictional premise of a race of eternal beings engaged in a long-running game of sudden-death elimination offers a different and valuable point of view. For how many centuries do you hold a grudge? How long do you hate? How do you behave when you can kill or not kill and nobody knows? Who and what are you? — and why? Renowned for its emphasis on ethics, learning and growing, in the world of an eternal warrior who must deal with the everyday griefs and joys of mortal life.

House of Games (Director: David Mamet, 1987)

He said "Son I've made a life out of watching people's faces, knowing what the cards are by the way they hold their eyes. — Kenny Rogers, The Gambler

A psychologist is drawn into a game of sleight-of-hand in the belief that she is studying the art and psychology of the con game. It is, in fact, observing and studying *her*. Superb illustrations of de Becker's summary of the verbal and psychological tools of the con, from "forced teaming," "tells" and body language, to our sad tendency to see and hear only what we want to.

Karate Kid (Director: John G. Avildson, 1984)

Famous for the training scene in which Daniel thinks he's there to become a lean mean fighting machine and learn esoteric martial secrets. Miyagi (Pat Morita) puts him to work painting fences and waxing cars. Source of the "wax on, wax off" line now heard at some point in every martial arts school. (The scene of attempting to catch flies with chopsticks comes in turn from Eiji Yoshikawa's novel *Musashi*). "Cobra Kai" has also entered the martial arts language to describe a *dojo* where abuse is mistaken for discipline, bullying and treachery for martial fervor.

Kentucky Fried Movie (Director: John Landis, 1979)

Raunchy but hilarious send-up of various American cultural icons including martial arts. "Fistful of Yen" is a good-natured spoof of Bruce Lee's classic *Enter the Dragon*, James Bond movies, spaghetti westerns, Disneyland and *The Wizard of Oz*. Still timely for its commentary on the now-obligatory "Really Spiritual Martial Arts Guy" segment — it's been done. In "Cleopatra Schwartz" ("She's 6 feet of fighting fury! He's a short Hassidic Jew!") this formula was intended to be completely absurd. And was.

Royal Wedding (Director: Stanley Donen, 1951)

Thin plot, but the source of the famous scene in which Fred Astair dances with a hatrack. As always he makes his partner look very very good. No clash. Only blending and flowing. Consider this in dealing with *uke*. Consider experimenting at home with the same partner or try the exercise with a *jo*.

Sanjuro (Director: Akira Kurosawa, 1962)

A rollicking tale of feudal Japan. In this sequel to *Yojimbo*, a gruff and rough wandering *samurai* (Toshiro Mifune) comes to the aid of a band of naive and hopelessly idealistic young noblemen. The young men see only yes and no, black and white. In their impatience they are determined to deal with every situation in a haste which results in death and destruction.

Mifune highlights the contrast between explosive action and relaxation, appropriate *in*action, the dangers of seeing everything in black or white, judging by surface appearances, and how insistence on Action Hero Solutions lead to tragic ends.

When enemy soldiers come to ambush the Boy Scout *samurai* at a secluded shrine, Mifune drives them off with a sheathed sword. The scene of the young men emerging from under the shrine floorboards reappears in Lucas' *Star Wars* when the rebels emerge from under the floorboards of the *Millenium Falcon*, following almost identical advice from a seasoned warrior that there are many ways to fight.

Shall We Dance? (Director: Masayuki Suo, 1997)

"In Japan," announces the opening lines, "ballroom dance is regarded with much suspicion." This leader was probably added by the distributor for the benefit of Western viewers who consider ballroom dancing to be hopelessly old-fashioned. Not so in Japan where a proper Japanese salaryman does the unthinkable: takes up ballroom dancing lessons. This charming tale offers unexpected insight into Aikido (leading, blending), teaching (*zengo*, *ma-ai*), and attitude towards others. Consider the images of the men practicing individually, moving through the steps of the "techniques" alone to practice flow, sequence and balance before working with *uke*. But what is the most important thing? Protecting your partner. The American remake completely missed the point.

Side Kicks (Director: Aaron Norris, 1993)

An asthmatic youth lost in a fantasy world is taken in hand by the canny and kindly Mr. Lee (Mako) who leads him out of the trap of fantasy into the world of real competence, true confidence, and genuine self-control. All the elements of the standard martial arts movie are here: Good Guy, Bad Guy, the opportunity to "take revenge" on one's opponent by beating him to a pulp — and they are all slyly lampooned and redirected. Who is the enemy? It isn't really the class bully; it is asthma. The Karate competition is won not by trashing an adversary but by "breaking," an exercise in concentration and self-control. The beautiful girl is not the prize won by defeat of a rival; she already liked him anyway. And "don't need karate *gi*," points out Mr. Lee (racing from kitchen to competition in an apron) "to break blocks."

Chuck Norris' all-time best movie pokes gentle fun at all his others. It suggests the value of hero-worship for setting direction and goals, but emphasis is firmly placed on the need to move beyond. For a sly commentary on "movie-*do*," watch the restaurant brawl scene carefully to see Chuck Norris made up in beard and black leather doubling as Biker Bad Guy.

Star Wars (Director: George Lucas, 1977)

George Lucas' world of *Star Wars* (inspired by Kurasawa's *Hidden Fortress*) has long been enormously popular with Aikidoists, inspiring many to begin training. Many of the concepts attributed to "The Force" come directly from Aikido. Darth Vader's hissing breath is a wonderful parody of *ki* breathing; his helmet is the traditional *samurai* helmet reinterpreted in black plastic. The inspiration for Yoda is believed to be Misao Shoji of Gardena, California. A superb Aikidoist, he is also renowned for his pixilated sense of humor. His favorite song, "Found A Peanut," is sure to be sung at his workshops.

Tatie Danielle (Director: Étienne Chatiliez, 1990)

A manipulative old woman terrorizes family and caregives. In theory, it's a comedy. It may not be amusing to anyone who has a similar relative but it should at least be educational on the end of *tenkan* and the time for *irimi*. For more subtle verbal attacks, observe the character Kai Winn (of Star Trek's *Deep Space 9*) whose unfailing sweetness and gentle manners cover an evil soul.

Ukemi: The Art of Falling (Director: Bruce Bookman, 2007)

Falls are a leading cause of accidental death and injury yet safe falling is rarely taught. Even in Aikido where it is a critical technique and teaching skill, it is rarely taught in a systematic manner. Bruce Bookman corrects that lack with two well-done videotapes. *Basic Ukemi* progresses from simple rocking chair rolls to breakfalls. Includes strategies for improving *ukemi* by effective blending with your partner. *Advanced Ukemi* continues to high-flying breakfalls. Compare with the falls seen in "pro-wrestling." (See *Exposed! Pro-Wrestling's Greatest Secrets*, page 262.

Glossary

—by Chizuko Suzuki

In Japanese, Chinese characters, *kanji*, can be read in two ways.

	Left	Right	Hand	Knee	Body	Technique
Chinese (ON)	*sa*	*yu̱*	*shu*	*shitsu*	*shin*	*gi*
Japanese (kun)	*hidari*	*migi*	*te*	*knee*	*mi*	*waza*

Single Chinese characters are often read in the Japanese manner; combinations may be read either way. For example, "left hand" and "right hand" are read in Japanese as *hidari-te* and *migi-te*, but the "left-right" exercise is read as *sayu* in Chinese.

Japanese has five short vowels; [a] art, [i] ink, [u] wood, [e] egg, [o] dog, and five long vowels; a̱, i̱, u̱, e̱, o̱ which should be pronounced as a continuous sound, equal in value to two identical short vowels such as *shomen*, document) and *sho̱men*, front) with a long "o" sound.

Double consonants: **kk, pp, ss**, and **tt** indicate a slight pause before them as in *ikkyo̱*, *bokken*, and *happo̱* (eight directions).

Sound changes occur when two Japanese readings are compounded: **k** becomes **g, s** becomes **z, t** becomes **d, h** becomes **b** or **p**. For example, *te*, hand + *katana*, sword = *te-gatana* or *tegatana*.

Japanese is rife with homonyms with the same sound but different meanings. (Because these words are written with different Chinese characters, Japanese often draw the the *kanji* in the palms of their hands while speaking in order to clarify the meaning of a word that may have as many as 10 different possible meanings). For example, *Shin-Shin To̱itsu Aikido̱* is "Aikido with Mind-Body Coordination" as *shin* can mean mind and also body.

It's conventional in Japanese-English dictionaries to write the *ON* (Chinese) reading of a *kanji* in all capital letters, to distinguish it from the *kun* (Japanese) reading. So you might see capital letters for *KI* (which is an ON reading), but not necessarily for other Japanese words and phrases.

1

ai n.— from *au*, to fit, suit, harmonize, agree, accord. Harmony, integration, unification, a coming together. In Aikido, it signifies the spirit of harmony and accord, hence Aikido is "the Way of Harmony."

ai pre. — each other. *Ai-te, from* "+ *te*, hand, a companion, a partner, an opponent. *Ai-hanmi* indicates *nage* with right foot forward and *uke* with right foot forward. See **gyaku** and **hanmi**.

ai n.—love, affection. *O-Sensei* said, "*Aiki* (harmony spirit) is *aiki* (love spirit)."

Aikido n.— the way of harmony, from *ai,* harmony + *ki,* spirit + *do,* way.

ashi n.— leg or foot.

atemi n.— a strike, from *ate*, strike, hit + *mi*, body. In Aikido, the strike is ideally a feint, not intended to injure but to distract, startle, and lead *uke's* mind.

bokken n.— wooden sword, from *boku*, wood + *ken*, sword. Originally *bokken* was a practice sword used to avoid damage by or to the razor-sharp and costly *katana*. Eventually it came to be considered as a weapon in its own right. Different schools use different styles for practice; some (such as the *suburito*) are extremely heavy; movement with tension or weight upperside is readily revealed by exhaustion and painfully sore muscles. See **shinken** (real sword).

budo n.— martial arts, from *bu*, power, bravery, military affairs + *do*, way. *Bushi* from budo + *shi*, warrior, leader, scholar, noble people. Bujin from budo + *jin,* person. See **samurai**.

-dachi n.— variant of *tachi,* from *tatsu,* to stand. See **tachi**.

dan n.— a level, a step. A rank above *kyu*. *Shodan* is first level; *nidan* the second, *sandan* the third, *yondan* the fourth.

do[(1)] n.— way, path, discipline, study with physical and spiritual implications. In the literal sense, a road or path; by extension, a course of study or a way of life but certainly not limited to martial arts. *Aikido* is The Way of Harmony; *Kendo* is The Way of the Sword; *Kyudo* is The Way of the Bow (archery); *Kado* is the Way of Flower [arranging]; *Sado* is the Way of the Tea [ceremony].

do[(2)] n.— rib area, from waist to shoulders. This term appears in the terminologies of Kendo and other sword arts as a target area for cuts.

dohai n. — equals, from *do*, same + *hai,* fellow. Typically refers to one's school mates or those entering a company in the same year. See **senpai** and **kohai**.

-dori n.— variant of *tori,* from *toru,* to grab. See **tori**.

dojo n.— place of practice, training hall, from *do*, way + *jo*, place. A *dojo* is a place to train in the way, *do*. *Dogi* or *dojogi* refers to the uniform or dress worn while practicing a given discipline. Dojo, "the place of enlightenment," is a word derived from the Sanskrit *bodhimanda*, the place where the ego self undergoes transformation into the egoless self. —Taitetsu Unn

dojo-sukui n.— *dojo*, loach + *sukui*, scooping. Appears in Taigi 8.

dosa n.— action, movement, from *do*, movement + *sa*, creation. Although sometimes mistaken for a wrestling contest, *kokyu dosa* is actually an exercise in breath movement and *ki* extension.

en n.— circle. *En-undo* describes a circular motion. *Kokyu-nage en-undo* and *kote-gaeshi en-undo* are named for their pronounced circular motion.

fudo-shin n.— the immovable-mind, from *fu*, not + *do*, moving + *shin*, mind, not in the sense of stubbornness or rigidity, but in the sense of calm, stability, and imperturbability. It is the calm and stability of a spinning top. While the mind cannot be tested directly, it can be tested through the body, as we do with various *ki* tests. Hence *fudo-tai* (immovable body) is considered to indicate the condition of *fudo-shin*.

---

1. a.= adjective adv. = adverb n.= noun v.= verb pref. = prefix suf. = suffix

fune-kogi n.— a boat rowing motion, from *fune*, boat + *kogi*, rowing, but very different from western-style rowing. Japanese boats were equipped with one oar which was sculled back and forth and also served as the rudder.

-gaeshi n. — variant of *kaeshi*, from *kaesu,* to turn out. See **kaeshi**.

gedan n.— lower level, from *ge*, low + *dan*, level. On the body, the area below the waist.

gi n.— *clothes*, but note that in Japanese this element does not stand alone; the use of *gi* to indicate practice uniform is an English usage. It is often used specifically like *Judo-gi, Karate-gi* or *Kendo-gi*. The uniform worn in class is *keikogi*, "practice clothes" or *dogi,* the clothing worn while you are practicing the "way."

gi n. — a technique. *Gi* [the Chinese reading], equivalent to **waza** [Japanese reading]. *Ken-gi* are sword techniques, *jo-gi* are stick techniques, *tai-gi* are "body" ("no-weapon") techniques.

-giri n. — variant of *kiri*, from *kiru*, to cut. *Happo giri* is a sword *kata* involving "cutting in eight directions." See **kiri**.

go n. — back, rear. [Chinese reading] See **ushiro** [Japanese reading]. Contrast with *zen*.

go-kyo n. — "fifth teaching," a painful pinning or immobilization technique.

gyaku n. — reverse; opposite. *Gyaku-hanmi* describes *nage* standing with right foot forward, *uke* with left foot forward. See **ai** and **hanmi**.

hachi-no-ji n.— figure eight, from *hachi*, eight + *no*, of, possessive particle + *ji*, figure or letter.

hagai-jime n. — pinion, from *hagai,* a part where feathers cross + *jime*, from *shime*, strangling.

hai adv.— yes. Pronounced in one sharp breath, not *hái-eee*, as in the English short form of hello.

hakama n. — the voluminous pleated pants or divided skirt worn over the *gi*. In Aikido, usually worn by (but not always limited to) advanced students.

hakucho-no-mizu'umi n. — *hakucho*, swan + *no*, of, possessive particle + *mizu'umi*, lake. Also known as the "Ghost Throw."

han n.— half, pertaining to physical position. *Zagi han-dachi* from *za*, seated + *gi*, techniques + *han*, half + *dachi* from *tachi*, standing, describes techniques in which a standing *uke* attacks a *nage* seated in *seiza*. *Nage* may rise to one knee, a half-standing position.

hanmi n.— *han*, half + *mi*, body is the basic Aikido stance in which the feet are placed to form two sides of a triangle, exposing only half the body to the attacker. Commonly garbled in English as "hamni." See **ai** and **gyaku**.

hantai n.— opposite, from *han*, reverse + *tai*, confront. In techniques involving a *hantai-tenkan*, *nage* reverses direction and turns.

happo-undo n.— The "eight direction exercise." Combines *zengo-undo* with *ikkyo-undo* to practice correct extension of *ki* and attention.

hara n. — the Center (One-Point) in the lower abdomen, thought of as physical and spiritual center of the body. *Hara kiri* (garbled into English as "harry-karry") was Japanese ritual suicide, involving a knife cut, *kiri* to the *hara*.

honbu n.— headquarters, from *hon*, base + *bu*, section, group. Garbled into English as "hombu."

hiji n. — elbow. *Ushiro hiji-tori* describes "elbows grabbed from the rear."

hikoki-nage n. — *hikoki*, airplane + *nage*, throw. Appears in Taigi 18.

hitori-waza n.— *hitori,* one person + *waza*, techniques. In Aikido, unpartnered single-person exercises to develop balance and coordination, and to pattern the basic movements of Aikido techniques. See **kumi-waza**.

ikkyo n.— first immobilization technique, from *ichi*, one, first + *kyo*, teaching. Also called *ikkajyo* or *ude osae* in different styles. See **katame**.

irimi n.— *iri*, from *ireru*, to put inside + *mi*, body. In Aikido, *irimi* is an entering motion, a stepping *inside* the line of attack. In Ki Society, *irimi* techniques are the equivalent of techniques designated as *omote* in other styles. Compare with **tenkan**.

jo n. — a wooden staff, stick. *Jo-nage* ("stick-throws") are techniques in which *nage* has the *jo* and uses it to throw an attacker. *Jo-tori*, ("*jo*-grabs") are the set of techniques used to disarm an attacker with a *jo*.

joho n. — upwards, from *jo*, up + *ho*, direction. See **kaho**, downwards.

juji n. — letter ten, from *ju*, ten + *ji*, letter. Appears in Taigi 13.

ju-jutsu n. — *ju*, soft, pliant + *jutsu*, art, craft, skill or discipline. An art of pliancy or strength through yielding, a Japanese form of unarmed combat which uses joint locks and throwing techniques.

-kaeshi suf.—from *kaesu*, to turn out, a change, reversal. (The suffixed **-*kaeshi*** often changes to *gaeshi* in compounds such as *kote-gaeshi*.) *Kote-gaeshi* describes "*turning the inside facing wrist, kote, to the outside.*" *Kiri-kaeshi* ("cut and reverse") involves complete reversal (180 degrees) of *uke's* motion. *Ura* ("back or reverse") + *gaeshi* turns him inside out, facing the other way.

kaho n. — downwards, from *ka*, down + *ho*, direction. See **joho**, upwards.

kaiten n.— revolving, rotating, from *kai*, turn, revolve + *ten*, roll. *Kaiten-nage* is a spinning throw; *uke's* body will revolve once before he is led down to the mat. In *zempo-kaiten-nage*, *uke* falls forward like a wheel.

kamae n. — posture, stance.

kata n.— shoulder. *Kata-tori* is a shoulder grab.

kata- pre. — one side, single. *Katate-tori* is a single-hand grab. See **ryo-**, both.

kata n. — form; hence a *jo kata* is a form done with the staff, intended to demonstrate flow and rhythm, an awareness of space and placement while perfecting technique.

katame n.— an immobilization, from *katameru*, to lock, to pin, or to harden. *Katame-waza* are immobilization techniques and include *ikkyo, nikyo, sankyo, yonkyo* and *gokyo* which mean "first," "second," "third," "fourth," and "fifth" techniques, respectively.

katana n. — a Japanese steel sword, slightly curved and single-edged. *Katana* is the Japanese reading. The Chinese reading is *to*. The wooden sword is a *bokken* (see **ken**). *Te-gatana*, hand-sword, refers to the use of the edge of the hand as if it were a blade or knife edge, a technique common in Karate.

kazu n. — number.

one — *Ichi*	Six — *roku*
two — *ni*	Seven — *shichi / nana*
three — *san*	Eight — *hachi*
four — *shi / yon*	Nine — *kyu / Ku*
Five — *go*	ten — *ju*

keiko n.— practice, training, study, lessons, from *kei*, to think + *ko*, old. *Keiko-suru* (v.) originally meant "to think of old things," later to "to learn or study old things such as arts, skills, and techniques." Learning these things requires *training*. Thus, *keiko* is "training" and *Keiko-gi* are "training clothes."

ken n.— a straight, two-edged sword. *Ken* is the Chinese reading. [The Japanese reading is *trurugi.*] *Kendo* is the "Way of the Sword" and its practitioners are known as *kendoka*. *Shinken* is a real sword. See **shinken** and **katana**.

kesa-gake n.— a diagonal cut from shoulder from *kesa*, surplice, part of monk's costume hanging from shoulder + *gake*, from *kake*, hanging, laying, putting over. Appears in Taigi 26.

ki n.— the universal spirit; life energy. In Japanese, *ki* appears in many contexts such as *gen-ki*, a spirit of health, *byo-ki*, a spirit of sickness, *ai-ki*, a spirit of harmony.

ki-ai n.— a piercing shout with *ki*, from *ki*, spirit + *ai*, harmony. The concept is that of an outpouring of *ki* energy from the One-Point, unifying body and spirit. In modern Japanese, it also refers to vigor. To put *ki-ai* into something (*kiai wo ireru*) means "to work at something with vigor."

kiri n.— from *kiru,* to cut. *Tekubi-kiri,* cut to wrist; *ude-kiri ,* cut to arm. The American *harry-karry* is a garbled version of *hara kiri,* a ritual cut to the *hara,* or Center (One-Point). This word also appears as *giri,* hence *happo-giri,* a sword *kata* involving "cutting in eight directions."

kohai n.— [one's] junior, from *ko,* back, later + *hai,* fellow. See **dohai,** equals, and **senpai,** senior.

koho n.— back; backwards, from *ko,* back + *ho,* direction. *Koho-tento undo* is the rolling backwards exercise. See **zempo.**

kokyu n.— breath, from *ko,* exhale, call + *kyu,* inhale, suck. A *kokyu-nage* is a breath throw, or, by extension, a timing throw, because it is done using only *uke's* momentum and *nage's* timing. *Kokyu-nage* techniques are a family of techniques which depend on timing, sensitivity, and *ki* extension rather than a joint lock. *Kokyu* is thought of as *ki* in motion, empowered by breath and its control. *Kokyu-nage* is known as *irimi nage* or as *ishi otoshi* in different styles.

kosa n.— cross, across from *ko,* cross, intersect + *sa,* finger crossing. *Tekubi- kosa-undo* is the "wrist-crossing-exercise." *Katate,* one hand + *kosa-tori* describes a "one-hand-grab." Compare with *katate-tori.*

koshi n.— hips. *Koshi-nage* is a "hip-throw."

koshin n.— moving backwards, from *ko,* backwards + *shin,* proceed. *Koshin-undo* is a series of exercises in which the student practices moving backwards while continuing to extend *ki* forward.

kote n.— hand, tips of hand, from *ko,* small + *te,* hand. *Kote-gaeshi* is a "wrist-bend" (wrist lock) which serves as a throw. *Kote* sometimes refers to the entire forearm. In *Kendo,* a *kote* strike is a blow, not to the wrist but to any point on the gauntlets covering the entire forearms.

kubi n. — neck. *Tekubi* is the wrist, that is, the "neck" of the hand (*te*).

Kubi-uchi is a strike to the neck. *Ushiro kubi-shime* is a one-armed neck choke from the rear. In medieval Japan, *uchi-kubi* was decapitation, a shameful and humiliating death.

kumi-waza n. — *kumi,* a pair, partners + *waza,* techniques. See **hitori-waza**.

kyu n.— level, quality. In martial arts, *kyu* designates any rank below *shodan (*first black belt. In other areas, *kyu* can refer to level or quality. For example, an "*ikkyu* restaurant" would be a restaurant of the first quality.

kyo n.— teaching. The standard wrist locks, *ikkyo, nikyo, sankyo,* and *yonkyo,* are the "first-," "second-," "third-," and "fourth-teachings."

ma-ai n.— the proper ("harmonious") distance between *nage* and *uke,* from *ma,* space + *ai,* fit, harmonize. *Ma-ai* depends on the reach of the partners and the types of weapons being used; it is closer for a pair of short opponents than for tall ones; it is closer for unarmed combat than for swordplay. Throughout Japanese culture, *ma-ai* is extremely important. In calligraphy, the space between the characters is just as important as the ink. In Japanese rock gardens the spaces between the rocks are just as important as the rocks themselves.

mae n.— front [Japanese reading]. See **zen** [Chinese reading]. Opposite is *ushiro.*

men n.— face, front of head; *men-uchi* is a head-strike. *Shomen-uchi* is a strike directly down to the head. *Yokomen-uchi* is a strike to the head or face with a diagonal component.

mi n.— body. *Mi* is Japanese reading. See **shin** [Chinese reading].

michibiki n.—, from *michibiku,* to lead or guide, guidance.

misogi n.— purification ritual.

mochi n.   from *motsu,* to hold, have, possess. *Ryote-mochi* is a hold with both hands [*te,* hand].

mune n.— chest, midsection, thorax. *Mune-tsuki* is a punch to the chest or midsection. Western fighting, particularly bar-room brawl variety, emphasizes a sock to the jaw; Eastern styles emphasize a blow to the *hara* or *ki* center.

nage n.— (1) A thrower, the person who performs techniques. (2) A throw. *Nage* is a common designation for the partner who performs the *nage-waza,* throwing techniques.

nido n. — twice from *ni,* two + *do,* a measure, a time, a degree

naname n.— oblique. *Kokyu-dosa* or *kokyu-ho* is sometimes called *naname kokyu nage* or the "oblique breath throw."

nikyo n. — "second" immobilization technique, from *ni,* two, second + *kyo,* teaching. See **katame**. Also known as *Nikajo* or *kote-mawashi* in different styles.

ojigi n. — bow, from *o,* an honorific + *ji* (originally came from time) + *gi,* greeting. Formerly, *ojigi* meant seasonal greeting. Now it means a bow. *Ojigi-nage* are throws down simply by bowing politely in response to an attack. Featured in *Taigi* 4 (known as "The Women's Taigi").

omote n. — front, forward. Usually equivalent to *irimi* techniques. See **ura**.

one-point n. — the English interpretation of *hara* or center point of the body, considered to be about two inches below the naval, roughly the point of the hip joints. Japanese sometimes use *itten* which literally means "one-point." See **seika-tanden**.

onshi-no-gyoi n.— *onshi,* receiving from the emperor + *no,* of, possessive particle + *gyoi,* honorific gift of clothes.

oroshi n.—, from *orosu,* to drop downward; to put down. The technique *ude-oroshi* involves dropping the arm-downward.

po n.— variant of *ho,* direction. See **ho**.

randori n.— a multiple-person attack; free-style sparring, from *randoru,* to spar, from *ran,* chaos, chaotic, random, or disorderly + *dori,* from *tori,* grab.

renzoku n.— continuance, succession, a series, from *ren,* link, join + *zoku,* continuance.

ritsugi n.— *ritsu,* standing + *gi,* techniques [Chinese reading]. Japanese reading is *tachi-waza.* See **zagi** [Chinese reading for sitting techniques] and **suwari-waza** [Japanese reading].

ritsurei n.— *ritsu,* standing + *rei,* bow. See **zarei** (sitting bow).

ryo- pre.— both; *ryote,* "both hands" from *te,* hand. *Ryo-kata-tori* is a "grab to both shoulders." *Katate ryote-mochi* is a "grab with both hands" (two hands grabbing one hand) and *ryote-tori* is an attack *to* both hands (two hands grabbing two hands). See **kata** (pre. indicating one side, single).

samurai n.— warrior. Originally, those who served the emperors with their lives. See **bushi**.

sankyo n. — the "third" immobilization technique, from *san,* three, third + *kyo,* teaching. Also known as *sanjakyo* or *kote-hineri* in different styles. See **katame**.

sayu n.— left and right, from *sa,* left + *yu,* right. *Sayu-undo* involves alternately shifting the arms to the right and left and dropping their weight underside to perform a throw.

seiza n.— the formal Japanese kneeling position, from *sei,* correct + *za,* sitting.

seika-tanden n. — *seika,* under the navel + *tanden,* the body part about 2 inches below the navel. *Seika-tanden* is the bodily source of *ki* energy.

sensei n.— instructor, teacher, from *sen,* before + *sei,* living or born, hence "one who was born before you."

senpai n.— from *sen* + *hai,* comrade, companion. The combination indicates anyone senior in a particular area. Hence, on the mat, you may be *senpai* to someone who joined the club before you did (regardless of *kyu* grade) but *kohai* to the same person who may be a "senior" at school, at work, or simply in age. See **dohai** and **kohai**.

shiho n.— four directions, all directions, from *shi,* four + *ho,* direction.

shikko n.— from *shitsu,* knee [Chinese reading] + *ko,* progressing. The Japanese reading of "knee" is *hiza.*

shinai n.— bamboo sword. A length of split and bound bamboo for sword practice. It makes a loud whack when it connects, but does not cause serious injury.

shin-shin n.— mind and body from *shin,* mind + *shin,* body. Both elements have the same pronunciation but different characters with different meanings. *Zan-shin* is the immovable mind, unbroken flow of *ki* and concentration on *uke* after the throw is completed; *fudo-shin* is the imperturbable mind. *Shin-Shin Toitsu Aikido* is literally "Aikido with mind and body coordinated" from *shin*, mind + *shin*, body + *toitsu*, coordination + *ai*, harmony + *ki*, spirit, energy + *do*, way.

shindo n. — shaking, swinging, oscillation, vibration from *shin*, shaking, waving + *do*, movement. *Tekubi-shindo-undo* is the "wrist-shaking-exercise."

shite n.— Yoshinkan style uses this term to designate what other styles call *nage*. Pronounced *shtey*, it is the word used for the principle actor in a *kabuki* play.

shomen n.— front from *sho*, correct, proper + *men*, face, mask, side. *Shomen-uchi* is an overhand strike (*uchi*) attacking the "front" of the head. See **yokomen**.

sode n.— sleeve. *Sode-tori* is a "sleeve grab."

suburi n.— *su*, origin, essence, true nature + *buri*, from *furi*, swinging. *Suburi* means sword swinging (exercise) without a partner or an opponent; it is also applied to practice with baseball bats and golf clubs.

sudori n.— a passing through, from *su*, origin, essence, true nature + *dori*, from *tori*, passing (*-dori* with long vowel is different from *dori* from *tori*, grab). *Sudori* is a type of forward throw in which *uke* passes through with no change in direction — then falls.

suwari n.— seated. *Suwari waza* pertains to exercises done from *seiza*.

tachi n.— long and big sword. Originally written "big sword," now written "thick sword." *Tachi-tori* techniques are those designed to take away an opponent's sword. See **tanto**.

tachi n.— standing, from *tachi*, to stand. *Tachi-waza* are "standing techniques." Also appears as *dachi*, hence *zagi han-dachi*.

taigi n.— *tai*, body + *gi*, techniques. *Taigi* generally refers to techniques without weapons in contrast to *ken-gi*, sword techniques or *jo-gi*, stick techniques. In the Ki Society, *taigi* refers to partnered exercises involving a series of attacks and defenses but intended to demonstrate flow and rhythm.

tanto n.— dagger, knife, from *tan*, short + *to*, sword. *Tanto-tori* techniques deal with knife attacks.

te n.— hand; *kara-te* is the way of the empty, hence weaponless hand; *kata-te* is the neck of the hand, that is, the wrist. *Katate-tori* are attacks to the wrist. *Tegatana* or *tekatana* is the "hand-blade" or "sword" edge (or knife-edge) of the hand.

tekubi n.— wrist, from *te*, hand + *kubi*, neck. *Tekubi-kosa*, wrists-crossing; *tekubi-kiri*, cut to wrist.

tenchi n.— *ten*, heaven + *chi*, earth. *Tenchi-nage* is "heaven and earth throw," based on being powerfully rooted to the earth while extending towards the heavens.

tenkan n.— *ten*, turn + *kan*, to interchange, reverse. *Tenkan* is a "turning" outside *uke's* line of attack. Compare with **irimi**.

tessen n.— *tetsu*, iron + *sen*, fan. It looked like any folding fan, but its skeleton was of steel. It had two main outside ribs of sword steel to fend off sword blows, thin and pointed inner ribs so that when opened and used to strike at throat of foe, at least one rib would pierce the silk cover and slit the attacker's throat. The steel fan was used where more overt weapons were forbidden, and even played a critical role (as a *fin*) in the art of swimming in armor (*tachi oyogi*).

tobikomi n.— *tobi*, to jump + *komi*, entering, into [something]. *Tobikomi* usually describes a jumping in behind *uke*, as in *Kokyu-nage* Basic (*katate-kosa-tori irimi tobikomi*).

toitsu n.— unity, unification, from *to*, reign, govern + *itsu*, one. *Shin Shin Toitsu Aikido* is Aikido with mind-body coordination or unification.

tori n.— from *toru*, to grab, take, pick. *Katate-kosa-tori* is a grab of the opposite [cross] wrist; *kata-tori* is a grab of the shoulder or, as we think of it, the lapel.

tsuki n.— from *tsuku*, to stick. A thrust, poke, stab, punch as with a fist, *jo*, or knife; *mune-tsuki* is a chest-punch; *ushiro-tsuki* can mean a stab from behind or a thrust to the rear.

uchi n.— from *utsu*, to strike. *Shomen-uchi* is a frontal attack [to the] head while *yokomen-uchi* is a diagonal attack [to the] head.

uchi n.— inside. Opposite is *soto*, outside. An *uchideshi*, from *deshi*, pupil, disciple, is an apprentice living in the home of his master.

ude n.— arm; *ude-furi undo* is the arm-swinging exercise.

uke n. — receiving, from *ukeru*, to receive. In Aikido the partner who *receives* (techniques). The opposite is **nage**. *Ukemi* is the art of receiving the technique and protecting oneself by falling safely. *Koho-ukemi* is a backwards roll or fall; *zempo-ukemi* is a forwards roll or fall.

undo n.— exercise, motion, movement from *un,* carry, transport + *do*, motion.

ura n. — behind, in back of [something]. In styles other than Ki Society Aikido, *ura* techniques are often the named equivalent to Ki Society *tenkan* techniques. See **omote**.

ushiro n.   back, backwards, behind. *Ushiro* techniques all involve an attack from the rear such as a bear-hug from behind (*ushiro-tori*). The opposite of *ushiro* is *mae*. *Ushiro tekubi-tori* describes a "wrist grab from behind." *Ushiro ryote-tori* describes "both hands attacked from behind." *Ushiro ryo-kata-tori* describes "both shoulders grabbed from behind."

waza n. — technique [Japanese reading]. *Hitori waza* refers to "single" person exercises such as *ikkyo-undo, funekogi-undo. Kumi waza* refers to "more than one person" technique, that is, throws involving an attacker and a defender. See **gi** [Chinese reading].

yoko n.— side, sideways, diagonally. *Yokomen-uchi* is a diagonal strike, *uchi* to the head, *men*. It actually begins as a straight forward strike, as does *shomen-uchi*, with an added diagonal component and a turning of the hips.

yonkyo n.— the fourth immobilization technique from *yon,* four, fourth + *kyo*, teaching.

yudansha n. — *yu*, from *yu-suru* to possess + *dan*, level + *sha*, person. Hence black-belt level students or "persons with *dan*."

zagi n.— *za,* seated, sitting + *gi,* techniques. Both *nage* and *uke* are seated in *seiza. Zagi-handachi* are techniques in which standing *uke* attacks kneeling *nage*.

zan-shin n.— the remaining or immovable mind. See **shin-shin**.

zazen n.— sitting meditation, from *za,* seated, sitting + *zen,* quietness, serenity. See **zen**.

zarei n.— a seated bow, from *za,* seated, sitting + *rei,* bow, etiquette, gratitude. See **ritsurei,** a standing bow.

zen n. — Originally this Chinese character meant that "emperors cleansed the earth and worshiped the heaven or heavenly God." It also meant "quietness" or "serenity". Nowadays, *zen* means to seek true senses or features by attaining a state of perfect self-effacement, and unifying spirit and soul.

zen n.— front [Chinese reading]. See **mae** [Japanese reading]. Opposite is *ushiro*. See **ushiro**.

zengo n.— *zen,* forward + *go,* backward, hence *zengo-undo*, "forward and backward exercise."

zenpo n.— forward, from *zen,* forward + *po,* from *ho,* direction. *Zempo kaiten* is a forward roll; *zenpo kaiten-nage* is a throw in which *uke* is projected into a forward roll. See **koho**.

Index

R

Also From Round Earth Publishing . . .

Ki in Aikido: A Sampler of Ki Exercises

Ki, the "Force" behind the Japanese martial art of Aikido, has much in common with *ch'i* (from Chinese), *prana* (from Sanscrit and yoga), and *pneuma* (from Greek) but all remain strange concepts to many Westerners. *Ki* exercises, derived from yoga, provide an unusual opportunity to actually test, measure, and evaluate traditional concepts of mind and body. Here are step-by-step instructions and illustrations of *ki* exercises and test techniques. This new edition expands the original chapters on breathing and meditation with additional information on modern biofeedback and science of breath.

　　Quality Paperback, 288 pages, 180 illustrations. $19.95

Range of Motion Testing Charts

Pain patterns can be highly diagnostic of problems in specific muscles and so the source of myofascial pain is often evaluated by observing the pain patterns alone. However, different muscles can produce confusingly similar and overlapping pain patterns. Range-of-Motion (ROM) testing allows therapists to:

- Distinguish between muscles with similar or overlapping pain patterns,
- Locate shortened or restricted areas where pain has not yet appeared,
- Effectively treat the actual source of pain—not just the symptoms.

The charts combine muscle testing information from Travell & Simons' *Myofascial Pain and Dysfunction* with fascial lines of Myers' *Anatomy Trains*. An invaluable resource for physicians, therapists, athletes, dancers—and anyone else with muscles.

　　Set of 2 charts (Upper and Lower Body) 22" x 34" on heavy coated stock: $60 per set.
　　US Shipping $7.00 per set, $3.00 each additional set.

Patterns for Martial Arts and Anime

Patterns for *hakama*, *dogi*, and more. Make real garments that will hold up to real practice by real martial artists. *Dogi* pants with traditional gussets. *Hakama* that fit. *Kimono*, *tabi*, vests, and other classic Japanese designs.

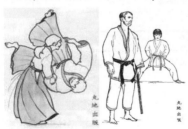

Not sure you're up to making your own uniform?

Meet our Budo Bear! Envelope includes patterns for jointed bear (will stand about 24" high), belt, jacket and *hakama* that will fit bear or other Small Person with hip/waist of about 20".

Learn the basics of *dogi* and *hakama* construction at a smaller, more manageable scale.

www.Round-Earth.com

Order Form	How Many?	Price	Total
Books Please specify if you wish your book autographed by the author			
Ki in Aikido—A Sampler of Ki Exercises		$19.95	$
Aikido Exercises for Teaching and Training		$19.95	$
Charts / Posters Note: Must ship separately from books and patterns			
Range-of-Motion Testing		$60.00	$
Trigger Points and Referred Pain Charts		$29.95	$
Patterns for Japanese Clothing $			
Adult Gi Pattern		$19.95	$
Hakama (include hip measurement)		$16.95	$
Budo Bear Pattern		$16.95	$
Total Merchandise:			$
US Shipping: Books/Patterns $6, Posters $7			$
Tax: PA residents please add 6%:			$
TOTAL:			$

Payment Check or Money Order

Ship to Name (Please print):

Ship to Address 1:

Ship to Address 2:

City: State: ZIP: Phone: (   )

Credit Cards Credit card purchases are shipped to billing address only.

Name as it appears on card (Please print):

Billing Address:

City: State: ZIP: Phone: (   )

__Visa __MasterCard __Discover __AmExpress

Expiration Date: /   3-digit code on back of card:_____

Card Number: -   -

Signature:

Mail check/money orders or phone/fax credit card orders to:

Round Earth Publishing
P. O. Box 157, Sewickley, PA 15143
E-Mail: Sales@round-earth.com (412) 741-7286 (voice) / (412) 741-7207 (fax)
For more items, sizes, information or on-line ordering visit www.Round-Earth.com